PLASTIC
SURGERY

CLINICAL PROBLEM SOLVING

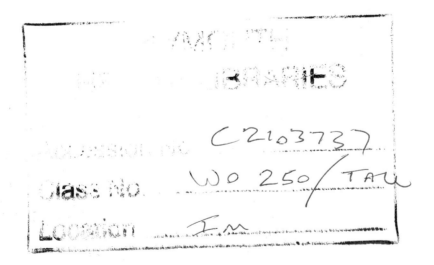

Notice

Medicine is an ever-changing science. As new research and clinical experience broaden our knowledge, changes in treatment and drug therapy are required. The authors and the publisher of this work have checked with sources believed to be reliable in their efforts to provide information that is complete and generally in accord with the standards accepted at the time of publication. However, in view of the possibility of human error or changes in medical sciences, neither the authors nor the publisher nor any other party who has been involved in the preparation or publication of this work warrants that the information contained herein is in every respect accurate or complete, and they disclaim all responsibility for any errors or omissions or for the results obtained from use of the information contained in this work. Readers are encouraged to confirm the information contained herein with other sources. For example and in particular, readers are advised to check the product information sheet included in the package of each drug they plan to administer to be certain that the information contained in this work is accurate and that changes have not been made in the recommended dose or in the contraindications for administration. This recommendation is of particular importance in connection with new or infrequently used drugs.

PLASTIC SURGERY
CLINICAL PROBLEM SOLVING

PETER J. TAUB, MD, FACS, FAAP

Associate Professor
Surgery and Pediatrics
Division of Plastic and Reconstructive Surgery
Mount Sinai Medical Center
New York, New York

R. MICHAEL KOCH, MD, FACS

Assistant Professor of Surgery
Division of Plastic and Reconstructive Surgery
New York Medical College
Valhalla, New York

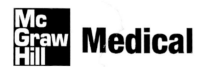 **Medical**

New York Chicago San Francisco Lisbon London Madrid Mexico City
Milan New Delhi San Juan Seoul Singapore Sydney Toronto

Plastic Surgery: Clinical Problem Solving

Copyright © 2009 by The McGraw-Hill Companies, Inc. All rights reserved. Printed in China. Except as permitted under the United States Copyright Act of 1976, no part of this publication may be reproduced or distributed in any form or by any means, or stored in a data base or retrieval system, without the prior written permission of the publisher.

1 2 3 4 5 6 7 8 9 0   CTP/CTP   12 11 10 9

ISBN 978-0-07-148150-2
MHID 0-07-148150-8

This book was set in Berkeley by Aptara®, Inc.
The editors were Marsha Loeb and Regina Brown.
The production supervisor was Sherri Souffrance.
The illustration manager was Armen Ovsepyan.
Project management was provided by Sumbul Jafri, Aptara®, Inc.
The designer was Eve Siegel; the cover designer was Mary McKeon.
China Translation & Printing Services, Ltd., was printer and binder.

This book is printed on acid-free paper.

Cataloging-in-Publication Data is on file for this title at the Library of Congress.

To my wife and family, whose love and support have been boundless—PJT

Contents

Contributors

Kodi K. Azari, MD, FACS
Assistant Professor
University of Pittsburgh
Pittsburgh, Pennsylvania

Stephen B. Baker, MD, DDS
Associate Professor
Department of Plastic Surgery
Georgetown University Hospital
Washington, District of Columbia

Michael L. Bentz, MD, FACS
Professor
Department of Pediatrics and Neurosurgery
University of Wisconsin at Madison
Madison, Wisconsin

Sean G. Boutros, MD
Diplomate
The American Board of Plastic Surgery
Houston Plastic & Craniofacial Surgery
Houston, Texas

Steven R. Buchman, MD, FACS
Professor
Division of Plastic and Reconstructive Surgery
University of Michigan
Ann Arbor, Michigan

Robert Buka, MD, JD
Clinical Assistant Professor
Department of Dermatology
Mount Sinai Medical Center
New York, New York

Charles E. Butler, MD, FACS
Associate Professor
Department of Plastic Surgery
The University of Texas MD Anderson Cancer Center
Houston, Texas

Courtney Carpenter, MD
Plastic Surgery Research Fellow
Montefiore Medical Center
Albert Einstein College of Medicine of
Yeshiva University

Paul S. Cederna, MD, FACS
Associate Chair and Associate Professor
Division of Plastic Surgery and Department of Surgery
University of Michigan Health System
Ann Arbor, Michigan

James Chang, MD
Chairman
Division of Plastic and Reconstructive Surgery
Stanford University Medical Center
Palo Alto, California

David T.W. Chiu, MD, FACS
Professor
Institute of Reconstructive Plastic Surgery
New York University
New York, New York

Jin K. Chun, MD
Associate Professor
Division of Plastic and Reconstructive Surgery
Mount Sinai Medical Center
New York, New York

Patrick Cole, MD
Professor
Department of Plastic Surgery
Baylor College of Medicine
Houston, Texas

Aaron Daluiski, MD
Professor
Hospital for Special Surgery
New York, New York

Rafael J. Diaz-Garcia, MD
Associate Professor
Department of Plastic and Reconstructive Surgery
University of Michigan Health System
Ann Arbor, Michigan

Gregory R.D. Evans, MD, FACS
Chairman
Division of Plastic and Reconstructive Surgery
University of California at Irvine
Orange, California

Evan Garfein, MD
Clinical Instructor
Surgery (Plastic Surgery)
Montefiore Medical Center
Albert Einstein College of Medicine of
Yeshiva University

Warren L. Garner, MD
Associate Professor
Division of Plastic Surgery
Children's Hospital of Los Angeles
Keck School of Medicine
University of Southern California
Los Angeles, California

Mark Gelfand, MD
Assistant Professor
Stonybrook University
Stonybrook, New York

Eric Genden, MD
Chairman
Department of Otolaryngology
Mount Sinai Medical Center
New York, New York

Richard Gilbert, MD
Clinical Assistant Professor
Mount Sinai Medical Center
New York, New York

Corey S. Goldberg, MD, BSc, MASc, FRCS
Professor
Division of Plastic Surgery
Children's Hospital of Los Angeles
Keck School of Medicine
University of Southern California
Los Angeles, California

Nicolas Guay, MD
Private Practice
Ottawa, Ontario, Canada

Adam H. Hamawy, MD, FACS
Chief Resident
Department of Plastic Surgery
Southwestern Medical Center
Dallas, Texas

Dennis C. Hammond, MD
Professor
Department of Plastic Surgery
Center for Breast & Body Contouring
Grand Rapids, Michigan

Marco Harmaty, MD
Assistant Professor
Mount Sinai Medical Center
New York, New York

Harvey Himel, MD
Assistant Professor
Division of Plastic and Reconstructive Surgery
Mount Sinai Medical Center
New York, New York

William Y. Hoffman, MD
Chairman
Department of Plastic and Reconstructive Surgery
University of California at San Francisco
San Francisco, California

Larry H. Hollier, Jr., MD, FACS
Associate Professor
Residency Program Director
Department of Plastic Surgery
Baylor College of Medicine
Houston, Texas

C. Scott Hultman, MD, FACS
Ethel F. and James A. Valone Professor
Chief and Program Director
Division of Plastic and Reconstructive Surgery
University of North Carolina School of Medicine
Chapel Hill, North Carolina

Jeffery E. Janis, MD
Assistant Professor
Department of Plastic Surgery
University of Texas Southwestern Medical Center
Dallas, Texas

Reza Jarrahy, MD
Assistant Professor
David Geffen School of Medicine
University of California, Los Angeles
Los Angeles, California

Neil Ford Jones, MD
Professor and Chief
Hand Surgery
University of California at Irvine
Orange, California

Henry K. Kawamoto, Jr., MD, DDS
Clinical Professor of Surgery
David Geffen School of Medicine
University of California, Los Angeles
Los Angeles, California

Timothy W. King, MD
Northwestern Children's Memorial Hospital
Chicago, Illinois

Ernest Kirchman, MD
Professor
Mount Sinai Medical Center
New York, New York

John Ko, MD
Clinical Assistant Professor
Mount Sinai Medical Center
New York, New York

R. Michael Koch, MD, FACS
Assistant Professor of Surgery
Division of Plastic and Reconstructive Surgery
New York Medical College
Valhalla, New York

Lily F. Lee, MD
Burn Fellow
Department of Surgery
Division of Plastic & Reconstructive Surgery
University of Southern California
Los Angeles, California

W.P. Andrew Lee, MD
Professor
Department of Surgery
University of Pittsburgh
Pittsburgh, Pennsylvania

Malcolm A. Lesavoy, MD
Clinical Professor
Division of Plastic and Reconstructive Surgery
David Geffen School of Medicine
University of California, Los Angeles
Encino, California

Joseph E. Losee, MD
Associate Professor
Department of Surgery
University of Pittsburgh School of Medicine
Pittsburgh, Pennsylvania

Donald R. Mackay, MD
Chief
Division of Plastic and Reconstructive Surgery
Pennsylvania State University
Hershey, Pennsylvania

Babak J. Mehrara, MD
Associate Professor
Department of Surgery
Memorial Sloan-Kettering Cancer Center
New York, New York

Michael W. Neumeister, MD
Professor and Chairman
Division of Plastic and Reconstructive Surgery
Southern Illinois University School of Medicine
Springfield, Illinois

Shelley Noland, MD
Resident
Department of Plastic Surgery
Stanford University Medical Center
Stanford, California

Pravin K. Patel, MD
Associate Professor
Feinberg School of Medicine
Northwestern University
Chicago, Illinois

David J. Pincus, MD
General Surgery Resident
Jackson Memorial Hospital
Miami, Florida

John F. Reinisch, MD
Clinical Professor
Division of Plastic and Reconstructive Surgery
Keck School of Medicine
University of Southern California
Los Angeles, California

Norman H. Schulman, MD
Clinical Professor
Department of Plastic Surgery
Lenox Hill Hospital
New York, New York

Joseph M. Serletti, MD
Professor and Chairman
Division of Plastic and Reconstructive Surgery
University of Pennsylvania School
of Medicine
Philadelphia, Pennsylvania

Lester Silver, MD, MS
Professor and Chief
Division of Plastic and Reconstructive Surgery
Mount Sinai Medical Center
New York, New York

Jessica Simon, BA
Medical Student
UMDNJ—New Jersey Medical School
Lyndhurst, New Jersey

Davinder J. Singh, MD
Attending Surgeon
Barrow Neurologic Institute
St. Joseph's Hospital and Medical Center
Phoenix, Arizona

Richard Skolnick, MD
Clinical Associate Professor
Mount Sinai Medical Center
New York, New York

Paul D. Smith, MD
Professor
Moffitt Cancer Center
Tampa, Florida

David A. Staffenberg, MD, DSc (Hon), FACS
Chairman and Associate Professor
Department of Plastic and Reconstructive Surgery
Albert Einstein College of Medicine of
Yeshiva University
Bronx, New York

Samuel Stal, MD
Professor
Texas Children's Hospital
Houston, Texas

Thomas P. Sterry, MD, MS
Clinical Assistant Professor
Division of Plastic and Reconstructive Surgery
Mount Sinai Medical Center
New York, New York

Mitchell A. Stotland, MD
Associate Professor
Department of Surgery and Department of Pediatrics
Dartmouth-Hitchcock Medical Center
Lebanon, New Hampshire

Peter J. Taub, MD, FACS, FAAP
Associate Professor
Surgery and Pediatrics
Division of Plastic and Reconstructive Surgery
Mount Sinai Medical Center
New York, New York

Seth Thaller, MD
Professor and Chief
Division of Plastic Surgery
University of Miami
Miller School Medicine
Miami, Florida

Mark M. Urata, MD, DDS
Professor
Division of Plastic Surgery
Children's Hospital of Los Angeles
Keck School of Medicine
University of Southern California
Los Angeles, California

Henry C. Vasconez, MD
Professor
Division of Plastic Surgery
University of Kentucky
Lexington, Kentucky

Jeffrey Weinzweig, MD, FACS
Chairman
Plastic and Reconstructive Surgery
Lahey Clinic
Burlington, Massachusetts

Bradon J. Wilhelmi, MD, FACS
Professor and Chief
Department of Plastic Surgery
University of Louisville School of Medicine
Louisville, Kentucky

Jack C. Yu, DMD, MD, MS ed, FACS
Professor and Chief
Department of Plastic and Reconstructive Surgery
Medical College of Georgia
Augusta, Georgia

Preface

Clinical Problem Solving in Plastic Surgery was conceived of as an exciting and interactive text designed to present clinical scenarios commonly encountered in the field of plastic and reconstructive surgery. Its format is unlike other sources of information in that an unknown visual problem is presented and the reader is guided through a logical and stepwise means to arrive at the correct diagnosis and recommend a logical treatment plan.

The 52 cases were chosen as they are felt to be clinical problems that every student of plastic and reconstructive surgery should understand and be comfortable discussing either in the office, on rounds, or during an oral examination. Each case begins with a full-color image of a clinical case and scant background information (much like real-life). The key questions to address in the history are outlined as well as the pertinent findings to identify during the physical examination. A review of commonly recommended preoperative studies and consultations is offered, followed by a discussion of the recognized operative and nonoperative management strategies. Finally, a list of potential complications is included so that the reader is aware of and prepared for potential problems following surgery. Each case is accompanied by a brief algorithm and selected schematic drawings are added to emphasize key points.

The authors who have contributed to this text were chosen by the editors for their recognition as leaders in the field of plastic and reconstructive surgery, not only for their clinical skills and academic publications but also for their dedication to teaching the next generation of surgeons.

Introduction

Dr. Taub and Dr. Koch present us with the book *Clinical Problem Solving in Plastic Surgery*. Initially, one asks, "Do we really need another plastic surgery book considering the volumes already written?"

In this case I would answer yes, since this book is structured in a way so as to encourage a "critical thinking pathway" and will, therefore, prove especially useful for residents, fellows, students, and surgeons who wish to refresh their approach to a particular clinical problem. This book will fit nicely between the large plastic surgery text volumes and the small resident handbooks (often found in the pocket of white coats) since, although it does not present essentially new material, it does offer a new approach. This is done by starting with the clinical problem and offering a schema as to how one would think through the problem so as to gain the information needed to decide upon treatment options.

The authors have selected a number of the entities frequently seen in plastic surgery practices and assembled well-known experts in the field to lead the reader through each clinical scenario almost as if it were a discussion at the bedside. The book was not planned to include all clinical problems in a comprehensive fashion. Rather, the chapters are selected to highlight some of the more common problems and to have the author guide the reader along the path to a solution. It is the approach that is emphasized. For this reason, I believe that *Clinical Problem Solving in Plastic Surgery* will occupy a useful niche among plastic surgery publications.

Lester Silver, MD
Professor of Surgery
Chief, Plastic Surgery
Mount Sinai School of Medicine and Medical Center
New York, NY

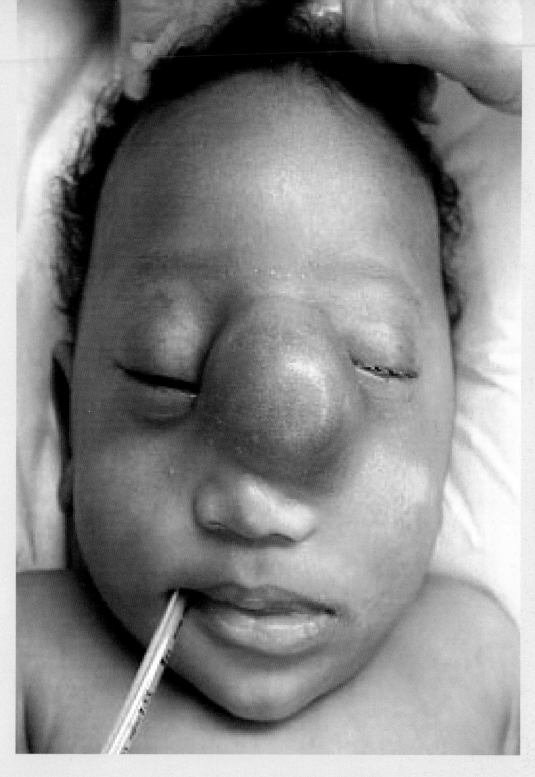

The neonatal intensive care unit requests your consultation for a 1-month-old infant with a lesion at the root of the nose.

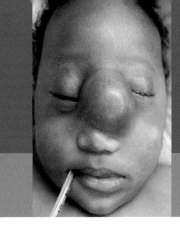

CHAPTER 1

Encephalocele

Reza Jarrahy and Henry K. Kawamoto, Jr.

1. Congenital midline facial masses are reported to occur in one out of every 20,000 to 40,000 births. Any request to evaluate a pediatric patient who presents with a superficial midline facial mass must prompt the examining surgeon to consider the possibility of an associated intracranial component. Making this determination at the outset is of paramount importance and must precede any surgical intervention. The differential diagnosis of a midline facial mass includes numerous acquired and congenital lesions. The most common of the latter group include nasal dermoid cysts, gliomas, encephaloceles, and vascular lesions. Acquired conditions include tumors, abscesses, and hematomas. **Nasal dermoid cysts** are lined by squamous epithelium and may contain variable adnexal structures and caseous material. They represent remnants of an embryological tract between the nasal ectoderm and neurocranium. **Gliomas** are tumors of mature glial tissue (astrocytes and connective tissue). They do not contain cerebrospinal fluid (CSF). Histologically, the tissue is reactive to glial fibrillary acidic protein and S-100 protein. On imaging, there is no defect in the base of the skull. **Encephaloceles** result from protrusion of cranial contents through defects in the skull base. The nomenclature is dependent upon the content of the lesion. Meningoceles contain meninges alone; meningoencephaloceles also contain brain; and cystomeningoencephalocele also contain portions of a ventricle. During early gestation a diverticulum containing dura and glial tissue extends either anteriorly through the *fonticulus nasofrontalis* (a temporary fontanelle between the paired nasal and frontal bones) or inferiorly into the prenasal space (a potential space between the nasal bones and underlying cartilage). This evagination typically obliterates during development. Failure to do so, however, results in a persistent neuroectodermal sinus. If neural tissue remains within the sinus, a glioma or an encephalocele will develop. If the diverticulum regresses and the sinus closes off, a cystic lesion results. With these embryological considerations in mind, obtaining a thorough history is the first step in establishing an accurate diagnosis.

   - **Was the lesion present at birth or did it appear sometime thereafter?** Midline masses may be diagnosed in the prenatal period during routine gestational ultrasound screening. It is possible to differentiate between masses with and without intracranial extension prior to birth. If the mass is present at birth, the likelihood of an acquired etiology is significantly diminished.

   - **Is there any history of respiratory distress?** The majority of newborns are obligate nose breathers for at least the first 6 months of life. Respiratory compromise in association with a midline facial mass suggests obstruction of the nasal airway.

   - **Is there any history of infection or rhinorrhea?** Any of the three common congenital causes of midline facial masses may present with external infection of the nasal skin or with meningitis, which would suggest an intracranial process. A nasal dermoid sinus may alternate between periods of quiescence and inflammation, characterized by erythema and drainage. An encephalocele may present with a primary CSF leak.

   - **Does the lesion change in character?** Temporary increases in intracranial pressure, as a result of normal crying, coughing, and/or straining, may cause the lesion to enlarge if there is an intracranial component.

   - **Are there any associated neurological or craniofacial anomalies or any family history of congenital craniofacial lesions?** Most lesions are sporadic in nature, but may be coincident with associated developmental aberrations of the craniofacial skeleton, such as cleft palate, or with more complex craniofacial syndromes. Moreover, hydrocephalus has been reported in up to 75% of all encephaloceles.

2. The physical examination should focus on the characteristics of the lesion, again with the goal of differentiating between superficial processes and those that are likely to contain an intracranial component.

   - **Where is the lesion located?** A nasal dermoid cyst may be located anywhere along the path of the sinus, from the glabella to the columella, with the former being the most common. Gliomas may be extranasal (60%), intranasal (30%), or both (10%). In the extranasal location, gliomas may occur anywhere from the glabella to the columella. Intranasal gliomas present as pale masses that may protrude from the nostril. The base of an intranasal lesion usually arises from the lateral nasal wall near the middle turbinate. Encephaloceles are most commonly occipital (75%). Those occuring in the frontal region may be subdivided into sincipital (60%) and basal (40%) lesions. Sincipital lesions are external nasal masses which occur in the nasofrontal, nasoethmoidal, and nasoorbital regions. The bony defect is in the anterior midline and may coexist with the rarer craniofacial clefts. Basal lesions are intranasal masses and are categorized as transethmoidal, sphenoethmoidal, transsphenoidal, and sphenomaxillary depending on their location. These manifest as smooth intranasal masses or in the areas of nasopharynx and pterygopalatine fossa.

- **How does the lesion appear?** When identified, a nasal dimple or pit associated with hair protrusion is considered to be pathognomonic for a nasal dermoid. In most cases, these are confined to the superficial tissues and terminate in a subcutaneous fistulous tract.

- **What does the lesion feel like?** Encephaloceles are typically soft, compressible lesions that may be pulsatile. The mass may increase in size with coughing, crying, or straining (positive "Furstenberg sign"). By comparison, dermoids and gliomas are firm, noncompressible, and do not change size with increased intracranial pressure.

- **Are the orbits in a normal position?** An encephalocele or, rarely, a glioma presenting in the fronto-orbital region may result in hypertelorbitism and/or vertical orbital dystopia. Often the interpupillary distance and lateral canthal distances are normal. A basic assessment of visual function, extraocular muscle excursion, and papillary response should also be performed. The normal intercanthal distance in adults is 28 to 32 mm (roughly equal to the palpebral fissure width). The normal intraorbital distance, as measured from lacrimal crest to lacrimal crest, is 24 to 32 mm in males and 22 to 28 mm in females. The normal interpupillary distance is 55 to 65 mm. Normal interorbital distance at 1 year averages 18.5 mm and increases to 22 mm by 5 years of age and approaches adult values by 12 years.
  — Orbital hypertelorism in the adult may be classified into degrees of severity. First degree is 30 to 34 mm, second degree is 34 to 40 mm, and third degree is >40 mm.

- **Is the nasal pyramid normal?** Lesions around the root of the nose may cause deviation or widening of the nasal pyramid. All patients should have an intranasal examination to identify any impact on nasal airflow. Intranasal masses may specifically cause septal deviation, nasal obstruction, and/or respiratory compromise.

- **What is the patient's neurologic status?** A thorough neurological examination should be performed, with specific attention to the signs and symptoms of hydrocephalus as a result of the high rate of association with an encephalocele. Excess CSF might require placement of a ventricular shunt on an urgent basis.

- **Are there associated anomalies?** Intraoral examination should look for evidence of cleft palate. Other malformations should be identified during a complete multisystem physical examination, including cardiac and extremity defects.

3. With open neural tube defects, prenatal diagnosis may be made on routine **ultrasound** or by measuring **alpha-fetoprotein** levels in amniotic fluid. Postnatally, one or more studies should be obtained to delineate the deformity and provide clues as to its location and nature. Additional intracranial abnormalities are not uncommon and should be sought.

- Radiologic studies are the most important diagnostic modalities.
  — An **ultrasound** is easy to obtain without sedation but yields less information than either a CT or MRI. It must also be performed through open fontanelles.
  — An **MRI** is perhaps the gold standard for evaluating the anatomy of an encephalocele. It is able to evaluate structures contained within the defect and the route of egress from the calvarial vault. Anteriorly, the cribriform plate may be displaced and the crista galli may be widened, duplicated, or absent. While no radiation is involved, it does require sedation for the child.
  — A **CT** scan is perhaps a better modality to evaluate the bony framework but less useful in delineating the soft tissues of the head and neck. 3-dimensional reconstruction of the bony windows of the CT scan yields a detailed topographical map of the abnormal craniofacial skeleton. The combination of CT scan

and MRI should give a complete picture of soft tissue and bony involvement and facilitate surgical planning. It also requires sedation for infants and younger children.

- Flexible **nasal endoscopy** should be an adjunctive part of the physical examination. It can be performed with relative ease and without the need for sedation in infants. However, it should be used for diagnostic purposes only: biopsy of any lesion with suspected intracranial involvement should not be performed as part of the physical examination.

4. Simple dermoid cysts or gliomas without any evidence of intracranial extension can in most cases be safely managed by the plastic surgeon independently. However, any evidence of an encephalocele with intracranial component, or any indication of associated craniofacial defects with or without syndromic presentation warrants multidisciplinary evaluation. This might occur in an established craniofacial clinic, but the actual setting is not as important as the participants:

- Patients should be seen by a **geneticist**, who may be able to provide clues as to any syndromic association.
- Eventual surgical correction will involve a combination of specialties, including the services of a **pediatric neurosurgeon**, who should evaluate the patient preoperatively. The need to address any issues related to hydrocephalus may dictate the timing of the initial surgical intervention.
- Prior to surgery, a consultation by the **pediatric ophthalmologist** will highlight any preexisting defects and will document a baseline examination.
- A **pediatric cardiologist** should be consulted if associated congenital heart anomalies exist.

5. Once the multidisciplinary preoperative assessment is completed and diagnostic studies obtained, an accurate diagnosis is made. Surgical intervention is customized to the patient and the lesions. In general, neurosurgical intervention is indicated in the setting of hydrocephalus and/or intracranial extension.

- Extracranial **dermoids** should be approached with the goal of complete excision, nasal reconstruction, and acceptable cosmetic outcome. Transverse and lateral rhinotomy as well as open rhinoplasty techniques with or without osteotomy have been described as effective in achieving these goals.
- Management of extranasal **gliomas** adheres to similar principles. Large lesions may require the use of a midline nasal incision or coronal approach. The use of transnasal endoscopy is indicated in the excision of intranasal gliomas. Any preoperative evidence of intracranial involvement, however, dictates a more involved approach, as discussed below.

- When a diagnosis of **encephalocele** is made, surgical planning in conjunction with a pediatric neurosurgeon should aim for removal of the anomalous sac and closure of the connection to the central nervous system. Early intervention helps minimize the risk of infection and significant cosmetic deformity. Definitive correction may be performed in two stages, particularly an associated fronto-orbital malformation is present. The exact surgical approaches are determined by the topography of the lesion.

  — Initial correction might involve a frontal craniotomy for access to and resection of the intracranial component with reconstruction and closure of the dura. A watertight seal is essential. The extracranial component can be removed at the same setting without undue morbidity; an extranasal location can be exposed via the same coronal incision used for the craniotomy. An intranasal extension may necessitate an additional transnasal approach, with or without endoscopy. Primary bone grafting of the nose, frontal bone, or cranial base can be performed as part of this first procedure.

  — When the child is older, the dystopia and hypertelorism may be addressed (e.g., via box osteotomy or facial bipartition). The frontal sinus often requires repeat bone grafting. In some cases, orthognathic rehabilitation may follow orbital reconstruction depending on the original caudal extent of the lesion and any subsequent effect on maxillary morphology.

6. Complications are more common with more extensive intracranial/extracranial procedures, as would be expected. These would include morbidities inherent to any major intracranial or orbital surgery, including hemorrhage, stroke, blindness, meningitis, and CSF leak. Families should be thoroughly counseled on the risks of these complications, including the risk of death, before a major neurosurgical/craniofacial procedure is planned.

- **Blindness** is rare and is best avoided rather than managed postoperatively. Any bleeding around the globes should be avoided and controlled if present. Osteotomies should be well visualized and supported with malleable retractors in front of any vital structures.
- Development of postoperative **meningitis** is best addressed with culture of the CSF and institution/continuation of appropriate intravenous antibiotics.
- Management of the **CSF leak** may include placement of a lumbar drain to diminish intrathecal pressure and/or return to the operating room.

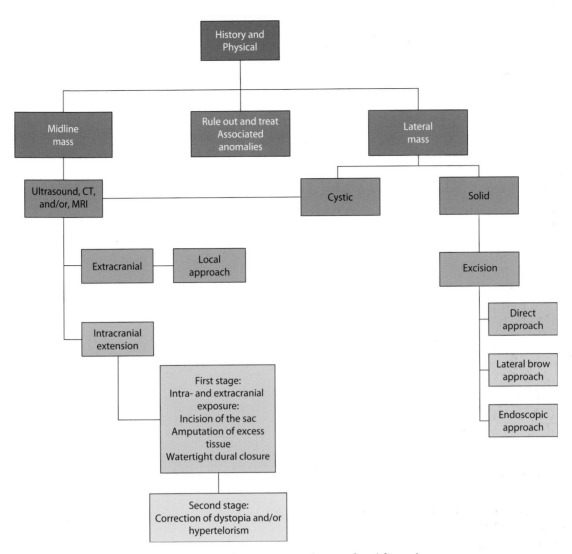

Algorithm 1-1 Management algorithm for patients with superficial frontal masses.

References

1. Bradley PJ. The complex nasal dermoid. *Head Neck Surg.* 1983;5:469.

2. Bui CJ, Tubbs RS, Shannon CN, et al. Institutional experience with cranial vault encephaloceles. *J Neurosurg.* 2007;107(1 Suppl):22-25.

3. De Biasio P, Scarso E, Prefumo F, Odella C, Rossi A, Venturini PL. Prenatal diagnosis of a nasal glioma in the mid trimester. *Ultrasound Obstet Gynecol.* 2006;27(5):571-573.

4. Frodel JL, Larrabee WF, Raisis J. The nasal dermoid. *Otolaryngol Head and Neck Surg.* 1989;101.

5. Lowe LH, Booth TN, Joglar JM, Rollins NK. Midface anomalies in children. *Radiographics.* 2000;20(4):907-922.

6. Pratt LW. Midline cysts of the nasal dorsum: Embryologic origin and treatment. *Laryngoscope.* 1965;75:968.

7. Rahbar R, Resto VA, Robson CD, et al. Nasal glioma and encephalocele: Diagnosis and management. *Laryngoscope.* 2003;113(12):2069-2077.

8. Rohrich RJ, Lowe JB, Schwartz MR. The role of open rhinoplasty in the management of nasal dermoid cysts. *Plast Reconstr Surg.* 1999;104(5):1459-1466.

9. Rosano A, Botto LD, Olney RS, et al. Limb defects associated with major congenital anomalies: Clinical and epidemiological study from the International Clearinghouse for Birth Defects Monitoring Systems. *Am J Med Genet.* 2000:17;93(2):110-116.

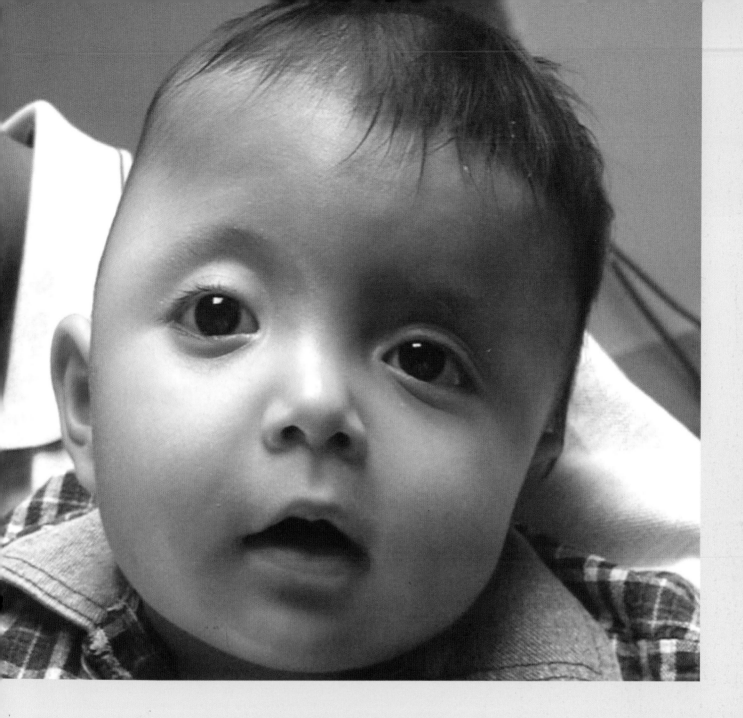

One of the pediatricians at your hospital asks you to evaluate a 6-month-old infant with facial asymmetry.

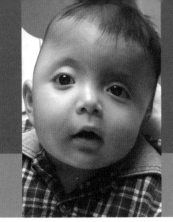

CHAPTER 2

Coronal Synostosis

Peter J. Taub

1. Congenital asymmetry around the orbits suggests a diagnosis of craniosynostosis, which may involve one of the paired coronal or lambdoid sutures. The coronal sutures run anterolaterally from the anterior fontanelle at the vertex of the skull, while the lambdoid sutures run posterolaterally from the posterior fontanelle. A thorough history is important to answer several important questions.

   • **Was the deformity present at birth?** Craniosynostosis often begins prenatally and presents with characteristic findings, such as an abnormal head shape, at birth. Postnatal changes may be the result of molding rather than synostosis. However, premature suture fusion after birth may produce similar findings.

   • **Was the child born preterm or admitted to the neonatal intensive care unit (NICU)?** Extended time in the NICU can be associated with positional head deformities, resulting from extended periods of restricted head posture in the crib.

   • **What is the age of the patient?** The age of the patient is important because surgical options differ not only by the experience of the surgeon but also by the age of the patient.

   • **Has the head shape changed over time?** Bony fusion, such as craniosynostosis, rarely, if ever, corrects itself over time. Molded bone does retain the ability to correct itself if the causative factor is removed, such as positioning or hydrocephalus.

   • **Has the child been meeting developmental milestones?** While there are studies arguing the physical implications of single and multiple suture synostosis, there is no definite indication that fusion of a single suture leads to developmental delay and that release of the suture will improve development in patients with delay.

2. Many times the diagnosis of synostosis can be made on physical examination alone. A thorough and complete examination of the child must be done to identify associated malformations.

   • **What is the shape of the skull?** Bone growth in the face of a rigidly fused suture occurs only parallel to the suture. In the case of a coronal craniosynostosis, the head takes on a trapezoid shape when viewed from above. The frontal and occipital areas on the side of the involved suture are closer together than they are on the contralateral side.

   • **Are the orbits symmetrical?** The hallmark finding in patients with a unilateral coronal synostosis is a "windswept" orbit on the affected side. Fusion of the suture holds the sphenoid wing more anterior, which contributes to the physical findings.

   • **Are there palpable ridges in the skull?** The stenosis is usually palpable beneath the scalp and runs in concert with the suture.

   • **Is the posterior fontanelle open?** While not usually as easily palpable as the anterior fontanelle, the posterior fontanelle may be prematurely closed in synostoses that affect the sagittal or lambdoid sutures.

   • **Is the anterior fontanelle open?** Premature closure of the anterior fontanelle is seen in adjacent synostoses (coronal, metopic, and/or sagittal).

   • **Do the sternocleidomastoid muscles feel similar and is there adequate and range of motion of the head to both the right and left?** Muscular torticollis may contribute to the synostosis since the muscle inserts on the mastoid prominence of the skull. Resultant interference with range of motion may lead to premature suture fusion.

   • **Is there papilledema?** Increased intracranial pressure is rare with single suture fusion. However, it is manifest by papilledema of the retina. The presence of papilledema may warrant earlier release to address the increased pressure.

   • **Are there other congenital anomalies elsewhere in the body?** Apart from limb anomalies, a search for associated congenital anomalies should be made. Syndromes that include craniosynostosis often involve genetic mutations in the fibroblast growth factor receptor (FGFR) family of proteins.

   — **Apert syndrome** is an autosomal dominant deformity that includes brachycephaly (bilateral coronal synostosis), midface hypoplasia, brachysyndactyly of the hands, and mental deficiency. The incidence of cleft palate in these patients is around 30%, and most have some degree of mental retardation.

— **Crouzon syndrome** is a similar autosomal dominant deformity that involves brachycephaly (bilateral coronal synostosis) and midface hypoplasia, but lacks the findings of syndactyly or mental retardation.

— **Pfeiffer syndrome** is also a similar autosomal dominant deformity that involves brachycephaly (bilateral coronal synostosis) and midface hypoplasia, but presents with broad thumbs and great toes rather than syndactyly.

— **Saethre-Chotzen syndrome** presents with craniosynostosis (often brachycephaly), midface hypoplasia, narrow or cleft palate, prominent ear crus, short clavicles with distal hypoplasia, and brachy- or syndactyly of the hands.

3. Radiographic studies are performed to confirm the diagnosis and to help give the parents a better image of the pathology.

- **Plain radiographs** are often sufficient to identify whether the coronal suture in question is patent or not. The resultant deformity includes asymmetry of the orbits as a result of malposition of the sphenoid bone. This has been termed as "harlequin deformity."

- **CT scan** is perhaps the gold standard to image the pathologic changes in craniosynostosis. It is best performed in the axial and coronal planes at 1.5-mm thickness so that the data can be reconstructed into a three-dimensional image. A CT scan does, however, expose the child to a higher dose of radiation than a plain X-ray series, which should be considered when deciding which studies to order.

- **MRI** is generally of little added benefit. In cases where a Chiari malformation, anomalous venous drainage, or parenchymal abnormalities of the brain are suspected, an MRI-based study (MRI or MRV) can be helpful and complementary to a CT scan.

4. Important consultations are required preoperatively to identify associated issues.

- Adequate evaluation of the optic discs by a **neuroophthalmologist** can often be challenging in an infant, but is exceedingly important when a diagnosis of craniosynostosis is suspected. A thorough neuroophthalmologic examination will help to determine the existence of papilledema as well serve as a baseline from which to compare all subsequent examinations as the child is followed postoperatively.

- A formal evaluation of the child and family by a **geneticist** to determine diagnostic evidence of a potential syndromic or a familial pattern of inheritance can be quite important in directing further testing, elucidating prognosis, and assisting with family planning.

- Thorough testing of the child's **neuropsychological** development can help to characterize underlying brain function and also serve as a baseline from which to compare subsequent developmental changes postoperatively.

- Patients with evidence of significant head tilt secondary to torticollis should be treated aggressively by a **physical therapist** to help treat the underlying positional head deformity as well as prevent relapse and abnormal head shape postoperatively.

5. There is no effective nonoperative therapy for synostosis. The parents may choose not to have the child undergo the procedure, but positioning and orthotic molding devices will not improve the child's appearance. Reconstruction should be performed to minimize the social implications of the deformity.

- **Fronto-orbital advancement** is the procedure of choice for patients with a coronal synostosis. It is generally performed around 8 to 10 months of age. Blood should be available at the beginning of the procedure. Preoperatively, donor-directed blood may be obtained for the patient from a parent. Alternatively, the patient may be given injections of erythropoietin starting 6 weeks before surgery to raise the blood count and minimize the need for transfusion. General anesthesia is required with the infant placed in a supine position. A neurosurgeon should be present for the uni- or bifrontal craniotomy used to access to the anterior fossa. The frontal bone plate ("bandeau") is protected in a moist saline dressing while the orbital bar is removed, recontoured, and replaced in a slightly overcorrected position. It may be held in place with resorbable polylactic plates and screws or dissolvable sutures. Metal wires or plates are no longer recommended because they tend to migrate intracranially with skull growth and remodeling. A drain may be left under the scalp

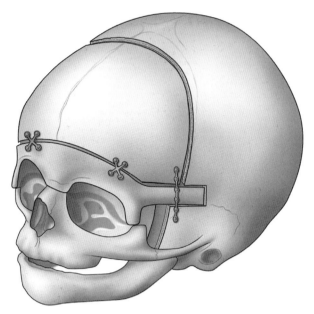

Figure 2-1 Schematic drawing of fronto-orbital advancement to reconstruct the orbital rim and forehead in patients with coronal synostosis.

and removed before discharge if the output is low. Patients are kept in an ICU for one or more nights and discharged when stable. Fronto-orbital advancement has been described using an endoscopic technique as well minimizing the need for a bicoronal incision.

6. Complications resulting from correction of craniosynostosis may be severe and therefore must be considered before, during, and after surgery to minimize their occurrence.

- Young children, with small circulating blood volumes, are prone to significant hemodynamic changes with even small volumes of absolute **blood loss**. Blood should always be available, even if preoperative erythropoietin is used.

- **Dural injury** may result from the craniotomy with adherence of either the stenosed suture or the normal dura to the undersurface of the skull. It is usually easily repaired at the time of injury with either direct approximation of the wound margins or a patch of pericranium or alloplastic material.

- The need to open the calvarial vault predisposes the patient to a small risk of **meningitis**. Perioperative antibiotics are advised.

- **Persistent deformity** will manifest as either undercorrection or temporal hollowing. Undercorrection may be owing to the large amount of advancement required at the initial procedure and reoperation may be indicated. Temporal hollowing results from atrophy or retraction of the temporalis muscle. Numerous techniques have been advocated to address this problem, including muscle resuspension and implants.

PRACTICAL PEARLS

1. Dissection in a supraperiosteal plane from the incision to the fronto-orbital rim will limit blood loss from small blood vessels to the bone.

2. All osteotomies should be carefully protected with a malleable retractor guarding the soft tissue around the saw blade or osteotome.

3. Grooves ("Kerfs") placed on the concave side of a curved piece of bone with a small round cutting burr will aid in contouring the bone, such as at the lateral orbital rim.

4. Slight overcorrection of the advanced segment is advisable since even some small amount of relapse is often seen because of the overlying soft tissue envelope.

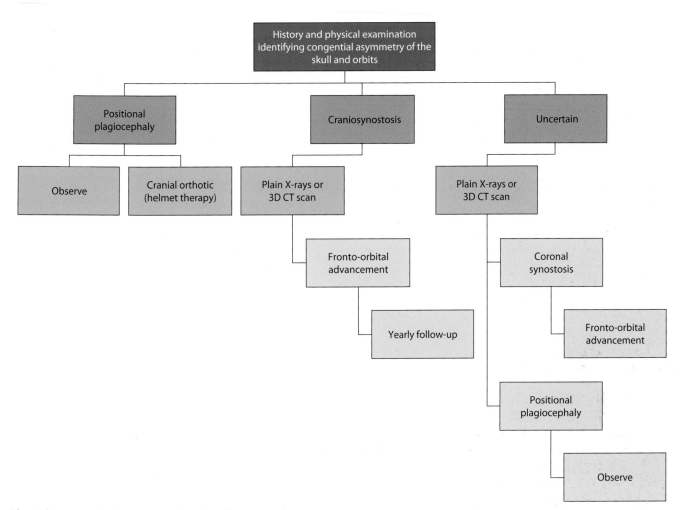

Algorithm 2-1 Management algorithm for coronal synostosis.

References

1. Cohen SR, Mittermiller PA, Meltzer HS, Levy ML, Broder KW, Ozgur BM. Nonsyndromic craniosynostosis: Current treatment options. In: Thaller S, Bradley JP, Gari J, eds. *Craniofacial Surgery*, Boca Raton, FL: Taylor and Francis; 2007: 83-102.

2. Lin KY, Jane J. Unilateral coronal synostosis. In: Lin KY, Jane J, eds. *Craniofacial Surgery: Science and Surgical Technique*. Philadelphia, PA: W. B. Saunders; 2002.

3. Cohen MM, McLean RE. *Craniosynostosis: Diagnosis, Evaluation, and Management*. London, England: Oxford University Press; 2000.

4. Hardesty RA, Marsh JL, Vannier MW. Unicoronal synostosis: a surgical intervention. *Neurosurg Clin N Am*. 1991;2:641-653.

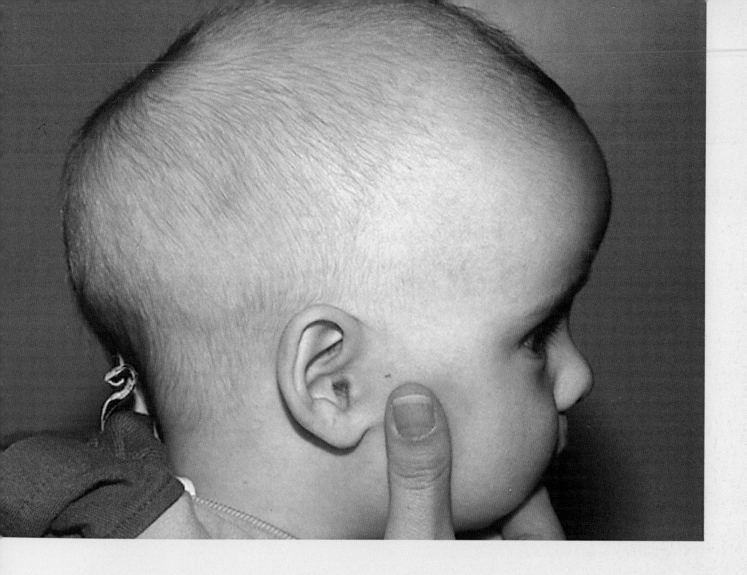

One of the pediatricians at your hospital

asks you to evaluate a 5-month-old child

for the deformity of the head seen

in this photograph.

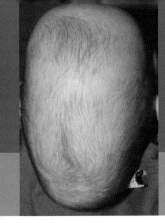

CHAPTER 3

Sagittal Synostosis

Steven R. Buchman, MD

1. The image shown illustrates a patient presenting with an abnormally shaped head. In such cases, it is important to determine whether the change in shape is secondary to a malformation or a deformation. A malformation is secondary to an intrinsic problem with the skull (such as craniosynostosis) while a deformation is secondary to an extrinsic process exerting an influence to deform the skull (such as molding or a positional head deformity). Questions aimed at discerning the differences between these two diagnoses are very important as the treatment varies considerably. In this case, the head shape could be described as scaphocephalic (boat or keel shaped) and a diagnosis of sagittal craniosynostosis should be seriously considered. The following questions should help to delineate better the diagnosis and possible treatment options.

- **Was the child born prematurely?** Premature children quite often demonstrate a dolichocephalic appearance that can be confused with sagittal craniosynostosis. In addition, extended time in the neonatal intensive care unit can be associated with positional head deformities as a result of lengthy times of restrictive head posture in their cribs.

- **Was the deformity present at birth?** Most commonly, craniosynostosis is a process that starts prenatally and the manifestations of abnormal head shape are present and severe at birth. Although molding can result from the birthing process itself, positional head deformities are often the result of postnatal extrinsic forces that function to hinder normal shape and contour of the skull.

- **Has the abnormal head shape been getting better, worse, or staying the same over time?** Craniosynostosis, rarely, if ever, corrects itself as it is caused by a fusion of the bones that prevent normal expansion of the brain leading to an abnormal head shape. Molding is a process of deformation caused by the birthing process and should self-correct over time. Positional head deformity is caused by extrinsic factors that predispose to abnormal head shape, when these extrinsic factors are removed, the deformity should start to self-correct.

- **What is the age of the patient?** The age of the patient is important as it will impact potential surgical options

(in the case of craniosynostosis), and the efficacy of nonsurgical options such as helmet therapy for positional deformities.

- **Does the child show any signs of developmental delay?** Increased intracranial pressure can be manifest by developmental delays. Delays can also signal more significant problems such as genetic syndromes or an intrauterine event leading to brain impairment. Physical delays may predispose a child to restrictive positioning and resultant abnormal changes in head shape.

2. The physical examination is an indispensable adjunct to the history as it guides both the diagnosis and treatment of the patient and serves to focus the surgeon on the specific findings to be addressed in the operating room. Often, the diagnosis of synostosis can be made on physical examination alone. A thorough examination of the child, however, must be done to identify associated malformations.

- **What is the shape of the skull?** Craniosynostosis presents with an abnormal head shape consisting of growth restriction perpendicular to the involved suture and compensatory growth in a parallel direction to the involved suture. In the case of sagittal craniosynostosis, the child will often demonstrate a scaphocephalic appearance, frontal bossing, bitemporal constriction, an occipital shelf, and a biaural width of the cranium that is greater than its biparietal width.

- **Are there palpable ridges in the skull?** A fused suture will often be raised and can frequently be palpated as a ridge running in the direction of the involved suture under the scalp.

- **What is the patient's head circumference?** Children with isolated sagittal craniosynostosis most commonly show an increased head circumference as a result of the shape of the skull and the conservation of the brain mass within the skull.

- **Is there evidence of papilledema?** The finding of papilledema on physical examination is a sign of increased intracranial pressure. Although rare in isolated cases of single suture craniosynostosis, increased intracranial pressure should prompt urgent intervention, including direct pressure monitoring and/or operative expansion and decompression of the skull. Increased intracranial pressure is rare with single suture fusion.

- **Are there other congenital anomalies elsewhere in the body?** A thorough search for associated congenital anomalies should be made. Findings of syndactyly, limb deformities, clefts, hypertelorism, midface retrusion, low hairline, low set ears, cardiac, and urologic deformities have all been associated with syndromic craniosynostoses.

- **Is there evidence of torticollis?** A tight sternocleidomastoid muscle and particular types of strabismus can result in a significant and persistent head tilt. An uncorrected head tilt can lead to a severe and enduring positional head deformity as well as negatively impact surgically corrected head shape.

3. Studies that are necessary for the workup of children suspected of sagittal craniosynostosis include:

- A **plain radiograph** skull series is often an adequate screening tool and adjunct to the history and physical examination to determine whether the child has craniosynostosis or a deformation of the skull. These plain films will often demonstrate fusion of the longitudinal sagittal suture on an AP view. The lateral view will highlight the distorted length of the skull, the frontal bossing, and the occipital shelf. Plain radiographic films may also reveal a "copper beaten appearance" that can be suggestive of increased intracranial pressure.

- If the diagnosis of craniosynostosis is still in doubt, after a thorough history and physical examination and the evaluation of plain radiographs, then a **CT scan** can be very helpful in determining the diagnosis. If the child has been diagnosed as having craniosynostosis then a CT scan can be very helpful to outline underlying anatomical findings to help guide the neurosurgeon and craniofacial surgeon. The head CT scan is best performed in the axial and coronal planes at 1.5 mm thickness so that the data may be reconstructed into a three-dimensional image.

- In cases where a Chiari malformation, anomalous venous drainage, or parenchymal abnormalities of the brain are suspected, an **MRI** (or MRV) based study can be helpful and complementary to a CT scan.

4. Important consultations can help to outline the nature of the child's malady as well as determine the need for other workup prior to determining a treatment strategy.

- Adequate evaluation of the optic discs by a **neuroophthalmologist** can often be challenging in an infant but is exceedingly important when a diagnosis of craniosynostosis is suspected. A thorough neuroophthalmological examination will help to determine the existence of papilledema as well serve as a baseline from which to compare all subsequent examinations as the child is followed postoperatively.

- A formal evaluation of the child and family by a **geneticist** to determine diagnostic evidence of a potential syndromic or a familial pattern of inheritance can be quite important in directing further testing, elucidating prognosis, and assisting with family planning.

- Thorough testing of the child's **neuropsychological** development can help to characterize underlying brain function and can also serve as a baseline from which to compare subsequent developmental changes postoperatively.

- Patients with evidence of significant head tilt secondary to torticollis should be treated aggressively by a **physical therapist** to help treat an underlying positional head deformity as well as prevent relapse and abnormal head shape postoperatively.

5. The treatment options for a documented scaphocephaly secondary to sagittal craniosynostosis are wholly surgical. There are no effective nonoperative therapies for craniosynostosis. Although the parents may choose not to have a surgical procedure to correct the problem, positioning and orthotic devices will not improve the child's appearance. In cases where the parents choose not to reconstruct their child's skull, close follow-up is mandated to continually assess the patient for signs of increased intracranial pressure. Surgical reconstruction is aimed at restoration of normal calvarial vault morphology, minimizing the social implications of the deformity, and preventing the development of increased intracranial pressure. Treatment options include:

- One of the earliest surgical procedures utilized to correct this malady is the simple **strip craniectomy**. This procedure removes the involved synostotic suture with

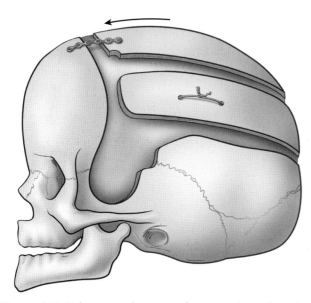

Figure 3-1 Schematic drawing of open calvarial vault reconstruction in patients with sagittal synostosis.

a margin of normal bone on either side. The procedure releases the growth restriction of the skull and relies on the growth and expansion of the underlying brain to correct the deformity over time. This procedure can be performed "open" or endoscopically.

- Because of the inability of the strip craniectomy procedure to predictably and reproducibly correct the scaphocephalic deformity, **barrel stave osteotomies** were often added to aid in molding the skull. Continued unpredictability led to the further addition of postoperative molding helmets to help "guide" the underlying brain in an attempt to attain improved and more predictable results.

- **Calvarial vault reconstruction** is the procedure of choice at most major medical centers for children with a sagittal synostosis. The specific types of calvarial vault reconstruction vary from center to center and from surgeon to surgeon.

  — Some surgeons approach the deformity posteriorly and place the child in the prone position for the operation. The occipital shelf and the narrowed occipital bone is the main focus of such an operation. The parietal and temporal bones are addressed within the limitations of the prone position. Those surgeons who utilize such an approach believe that the bossing of the frontal bone and the bitemporal narrowing will then self-correct. In cases where such self-correction is in doubt or in cases where the frontal deformity is severe, many surgeons would then consider a second-stage operation to address the frontal abnormality.

  — Surgeons that utilize the supine position perform a procedure that is most often aimed at complete restoration of normal calvarial shape and frontal appearance at the time of the operation. This total or subtotal calvarial vault reshaping may have

limitations at the most posterior level of the occipital bone. Gentle flexing of the cranium at the time of surgery, however, will often allow access to the occiput enabling a total calvarial vault reconstruction. In these cases, the anterior–posterior (AP) dimension of the skull may be shortened and the biparietal width is expanded to effect an immediate change in the appearance of the skull. In cases where access to the total cranial vault is thought to be difficult and a single-stage procedure is desired, the patient can be placed in a "Sphinx" position.

- In severe cases of frontal bossing where the deformity may preclude the ability to effect a normal contour, a **frontal orbital advancement** can be added to the calvarial vault reconstruction allowing a more normalized relationship between the frontal orbital bar and the forehead. Such an approach may often be necessary in children that present late with the deformity and are much older at the time of surgery. In all these cases, the procedures may often be carried out as early as 3 months of age. It is recommended that a neurosurgeon be present to perform the craniotomy to afford access to the cranial vault. General anesthesia and advanced monitoring is required and the children are usually kept in the intensive care unit overnight. Transfusion is not uncommon and therefore blood should be available at the beginning of the procedure. Donor directed blood may be possible although blood obtained from the patient's parents is usually not advised as they could be utilized as potential transplant donors for other needs of the child in the future. Strategies for decreasing transfusions can also be employed such as the use of Aprotinin at the time of surgery or alternatively, the patient may be given injections of Epogen starting 6 weeks before surgery to raise the blood count.

6. The potential complications resulting from calvarial vault reconstruction for sagittal synostosis are significant, including injury to vital surrounding structures. All must be considered before, during, and after surgery to minimize their occurrence.

- The sagittal sinus and torcular Herophili are large venous channels that, if violated, can lead to life-threatening **bleeding**. **Blood loss** from osteotomies and from dural vessels need to be controlled and careful monitoring of fluid status and blood volume is imperative.

- The covering of the brain can be damaged during any osteotomy and particularly at the time of craniotomy as the adherent dura is dissected free from the underlying skull and stenosed suture. The **dural injury** should be directly repaired at the time of injury with either direct approximation of the wound margins or a patch of pericranium or alloplastic material.

- As is the case with most surgical procedures the risk of **infection** is ever present. The sterile confines of the cranial cavity are particularly at risk in these cases where the unclean regions of the face and ears and

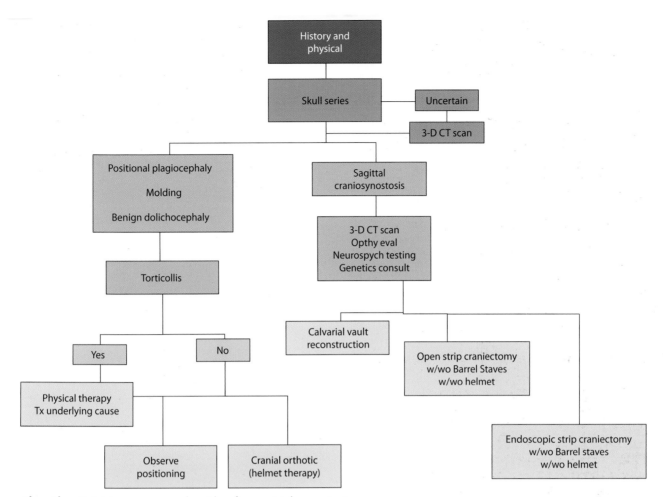

Algorithm 3-1 Management algorithm for sagittal synostosis.

1. In general, the earlier repair the easier the operation and the better the results. We rarely will perform surgery on these children before the age of 3 months but somewhere between 3 months and 6 months is ideal.

2. Head tilt secondary to torticollis can have profound effects on head shape and facial form. In cases where the head tilt is found in patients with craniosynostosis that undergo surgical correction, the consequences of the condition can be profound and may act to destabilize and thwart the potential for an excellent outcome. Vigorous physical therapy and persistent exercises by the parents is warranted for habitual torticollis and treatment for any underlying causes are paramount before moving forward with craniofacial surgery.

3. The "memory" of the enveloping scalp will often work toward relapse back to the original skull shape. The best ways to counteract these forces are to stabilize, firmly fix, and overcorrect areas of advancement and expansion of the surgical reconstruction.

4. There is often fluid that builds up in the subgaleal space after a craniofacial operation. Some surgeons place a drain for this fluid while others consider tapping residual fluid sometime after surgery. We perform a serpentine bicoronal incision that starts and ends behind the ears and leave a 5 to 6 mm opening the very base of the incision to drain. Reinforced gauze left at those areas does absorb the drainage and the areas close by themselves without difficulty.

5. When operating on young children that still have significant growth of the skull ahead of them, "tactical" openings of the skull should be used. The open areas should allow preferential brain growth in a direction that is reinforcing and salutary to the repair and preferentially left at the base of the skull adjacent to intact native bone as the bone edge as well as the dura will function to fill the bone gap over time lessening the likelihood of a long-term cranial defect.

scalp can contaminate the operative field. The potential for meningitis is increased even further if the dura is violated during the case. Surprisingly, the incidence of infection in the cases is quite low.

- In cases where self-correction is required for normalization of shape and contour, a **persistent deformity** may prompt the need for reoperation of some or all of the involved areas. In cases where total reconstruction is performed at the time of the operation, undercorrection or malpositioning could also warrant revisions. It should be remembered that the child will undergo considerable growth after surgery and that the surgical reconstruction should take that into consideration. The "memory" of the scalp and soft tissue envelope should not be underestimated during the postoperative period.

- Although the procedures for correction of scaphocephaly secondary to sagittal craniosynostosis are much safer than they have ever been, they still carry with them the risk of **death**. Craniofacial procedures involving the cranial cavity pose many of the same risks to the patient's life as other neurosurgical procedures.

References

1. Buchman SR, Murazsko KM. Syndromic craniosynostosis. In: Lin, Ogle, Jane, eds. *Craniofacial Surgery A Multidisciplinary Approach to Craniofacial Anomalies*. Philadelphia, PA: W. B. Saunders; 2002:252-271.

2. Shin JH, Persing JA. Sagittal craniosynostosis. In: Lin, Ogle, Jane, eds. *Craniofacial Surgery A Multidisciplinary Approach to Craniofacial Anomalies*. Philadelphia, PA: W. B. Saunders; 2002:225-232.

3. Buchman SR, Murazsko K: Fronto-orbital reconstruction: *Atlas of the Oral & Maxillofacial Surgery Clinics of North America* 2002;10(1):43-56.

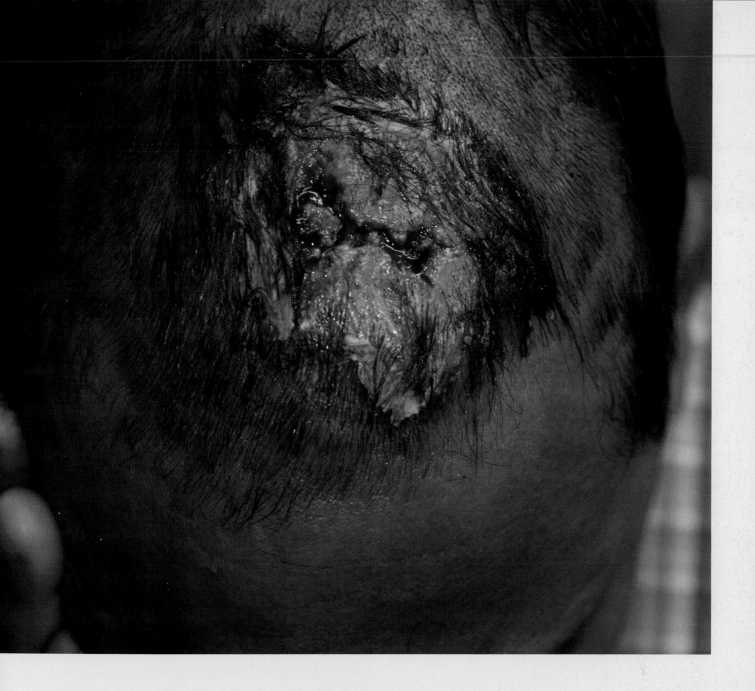

A 55-year-old man is found unconscious following a lightning storm and brought to the emergency department for evaluation of a wound at the top of the head.

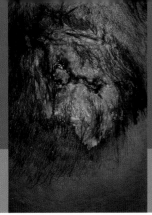

CHAPTER 4

Scalp Wound

Bradon J. Wilhelmi, MD, FACS

1. In evaluating a traumatic wound of the scalp, it is critical to determine the inciting cause of the injury by obtaining an adequate history of the event. By report, the wound in question resulted from an electrical current. Similar defects can follow acute or chronic blunt trauma or tumor resection. An electrical insult results in progressive tissue necrosis in excess of the originally apparent trauma, and somewhat resembles a crush injury. Controversy exists as to whether this is a slow manifestation of irreversible muscle damage secondary to the original current of passage, or if is actively progressive ischemic necrosis secondary to ongoing macrovascular or microvascular compromise. Passage of the electric current through a solid conductor can result in conversion of electrical energy into heat. The extent of injury depends on the type of current, the pathway of flow, the local tissue resistance, and the duration of contact. Because high-voltage burns can result in a fall from a height or throw from the inciting source, these patients should have a proper level I trauma evaluation with attention to the ABCs with a primary and secondary survey. If the injury is acute but there is no antecedent burn injury, this could be a traumatic avulsion which could be replanted. If the injury is chronic, tumor or pressure may be the cause for the tissue damage. Specific information in the history can point to pressure, such as loss of consciousness or a long operation.

- **When did the injury occur?** Wounds that are fairly recent may not have demarcated fully and may further demonstrate areas of necrosis or viability with time. In some instances, it is prudent to wait some time before performing definitive coverage.

- **How much voltage was the patient subjected to?** Injury resulting from an electrical burn can be divided into high and low voltage injuries as determined by the amount of voltage to which the patient is exposed. Low voltage burns occur with exposures below 1000 V and behave similar to thermal burns, having zones of injury from the surface extending into the tissue. Households in the United States have currents between 100 to 220 V that alternate current (AC) at a cycle of 60 Hz. High voltage electrical injuries (industrial or power line) occur when patients are exposed to greater than 1000 V. A high voltage electrical injury

is more of a syndrome than a specific injury, because several organ systems can be involved. The high voltage burn injury involves the cutaneous skin as well as hidden destruction of deeper tissues and sometimes other organs such as the kidneys, brain ("**Is the patient coherent and reasonable**"), spinal cord ("**Is the patient able to move all four extremities**"), peripheral nerves, intra-abdominal organs ("**Does the patient have abdominal pain**"), fractures, vascular system ("**Is there evidence of circumferential burns or a compartment syndrome**"), and eyes ("**Is the patient's vision similar to his preinjury state**").

- **What was the duration of contact?** A current of 10 milliamperes (mA) that enters the head and travels through the forearm may produce static contracture of the muscles not allowing the patient to let go of the electrical source.

- **Did the patient lose consciousness?** Loss of consciousness can be related to current strength or concomitant head trauma or an inciting event prior to the scalp injury. A current of 50 mA for longer than 2 seconds may produce ventricular tachycardia.

- **Where was the patient found and was there associated trauma?** If the patient has an acute injury in association with a high voltage electrical burn, fall from a height, throw a significant distance, or occur in association with motor vehicle accident or industrial injury, a level I trauma evaluation should be performed.

- **Does the patient have preexisting medical problems?** Many patients with cardiovascular disease have other comorbid conditions that preclude major reoperative surgery. In such cases, drainage/debridement and extended wound care may be a more prudent strategy.

- **Is there a history of radiation exposure?** Radiation adversely affects skin vascularity and flap viability and can lead to further necrosis of random and axial patterned flaps.

- **Does the patient smoke?** This is important to note since smoking affects the vascular anatomy and can impair circulation to pedicled flaps.

2. After obtaining the history, the extent and stage of the disease can be determined through performing the direct physical examination. A thorough physical examination should address the specific complications of electrical injury as well as the wound itself to dictate the reconstructive options. In severe electrical injuries, death of large volumes of muscle will occur, and this results in extremely large fluid loss. Significant blood loss may occur as a consequence of vascular injury or from associated fractures or chest or abdominal trauma. Shock should not be attributed to an uncomplicated electrical injury.

- **Where is the entry wound? Where is the exit wound?** Contact area wounds should be located on careful full-body examination. This requires careful examination of the scalp, as well as the soles of the feet. Tissue resistance progressively increases from nerve to blood vessels, muscle, skin, tendon, fat, and bone. Bone, having the greatest resistance, generates the most heat. Any burn injury should be evaluated for depth/degree realizing that determination is difficult because much of the injured tissue is hidden beneath the apparently less injured skin. The injury should be documented with photos and designated on a Lund-Browder chart.

- **What is the patient's neurologic status?** In addition to the mental status, a cursory neurological examination should be performed to check for focal motor and sensory deficits. Later, a detailed examination of the nervous system will be necessary, for diagnosis of hemiplegia, aphasia, cerebellar dysfunction, and epilepsy which can complicate high voltage electrical injuries.

- **Does the patient have signs of ocular injury?** Higher than normal current passing through the lens of the eye may produce cataracts, but these usually develop 6 months after injury.

- **Is there spine tenderness?** Cervical or lower spine injury should be managed with prompt placement of a rigid collar and then ruled out by physical examination by noting the patient's level of distal motor function and sensory awareness. If the history suggests a chronic etiology the systemic examination is performed to assist with the diagnosis. In performing the examination of a patient with a scalp wound that may be a pressure sore, the patient may be found to have sores in other supine, pressure bearing areas such as the sacrum or heels.

- **Does the patient have a regular heart rate and rhythm?** Electrical injury can affect conduction through the heart. Ventricular fibrillation is not uncommon with high voltage electrical injury.

- **Does the patient have abdominal tenderness or signs of peritoneal irritation?** The possibility of associated hemorrhage or perforation of an intra-abdominal viscus should always be considered, especially in the presence of peritoneal findings, nausea, and/or vomiting.

- **Is there deformity of the extremities?** In addition to exit wounds, a full extremity examination should be performed to identify associated dislocations and fractures as a result of violent titanic muscular contractions seen with high voltage electrical injuries or a secondary fall.

- **Is there evidence of distal extremity compromise?** The peripheral circulation is assessed to determine the presence of compartment syndrome and the need for escharotomy or fasciotomy. Muscle compartment pressure recording may be a necessary adjunct to making this determination. A compartment syndrome can be seen at the point of contact or at the exit site of a high voltage electrical injury. Increased pressure can result from muscle damage within a confined fascial compartment with a high voltage electrical injury which ultimately occludes arterial flow. The classic signs of acute arterial occlusion are pain, pallor, absence or diminished pulse, paralysis, and/or paresthesia (the 5 P's). The first indication of compartment syndrome is pain on passive motion causing stretching of the muscles within the compartment. Direct measurement of the pressure within a given muscle compartment using a pressure-sensitive needle may be performed if there is concern. An elevated pressure (>30 mm Hg) would necessitate emergent fasciotomy. There are four compartments of the leg (anterior, lateral, superficial, and deep posterior), three compartments of the forearm (flexor, extensor, and mobile wad), and ten in the hand. Because pressure changes in these compartments over time, in high voltage electrical injuries, these patients have to be serially monitored for compartment syndrome over time. Muscle viability can be evaluated at the time of fasciotomy by direct inspection for bleeding and contractibility.

- **Are there similar lesions?** If the wound is the result of excision of a cutaneous carcinoma, a full body skin and nodal examination should be performed.

3. Specific studies offer little in confirming the diagnosis if caused by trauma. However, several studies are indicated depending on the etiology of the injury. Specific concern in the electrical burn patient is cardiac and renal injury.

- A full admission panel, including electrolytes should be obtained in the trauma patient. Increased potassium levels and acidosis suggest extensive muscle injury. High creatinine levels suggest renal impairment. Elevated potassium levels may require treatment with calcium and dextrose/insulin in addition to the bicarbonate to prevent cardiac complications from hyperkalemia such as "torsades de pointes" and cardiac arrest.

- A routine series of radiographs, including chest, pelvic and cervical spine, should be obtained in cases of trauma.

- Scalp wounds resulting from acute trauma can occur in patients as a result of loss of consciousness or a cardiac event. This should be appropriately evaluated with a **head CT and EKG**.

- Patients should have **cardiac monitoring** and pharmacologic treatment for dysrhythmias.

- Initial and serial **urine myoglobin** levels should be obtained to identify the risk for acute tubular necrosis. The level should be followed to document a continual decline to normal.

- Muscle necrosis within a wound can be evaluated with a **Technetium-99m pyrophosphate muscle scan**. However, if compartment syndrome is suspected fasciotomy should be performed without delay to minimize risk for irreversible muscle loss.

- If the wound is suspicious for cutaneous carcinoma, either an incisional or excisional **biopsy** of the lesion is warranted. If the lesion appears fixed and suggestive of bone involvement, a CT scan or MRI can be helpful.

4. Consults should be arranged as necessary. Traumatic injuries may require the services of other specialists such as cardiology, nephrology, orthopedics, ophthalmology, neurosurgery, etc.

- If the etiology of the defect is tumor excision, an oncologist should be consulted for adjuvant treatment and follow-up. The staging for cancer of the head and neck is as follows:

— Primary tumor (T)

a. TX - Primary tumor cannot be assessed.

b. T0 - No evidence of primary tumor.

c. Tis - Carcinoma in situ.

d. T1 - Tumor 2 cm or less in greatest dimension.

e. T2 - Tumor more than 2 cm but not more than 4 cm in greatest dimension.

f. T3 - Tumor more than 4 cm.

g. T4 - Tumor invades adjacent structures.

— Regional lymph nodes (N)

a. NX - Regional lymph nodes cannot be assessed.

b. N0 - No regional lymph node metastasis.

c. N1 - Metastasis in a single ipsilateral lymph node, 3 cm or less in greatest dimension.

d. N2 - Metastasis in a single ipsilateral lymph node, more than 3 cm but not more than 6 cm in greatest dimension or in multiple ipsilateral lymph nodes, none more than 6 cm in greatest dimension, or in bilateral contralateral lymph nodes, none more than 6 cm in greatest dimension.

e. N2a - Metastasis in a single ipsilateral lymph node more than 3 cm but not more than 6 cm.

f. N2b - Metastasis in multiple ipsilateral lymph nodes, none more than 6 cm.

g. N2c - Metastasis in bilateral or contralateral lymph nodes, none more than 6 cm.

h. N3 - Metastasis in a lymph node more than 6 cm.

— Distant metastasis (M)

a. MX - Presence of distant metastasis cannot be assessed.

b. M0 - No distant metastasis.

c. M1 - Distant metastasis.

— Stage grouping

a. Stage 0: Tis,N0,M0

b. Stage I: T1,N0,M0

c. Stage II: T2,N0,M0

d. Stage III: T3,N0,M0 and T1,N1,M0, and T2,N1,M0 and T3,N1,M0.

e. Stage IV: T4,N0,M0 and T4,N1,M0 and any T,N2,M0 and any T,N3,M0, and any T,any N,M1.

5. Treatment will vary by etiology. Burn injury warrants fluid resuscitation cognizant often in excess of the calculated Parkland formula. Initially, the IV fluid rate should be titrated carefully to promote 70 to 100 mL/h urine output to reduce the risk of developing acute tubular necrosis from myoglobin deposition. Mannitol (50 g every 8 hours) can be used to promote diuresis and bicarbonate can be added to reduce the precipitation of myoglobin.

- Circumferential constricting burns on the extremities require at least escharotomies and consideration for fasciotomies, when indicated or compartment syndrome is suspected. Because major nerves are susceptible to increased pressure in closed compartments, escharotomy and/or fasciotomy alone may not be sufficient to decompress nerves in an upper extremity. Therefore, decompression of the median and ulnar nerves as an emergency procedure in high voltage injuries may be required at the time of the fasciotomies.

- Patients with open wounds should also receive tetanus prophylaxis with the goal being to avoid life-threatening clostridial infection. For tetanus prone wounds (yard and farm injuries with devitalized tissue) that occurred more than 12 to 24 hours from the time of injury, treatment depends on the patient's vaccination history. Patients who were fully immunized in the past but have not received a booster for more than 5 years should receive 0.5 mL of tetanus toxoid IM. Patients who have not received a full course of immunization should not only receive tetanus toxoid but also passive immunization with 250 units of human tetanus immune globulin IM. The pediatric dose is 4 U/kg.

- If the electrical burn wound is from a low voltage (<1000 V) household injury the wound can be managed similar to a thermal injury with a topical antimicrobial to control bacterial contamination and minimize risk of infection. *Silver sulfadiazine* (Silvadene) is the most frequently used topical agent for thermal burn wounds because it cases minimal pain. When the wound is a result of a high voltage burn, *Mafenide acetate* (Sulfamylon) is particularly well suited for these wounds since it can penetrate to the deep levels of the injury.

- Early wound debridement of devitalized necrotic tissue may lower the burden on the immune system against infection as the most frequent cause of death in this patient population is from systemic infection (7%). Debridement of skin, soft tissue, and bone (outer table followed by full thickness) may be necessary, if any of these tissue layers are not viable. Only viable tissue margins should remain.

- Reconstruction should be planned even if not possible at the time of the initial debridement or resection. The scalp and skull are the primary tissue types covering the brain and meninges. The scalp contains skin, fat, and galea. The underlying calvarium is covered with periosteum. Bone requires soft tissue coverage and the brain requires rigid protection. Early coverage may be necessary if there is exposure of bone to avoid full thickness calvarial desiccation and loss. A negative pressure sponge dressing may be utilized on exposed bone to minimize bone desiccation until ultimate reconstruction can be safely performed.

  — Skin grafts may be used over pericranium (periosteum of cranium) but require a well-vascularized bed. Skin grafts survive initially by plasmatic imbibition but ultimately inosculation and angiogenesis must occur for the graft to survive. If the pericranium is deficient or absent, grafts can revascularize on granulation tissue formed over the calvarium, but not on bare bone. Granulation tissue can form on the bare calvarium by burring the outer table and allowing tissue to develop from the openings.

  — Local and regional flaps are useful for limited defects since the scalp is fairly immobile and difficult to rotate over the convexity of the calvarium. The advantage of using flaps for scalp reconstruction, is the ability to provide skin, dermal elements (such as hair and moisturizing glands) and subcutaneous fat to provide more reliable and aesthetically matching tissue.

    a. The temporoparietal flap (superficial temporal fascial flap, STF) is based on the frontal and parietal branches of the superficial temporal artery. The fascia of STF is an extension of the galea. The axis of rotation of the STF is immediately anterior to the base of the helical crus at the scalp, which limits its arc of rotation.

    b. The temporoparieto-occipital flap (Juri) may be used for frontal or frontoparietal defects. The base is 2 to 3 cm above the zygomatic arch and the flap extends posteriorly. The normal width of the Juri flap is 4 cm and the flap should be delayed to optimize its reliability, since it is 32 cm long. It is raised in a subgaleal plane at the second stage.

    c. The more commonly used Orticochea flap is useful for covering defects that encompass up to 30% of the scalp. These flaps are elevated deep to the galea and incisions within the galea may be used to allow for stretch of the flaps. The anterior pedicle arises from the ophthalmic vessels, the lateral pedicle from the superficial temporal vessels, and the posterior pedicle from the medial and lateral occipital vessels. In the high-voltage burn wound patient, these flaps may not be useful because of the risk of worsening the circulation to adjacent tissues with marginal blood supply from the inciting injury, as contiguous injury as far as 25 cm from the point of current entry has been described. Other pedicle flaps used for head and neck reconstruction including the latissimus, pectoralis, and trapezius muscles, may be too bulky and have a limited arc of motion for most scalp wounds.

  — Tissue expanders may be used to advance surrounding skin and scalp when a two-stage reconstruction is preferred. If the wound is acute and open with desiccating bone, as is encountered in high-voltage electrical burns, tissue expansion is not an immediate option for reconstruction. Tissue expansion is useful if the wound has been temporarily covered with a skin graft and the goal is to replace the skin grafted areas with more durable soft tissue coverage. Tissue expanders should be placed in the subgaleal plane. Rectangular or crescent-shaped expanders provide a greater expansion over round expanders. Tissue expanders are contraindicated for scalp reconstruction in children younger than 3 years of age because of

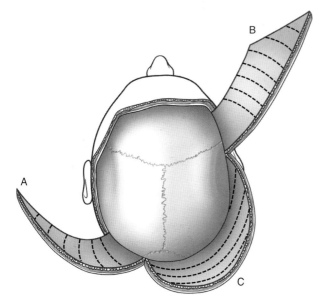

Figure 4-1 Schematic drawing of subgaleal scalp flaps useful for scalp reconstruction. Note the option for galeal scoring to increase the dimensions of the flap.

the presence of open calvarial sutures. Also, the patient has to be amenable to the disfigurement of the head during the expansion process which requires frequent office visits. Complications of tissue expansion are common (50%) and include deflation, thinning alopecia, exposure, infection, skin erosion from folds or thin skin, and pain. As much as 50% of the scalp can be resurfaced with staged tissue expansion.

— Free tissue transfer is reserved for larger, complex defects. Recipient vessels can be challenging to select and use. The superficial temporal and occipital vessels are of small caliber and difficult to expose. Smaller vessels are prone to spasm and occlusion. The external carotid artery and internal jugular vein are usually remote enough from the wound to necessitate the use of vein grafts to reach the defect. Several free flaps have been described for scalp reconstruction. The most commonly used free flaps for scalp reconstruction include the latissimus dorsi (with sheet skin graft), omentum, scapular, and radial forearm flaps.

— Replacement of bone is required for protection if there is a full-thickness skull defect after resection of necrotic bone or bone involved with tumor. Reconstruction may be performed solely with titanium mesh, or with an acrylic implant, methylmethacrylate, or autogenous bone.

— Replantation of an avulsed scalp may be considered for immediate reconstruction when the amputated part has minimal injury and a short ischemia time (<24 hours). The entire scalp can survive on a single artery and vein because of the extensive collateral flow in the scalp. The most commonly used vessels for scalp replantation include the

superficial temporal artery and vein. Because these lateral vessels may be difficult to expose in a patient with a rigid cervical collar, vein grafts can be used. These vein grafts have to be reversed appropriately to avoid obstruction of flow by the valves. Once the vein grafts are repaired to the scalp vessels, the amputated part is brought to the patient and repaired to the donor vessels. The hair in the replanted scalp, when successful, can be expected to grow and densely populate after a period of telophase (resting phase for the hair follicles).

6. The complications of an electrical burn are numerous. They include cardiac arrhythmias, renal failure from myoglobinuria, and intestinal bleeding. The latter was formerly a common complication in burn patients, but it is less commonly encountered today. Gastric and duodenal mucosal lesions have been shown to occur within 48 hours postinjury, and previously led to hemorrhage, ulceration, perforation, and death. Because antacid prophylaxis is a routine part of therapy in burn patients, this complication has declined. Those resulting from scalp reconstruction are similar to other areas of the body but unique in the need for hair-bearing tissue in children and many adults.

• **Flap loss** may occur in any area of the body. The more reliable the flap, the better will be the chance of success. Local wound care should precede aggressive reconstructive efforts. Reconstruction with split thickness skin grafts may be performed for secondary wound closure and then removed following tissue expansion of the lateral hair-bearing scalp.

• **Alopecia** is a noticeable but minor complication of scalp reconstruction. It will certainly result from skin grafting over an area of burred calvarium. Once stable, the wound may be revised either with single-stage scar revision or with multistaged tissue expansion.

PRACTICAL PEARLS

1. In treating high-voltage electrical burns, life-threatening and limb-threatening problems should be operatively managed acutely and definitive wound closure delayed at least 72 hours until the progressive injury is complete.

2. Waiting for all the signs of compartment syndrome to appear (pain, pallor, absence or diminished pulse, paralysis, and paresthesia) in patients with suspected compartment syndrome may be too late. Fasciotomies should be performed without delay to minimize risk for irreversible muscle loss.

3. Moderate length can be achieved with scalp flaps by incising the underlying galea but being careful not to injure the axial (or random) blood supply.

4. Incisions in the scalp should be beveled to minimize injury to developing follicles.

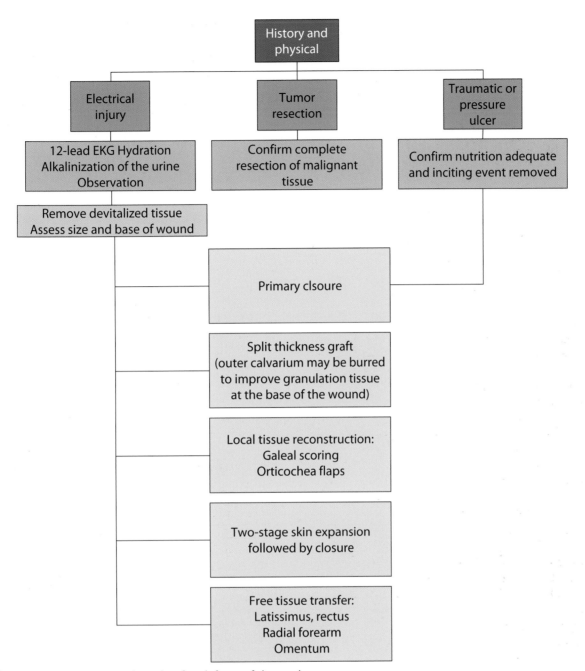

Algorithm 4-1 Management algorithm for defects of the scalp.

Boxes in the figure:

- History and physical
- Electrical injury
- Tumor resection
- Traumatic or pressure ulcer
- 12-lead EKG Hydration Alkalinization of the urine Observation
- Confirm complete resection of malignant tissue
- Confirm nutrition adequate and inciting event removed
- Remove devitalized tissue Assess size and base of wound
- Primary clsoure
- Split thickness graft (outer calvarium may be burred to improve granulation tissue at the base of the wound)
- Local tissue reconstruction: Galeal scoring Orticochea flaps
- Two-stage skin expansion followed by closure
- Free tissue transfer: Latissimus, rectus Radial forearm Omentum

References

1. Young DM. Burn and electrical injury. In: Mathes SJ, ed. *Plastic Surgery*. Vol I. Philadelphia, PA: Saunders Elsevier; 2006;811-834.

2. Fordyce TA, Kelsh M, Lu ET, Sahl JD, Yager JW. Thermal burn and electrical injuries among electric utility workers, 1995–2004. *Burns*. 2006;33(2):209-220.

3. Dalay C, Kesiktas E, Yavuz M, Ozerdem G, Acarturk S. Coverage of scalp defects following contact electrical burns to the head: A clinical series. *Burns*. 2006;32(2):201-207.

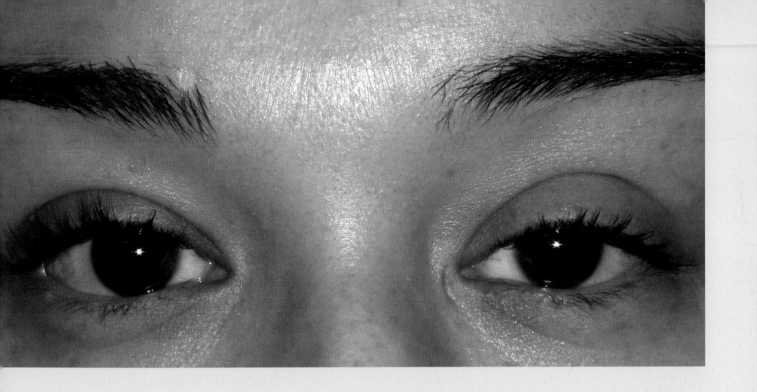

A 30-year-old woman presents with complaints of heaviness of her eyelids and visual obstruction.

CHAPTER 5
Eyelid Ptosis

Marco Harmaty

1. Patients on various ages may present with a complaint of inability to fully open one or both eyelids, sagging of the eyelids, or difficulty holding their eyes open. For these patients, a careful history should elucidate one of several clear etiologies so that the appropriate treatment may be offered.

   - **Was the deformity present at birth?** Congenital ptosis is caused by maldevelopment of the levator muscle. Opening of the upper eyelid is controlled by the levator palpebrae superoris muscle which originates from the apical cone of the orbit immediately superior to the superior rectus muscle. It is innervated by the oculomotor nerve (CN III). The muscle runs anteriorly within the orbit to become an aponeurosis at the superior equator of the globe. The superior transverse ligament of Whitnall travels from the lacrimal gland fossa laterally to the trochlea medially. It is thought to act as a clothesline over which the levator hangs and changes from a horizontal structure to a vertical one. The aponeurosis divides into an anterior–portion, which inserts into the lower third of the anterior surface of the tarsal plate, and a posterior portion, which inserts into the superior edge of the tarsal plate as Muller's muscle. The striated muscle fibers of the levator become replaced with fibrous tissue and fat.

   - **How old is the patient and what is the quality of the skin?** Disinsertion or laxity of the levator aponeurosis is the most common cause of eyelid ptosis and is seen with increasing age. The course is more often progressive over time rather than presenting in an acute fashion.

   - **Does the patient have trouble with vision?** Adults usually present with aesthetic concerns about the appearance of the eyelids or with problems related to their vision. However, in neonates, eyelid ptosis is more critical and interference with vision needs to be corrected urgently to allow normal development of the visual axis and prevent the occurence of strabismus in which the eyes are not properly aligned with each other. This may result from problems with the brain coordinating the movement of the eyes or of the ocular muscles themselves.

   - **Do the patient's symptoms have a temporal quality during the day?** Eyelid ptosis may be the first signs of myasthenia gravis. In this instance, myopathy of the levator muscle causes the eyelid position to be high in the morning and low in the evening as the muscle fatigues.

   - **Does the patient have associated symptoms of miosis and anhydrosis?** Disruption of the sympathetic nervous system leads to ptosis of the eyelid, miosis of the pupil, and anhydrosis of the skin, whose constellation of findings is termed Horner syndrome. In this case, the sympathetically innervated Mueller's muscle is responsible for initiating eyelid retraction during eyelid opening and is involved with the ptosis. Sympathetic innervation to the eye originates in the hypothalamus and travels through the brain stem and cervical spinal cord to the T1 and T2 nerve roots. Neurons synapse with preganglionic sympathetic fibers to exit the cord and travel to the sympathetic chain and superior cervical ganglion. There they synapse with postganglionic sympathetic fibers, which travel along the internal carotid artery to the orbit and Mueller's muscle. Causes of Horner syndrome include a defect in the pre- or postganglionic neuron, a tumor or cerebrovascular injury in the brainstem, trauma to the brachial plexus, a tumor or infection in the apex of the lung, and a dissecting aneurysm of the carotid system, among others.

   - **Does the patient have a history of prior surgery to the eyelids?** Iatrogenic injury from prior surgery can lead to scarring and poor levator function.

   - **Does the patient have concerns about the aging appearance of the eyelids?** The approach to the standard blepharoplasty lends itself to simultaneous correction of the rhytids and the ptosis since both procedures may be performed through an upper eyelid crease incision.

2. Physical examination of the patient with ptosis of the eyelid(s) is directed to the structures around the orbit but should consider other organ systems.

   - **Does the frontalis muscle function adequately on each side?** Frontalis muscle function has implications for treatment as it is used in the case of minimal to no levator function.

   - **What is the position of the eyebrow?** The normal position of the upper eyebrow is 22 mm to the central eyelid and roughly 10 mm from temporal and nasal areas. Often, patients have "compensated brow ptosis" in which the frontalis muscle compensates for eyelid ptosis by raising the brow and the eyelid. Blepharoplasty will correct the eyelid position, but fail to improve the appearance of the periorbit long-term since the brow will return to its normally low position once the visual obstruction is removed.

- **Are the palpebral fissures of normal width and symmetrical?** The normal palpable fissure width is 10 mm. In downward gaze with brow held fixed, the width is approximately 2 mm.

- **What is the level of functioning of the upper eyelid?** Function of the levator palpebrae superioris may be measured by blocking movement of the eyebrow and observing the excursion of the upper lid from downward to upward gaze behind a clear ruled instrument. More than 8 mm of movement indicates good function, 5 to 7 mm indicates moderate function, while less than 4 mm indicates poor function. At rest, the eyelid should lie 1 to 2 mm below the superior limbus. Eyelid closure is mediated by the facial nerve which innervates the orbicularis muscle.

- **Does the pupil dilate and constrict appropriately?** Miosis of the eye is a component of Horner syndrome and adequate pupillary function should be noted on examination.

- **Where does the upper eyelid crease fall?** The upper eyelid crease is measured from the lash line, as the patient looks downward (normal is 9 to 12 mm, tapering temporally to 5 to 6 mm above the lateral canthus and medially 6 to 7 mm above the punctum). This line corresponds to the superior border of the tarsal plate.

  — The **margin reflex distance** (MRD) may be used to assess the presence and degree of eyelid ptosis. It is measured as the distance between the eyelid margin and the light reflex on forward gaze. It quantifies ptosis without considering the palpebral fissure width since the lower eyelid muscle also responds to phenylephrine if administered. If the MRD is less than 4 to 5 mm, ptosis should be considered.

  — The **margin crease distance** (MCD), is the distance from the upper eyelid margin to the lid crease. In women, a central measurement of 10 to 11 mm is considered normal, and in men, 8 to 10 mm is considered normal.

- **Where is the lacrimal gland located?** The lacrimal gland is normally located within the superolateral orbit just behind the rim. Prolapse may be noted temporally where there is an absence of fat.

- **Is a tumor palpable within the eyelid?** Sometimes a tumor may be present that causes a mass effect on the function of the eyelid.

3. No specific radiologic tests or laboratory studies need to be obtained in these patients.

- Imaging studies of the head may be indicated in patients suspected of intraorbital or CNS lesions producing the ptosis. In this case, MRI is the study of choice. A solution of **10% phenylephrine**, a sympathomimetic agent can be used to stimulate Mueller's muscle.

- It may be instilled between the upper eyelid and globe with the head tilted backward and the cannaliculi compressed for 10 seconds. This is repeated two times and the patient is allowed to sit for 5 minutes. Ptosis caused by myasthenia gravis should be improved with phenyephrine. Side effects include hypertension and myocardial ischemia.

4. An **ophthalmology** consultation should be requested to identify any associated problems with the globe or extraocular muscles.

5. Treatment of eyelid ptosis depends on the etiology of the problem. In the case of myasthenia gravis, medication should improve the ptosis. For other causes of ptosis, there is a little role for pharmacologic management. Surgical correction involves rearrangement of the levator mechanism, if possible, and replacement if not. Awake analgesia is perhaps the best technique for anesthesia since the patient is able to cooperate with eyelid opening during the procedure to confirm the correct height of the eyelid. The type of the reconstruction is often determined by the degree of impairment.

- 8 to 12 mm of movement (good) warrants simple advancement of the levator muscle. Without dividing the muscle, the inferior edge of the levator aponeurosis

29

is sutured to superior border of tarsal plate. The position is placed 1 to 2 mm higher than ideal using 5-0 Vicryl and the patient upright to account for settling. In such cases, it is aways safer to overcorrect.

- 5 to 7 mm of movement (moderate) warrants levator resection and resuspension. This procedure is also performed if more than 4 mm of aponeurosis must be advanced over the tarsal plate.

  — A **Muller's muscle-conjunctival resection** can be performed as an alternative procedure in patients whose eyelids respond appropriately to phenylephrine. Unlike the Fasanella-Servat operation for mild ptosis and good levator function, the levator palpebrae superioris, is not excised along with Muller's muscle and conjunctiva. Here, the upper lid is everted and a specially designed clamp placed across the conjunctiva and Mueller's muscle a preset distance from the superior tarsal border (6.5 to 9.5 mm), sparing the more anterior levator mechanism. The distance can be determined following phenylephrine testing: 4 mm of resection for 1 mm of ptosis, 6 mm of resection for 1.5 mm of ptosis, 10 mm of resection for 2 mm of ptosis, and between 11 and 12 mm of resection for greater than 3 mm of ptosis. The intervening tissue is removed and the resultant defect closed. The technique can be combined with a simultaneous upper blepharoplasty.

- 0 to 4 mm (poor) warrants suspension of the levator mechanism from the frontalis muscle. Numerous materials, both autogenous (fascia lata graft and frontalis muscle flap) and allolastic (acellular dermis, nonabsorbable suture, frozen dura mater, and silicone) have been used with success to suspend the upper eyelid from the eyebrow or frontalis muscle. The eye then opens with contraction of the frontalis muscle and closes with action of the orbicularis oculi muscle.

- Postoperatively, cold compresses are important to minimize immediate swelling and lubricating drops/ointment are important to moisturize the eyes if eyelid closure is not immediately complete.

6. Complications common to all surgical procedures include bleeding and infection. **Bleeding** is worrisome following ptosis repair but may be averted by careful perioperative maneuvers, such as blood pressure control during induction and emergence and care hemostasis. **Infection** is uncommon. Specific complications following ptosis repair are related to the position and function of the eyelid.

- Mild **lagophthalmos** is important since it may lead to exposure keratitis. It is treated with topical lubricants and usually resolves in time and with gentle massage.

- **Exposure keratitis** results from abrasion or other injury to the sensitive cornea. Every effort should be made to minimize inadvertent contact with the globe. Intraoperative lubrication is helpful. Corneal shields prevent inspection of the pupil and iris to gauge proper lid placement.

- **Overcorrection** generally responds to massage for five to ten minutes four times per day. Significant overcorrection noted in the first ten days can be managed with removal of one or more Vicryl elevation sutures.

- **Undercorrection** less than 2 mm may be observed until the resolution of edema. If it is more than 2 mm, reoperation is best performed in the first postoperative week. This requires repeating the suspension of the aponeurosis.

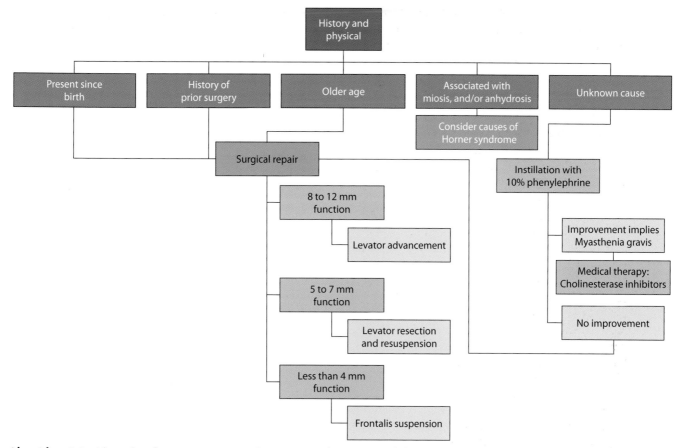

Algorithm 5-1 Algorithm for management of patients with upper eyelid ptosis.

PRACTICAL PEARLS

1. Consider myasthenia gravis as a cause since improvement may be obtained with medical therapy alone.

2. In the lateral portion of the eyelid, the position of the lacrimal gland should be noted so that it is not misidentified as herniated lateral fat.

3. Sutures into the tarsal plate should be placed at the superior edge so as not to create an ectropion.

4. When readvancing the levator aponeurosis, Mueller's muscle may be left alone.

References

1. Arslan E, Demirkan F, Unal S. Enhanced frontalis sling with double-fixed, solvent-dehydrated cadaveric fascia lata allograft in the management of eye ptosis. *J Craniofac Surg.* 2004;15(6):960-964.

2. de la Torre JI, Martin SA, De Cordier BC, Al-Hakeem MS, Collawn SS, Vasconez LO. Aesthetic eyelid ptosis correction: A review of technique and cases. *Plast Reconstr Surg.* 2003;112(2):655-660.

3. McCord CD, Seify H, Codner MA. Transblepharoplasty ptosis repair: Three-step technique. *Plast Reconstr Surg.* 2007;120(4):1037-1044.

4. Ramirez OM, Pena G. Frontalis muscle advancement: A dynamic structure for the treatment of severe congenital eyelid ptosis. *Plast Reconstr Surg.* 2004;113(6):1841-1849.

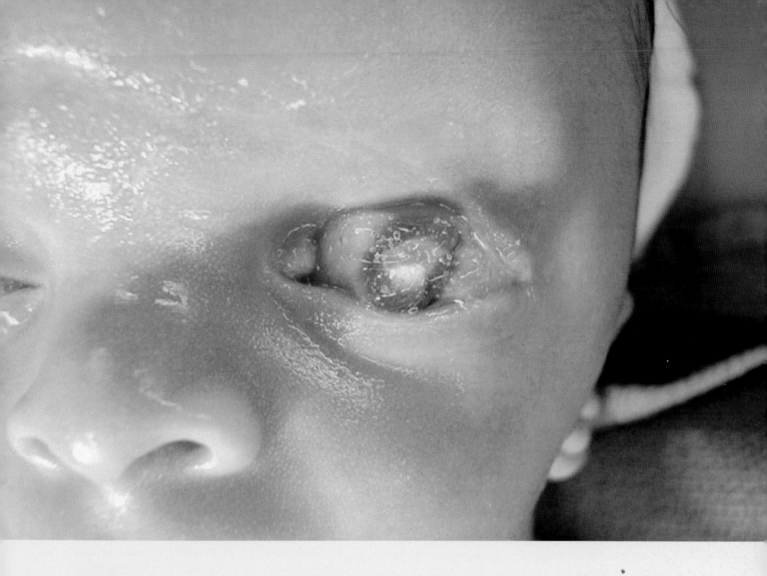

The neonatal intensive care unit requests a plastic surgery consult in order to evaluate and manage an eyelid defect in a newborn.

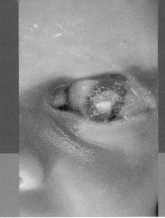

CHAPTER 6

Upper Eyelid Defect

David Staffenberg, Evan Garfein, and Courtney Carpenter

1. The patient shown here demonstrates near complete absence of the upper eyelid (a generous amount of ocular lubricant protecting the cornea is visible). This may be a rare congenital finding, as depicted above, or be more commonly seen in the setting of trauma or malignancy. In some cases, the history may not yield much useful information other than the suitability of the patient for surgical reconstruction. In adult patients with lesions of suspicious pathology or known malignancy, a thorough history should yield information about the nature of the lesion (if known), prior interventions (if any), and existing medical conditions (if relevant).

   - **What is the etiology of the defect** (congenital, traumatic, neoplastic, or other)? Patients are commonly seen with lesions of the upper eyelid that have been referred for further diagnosis and treatment. Some have been referred for reconstruction alone. All should be adequately evaluated prior to intervention. Existing defects may require more urgent treatment to minimize complications such as corneal exposure.

   - **How long has the lesion been present?** Chronic non-healing wounds should be suspect for malignancy, while chronically open lesions develop scar formation at the margins that prevents timely closure.

   - With significant loss of the upper eyelid, particularly in the middle third, an intact Bell's phenomenon will not be able to protect the cornea from exposure so generous application of and ocular lubricant is necessary. A shield should also be placed to protect the globe from direct injury. Pain in the region of the eye may indicate corneal exposure.

   - **Are there any other congenital anomalies or preexisting medical conditions?** Patients with isolated congenital anomalies should be worked up for associated anomalies of other organ systems. More common associations include those of the cardiac and/or genitourinary systems as well as anomalies of the hands and feet.

2. The physical examination should be thorough with regards to the periorbital structures and include other organ systems that might be involved.

   - **Is the Bell's phenomenon intact?** It must be reemphasized that if the defect is located in the middle third of the upper eyelid (overlying the cornea) the cornea will remain exposed even when the Bell's phenomenon is intact; additional lubrication and protection must be assured. As a means to protect the cornea, patients with exposure have a reflex mechanism in which the eyeball rotates superiorly so that only sclera is visible. This may be seen when the patient is sleeping.

   - **Where on the eyelid is the lesion or defect located?** In general, exposure of the cornea is more of a concern with upper eyelid defects than lower eyelid defects. Defects involving the middle third leave the cornea less protected. When exposure is significant, aggressive protection is essential and urgent correction is indicated.

   - **Is the patient's vision intact?** A baseline examination by the craniofacial team should include a thorough examination by a pediatric ophthalmologist.

   - **Which lamellae are involved?** Lesions involving the eyelid margin will likely lead to a full-thickness defect when excised. Reconstruction of the defect (analogous to nasal reconstruction) should be considered in terms of inner lamella (conjunctive), middle lamella (tarsus in the leading edge of the lid), and outer lamella (full-thickness skin).

   - **How much of the eyelid is involved or anticipated to result from excision?** A small defect may allow a primary repair. A defect of up to one-third of the eyelid may require additional maneuvers. Larger defects typically require lid-switch or lid-sharing flaps from the lower eyelid. A lid-switch flap has the advantage of transferring lashes along the margin.

   - **Are there any indications of other congenital anomalies?** Associated anomalies of the heart and great vessels, indicated by the presence of murmurs, or of the extremities and other organ systems, are seen in conjunction with craniofacial anomalies.

3. The etiology of any lesion of the eyelid should be known prior to proceeding with the final reconstruction. In general, benign lesions require less aggressive margins, have a better prognosis, and thus allow for a less frequent follow-up schedule. The converse is true for malignant lesions. The most common skin malignancy is basal cell carcinoma, followed by squamous cell carcinoma

and malignant melanoma and should be identified if present.

- Permanent **biopsy** will show the histopathologic details at the periphery of the lesion better than frozen sections. **Mohs' chemosurgery** provides for evaluation of margins during the resection. It is beneficial in areas where tissue conservation is important. For malignant melanoma, the greatest depth of the tumor needs to be ascertained prior to Mohs', which lacks the ability to provide an adequate measure of the lesion's depth.

- To adequately stage some more aggressive lesions, imaging studies consisting of a chest X-ray, CT scans of the head, neck, abdomen, and pelvis, or MRI may be required.

- **Classification of basal cell carcinoma** is as follows:

  — Primary tumor TX: Primary tumor cannot be assessed.
    a. T0 - No evidence of primary tumor
    b. T1 - Tumor 2 cm or less in greatest dimension
    c. T2 - Tumor more than 2 cm but not more than 5 cm in greatest dimension
    d. T3 - Tumor more than 5 cm in greatest dimension
    e. T4 - Tumor invading deep extradermal structures

  — Regional lymph node NX: Regional lymph node cannot be assessed.
    a. N0 - No regional lymph node metastasis
    b. N1 - Regional lymph node metastasis

  — Distant metastasis MX: Presence of distant metastasis cannot be assessed.
    a. M0 - No distant metastasis
    b. M1 - Distant metastasis

- The following outline may be used for the **staging of nonmelanomatous skin cancers** (basal cell and squamous cell):

  — Stage 0 (carcinoma in situ): Malignant cells are confined to the epidermis.
  — Stage I: The lesion is 2 cm or smaller.

  — Stage II: The tumor is larger than 2 cm.
  — Stage III: Cancer has spread below the skin to cartilage, muscle, or bone and/or to nearby lymph nodes, but not to other parts of the body.
  — Stage IV: Cancer has spread to other parts of the body.

- A number of different systems have been used for **staging of melanoma**. The TNM system describes the thickness of the lesion and whether there is any spread to lymph nodes or other parts of the body.

  — Tumor size (T)
    a. T1 - The melanoma is less than 1 mm thick
    b. T2 - The melanoma is between 1 mm and 2 mm thick
    c. T3 - The melanoma is between 2 mm and 4 mm thick
    d. T4 - The melanoma is over 4 mm thick or there are clusters of melanoma cells in the surrounding skin less than 5 cm from the primary melanoma

  — Lymph node status (N):
    a. N0 - There are no positive lymph nodes
    b. N1 - There is one positive lymph node
    c. N2 - There are two to three positive lymph nodes
    d. N3 - There are four or more positive lymph nodes

  — Metastasis (M):
    a. M0 - There is no sign of cancer spread anywhere else
    b. M1 - There is melanoma in another part of the body

- Using the TNM classification, melanomas are grouped into four number stages.

  — Stage I: Lesions are less than 2 mm thick or less than 1 mm thick and ulcerated. There are no positive lymph nodes and no sign of cancer spread.
  — Stage II: Lesions are either more than 2 mm thick, or more than 1 mm thick and ulcerated. There are still no signs of spread or positive lymph nodes.

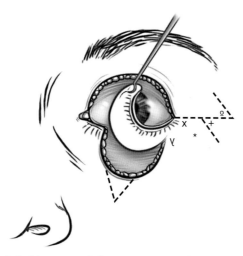

Figure 6-1 Upper eyelid reconstruction by transposition of lower eyelid elements. The donor defect is closed by lateral canthal release and z-plasty of the skin.

— Stage III: Lesions are any size and have spread to the lymph nodes, but possess no evidence of more distant metastasis.

— Stage IV: Lesions are any size and have spread to remote sites in the body.

4. A broad assessment is performed. The large coloboma of the upper eyelid in the case pictured is a component of Goldenhar syndrome (preauricular appendages are seen on the cheeks).

- An **ophthalmology** evaluation is obtained as well as genetics. Continued follow-up with plastic surgery, ophthalmology and a multidisciplinary craniofacial team is essential.

- In cases of carcinoma, an **oncologist** should be consulted if the event adjuvant therapy is required.

5. The final reconstruction is ultimately directed by the characteristics of the defect. To achieve a satisfactory result, it is essential to restore both form and function. The upper eyelid must protect the cornea so lagophthalmos is to be avoided. A smooth mucous membrane on the inner surface of the eyelid without suture knots.

- Even in the presence of an adequate Bell's phenomenon, protection of the cornea is imperative. As such, the surface of the eye should be covered with ointment as a means of lubrication.

- For upper eyelid defects involving only the skin, ones that are relatively small can be closed primarily, while larger ones require skin grafts or local flaps. Local flaps can be designed from adjacent intact eyelid, temporal or glabellar skin. When feasible, flaps of adjacent eyelid skin provide the best color and texture match. Flaps from the glabella and forehead are thicker and less favorable flaps. When the flap needs more laxity, the upper limb of the lateral canthal tendon can be released. Additional release is achieved by extending an incision from the lateral canthus toward

the temporal area in a semicircular fashion (i.e., an upside-down Tenzel flap). A Z-plasty lateral to the canthus may be added for further release. When the orbicularis muscle is intact, skin grafts may be utilized. Full-thickness grafts are chosen because of their lack of secondary contracture. The superior skin graft donor site will provide a graft with favorable skin color and texture. The first-line choice for full-thickness grafts, particularly in older patients with lax skin, is the contralateral upper eyelid, which undergoes a blepharoplasty to yield the graft. When the excess skin of the contralateral upper eyelid is not enough a more remote donor site is needed. Such sites include postauricular skin or preauricular. Primary closure of these donor sites requires adequate undermining.

- For more extensive defects involving the full thickness of the eyelid, a multilayered reconstruction is required.

— A **composite graft** of nasal mucosa and underlying rigid septal cartilage may be used to replace the conjunctiva (inner lamella) and tarsus (middle lamella). The septal cartilage can be thinned if needed. Another option is the hard palate mucosa which is lubricated and rigid enough to provide support. A vascularized surface for the graft is required. A skin flap may be advanced from adjacent eyelid. The donor defect is then covered with a full-thickness skin graft from the opposite upper eyelid or ear.

— The lower eyelid can also be shared providing a **tarsoconjunctival flap**, which is then covered by a full-thickness skin graft. The caudal border of the tarsal plate is transferred up to the defect as a rectangular flap that is divided about a week later.

— A **lid-switch flap** (like the one seen in figure 6-1) is another technique that transfers a full-thickness pedicled flap from the lower eyelid. This is similar to an Abbe flap for upper lip reconstruction and requires a division and inset as a second procedure at least a week later. The flap is slightly narrower than the defect and the lower eyelid is repaired primarily. The lower limb of the lateral canthal tendon may need to be divided and an advancement flap from the temporal area may be required to close this donor site. The advantage of this technique for a full-thickness defect is that it provides all three lamellae as well as eyelashes and scars are limited to the eyelids. Disadvantages of this technique include the need for a second procedure.

6. The complications of treating patients with lesions of the upper eyelid are largely related to delay in treatment with inadequate protection or to the repair itself and injury to the underlying eye.

- **Bleeding** may occur from injury to the vascular arcade that transverses the upper eyelid superior to the tarsal plate. Retrobulbar bleeding is rare but should be considered in the patient with excessive edema and periorbital pain in the postoperative period.

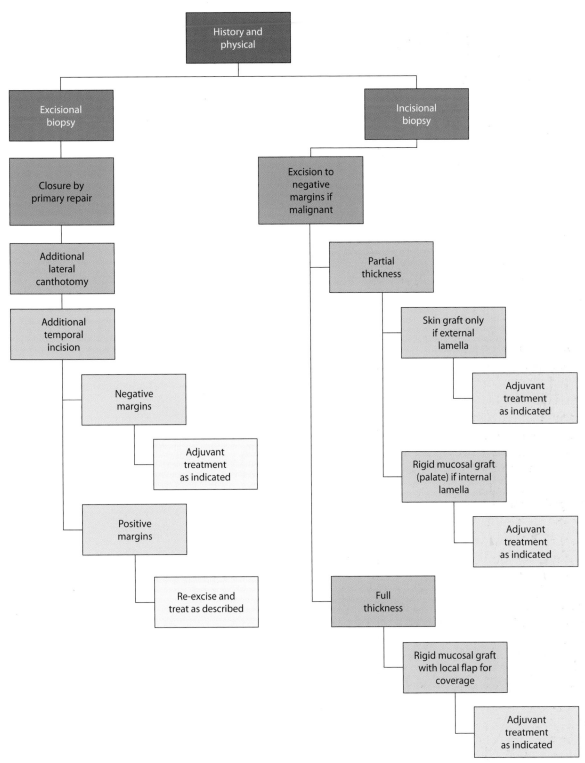

Algorithm 6-1 Management algorithm for defects of the upper eyelid.

- **Infection** of the periorbital structures should be treated aggressively with topical and possibly parenteral antibiotics.

PRACTICAL PEARLS

1. It is important to keep the cornea protected and lubricated pre-, intra-, and postoperatively. Care should be exercised that sutures do not come in contact with cornea. Avoid lagophthalmos by considering it as a postoperative possibility.

2. Reconstruction should be thought of in a stepwise fashion, dictated by size of the defect as well as the layers (lamellae) involved: direct closure should be considered first, followed by skin grafts, and then local flaps.

3. For cases of primary closure, a shield excision pattern minimizes the risk of notching at the lid margin. When a full-thickness resection is indicated, perpendicular incisions are best so that closure allows a properly aligned closure.

4. If a skin graft is required, skin from the contralateral lid provides the best replacement.

5. If a cross-lid flap is chosen, the reliability of a medial pedicle appears to be better than that of a lateral one and the rotation point of the flap should be designed so as to lie at the junction of the middle and lateral thirds of the defect.

- **Lagophthalmos** can be a serious condition. The inability to close the eyelid causes problems with the distribution of the surface film necessary to maintain lubrication and proper eye health. Initial lagopthalmos may be managed with frequent massage. Causative scarring may need to be released and/or replaced with more adequate tissue for reconstruction.

- **Corneal injury** may result from lagopthalmos or from inadvertent contact during surgical intervention. It is best diagnosed by examination of the cornea with a Woods lamp following application with fluorescein. Treatment involves antibiotic lubrication and careful observation.

References

1. Erdogmus S, Govsa F. The arterial anatomy of the eyelid: Importance for reconstructive and aesthetic surgery. *J Plast Reconstr Aesthet Surg.* 2007;60(3):241-245.

2. Ito R, Fujiwara M, Nagasako R. Hard palate mucoperiosteal graft for posterior lamellar reconstruction of the upper eyelid: Histologic rationale. *J Craniofac Surg.* 2007;18(3):684-690.

3. Fujiwara M. Upper eyelid reconstruction with a hard palate mucosa-lined bipedicled myocutaneous flap. *J Craniofac Surg.* 2006;17(5):1011-1015.

4. Lalonde DH, Osei-Tutu KB. Functional reconstruction of unilateral, subtotal, full-thickness upper and lower eyelid defects with a single hard palate graft covered with advancement orbicularis myocutaneous flaps. *Plast Reconstr Surg.* 2005;115(6):1696-1700.

5. DiFrancesco LM, Codner MA, McCord CD. Upper eyelid reconstruction. *Plast Reconstr Surg.* 2004;114(7):98-107e.

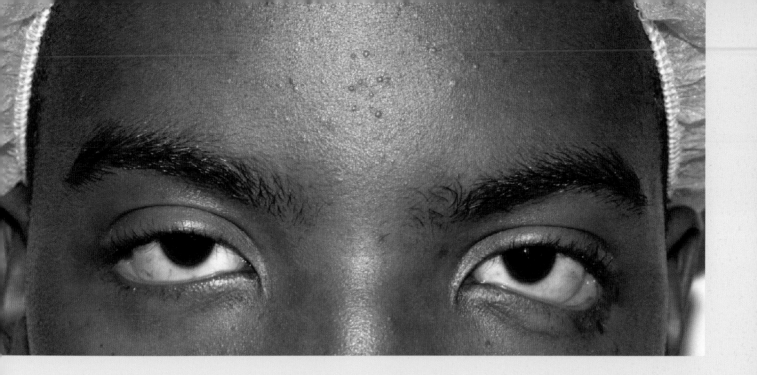

A 20-year-old male patient presents with complaint about the appearance of his eyes following fracture repair.

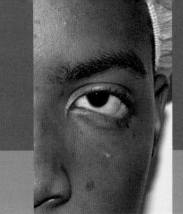

Ectropion

Peter J. Taub

1. The patient in question has malposition of the lower eyelid noticeable by the increase in lateral scleral show. This may be caused by retraction of the eyelid or true ectropion rather than the eyelid simply being pulled inferiorly. Ectropion implies an outward *eversion* of the lower eyelid. Patients usually have concerns about one or more of the following: their appearance, excessive tearing ("epiphora"), and/or irritation of the globe and/or conjunctiva. In order to make the treatment successful, it is important to understand the etiology of problem. Several causes of ectropion exist and must be sought in obtaining a thorough history:

- **How old is the patient?** Senile ectropion refers to the rare case of ectropion as a result of the downward pull of the malar structures as they are affected by gravity with aging. This is less common in younger patients.

- **Does the patient have a chronic history of sun exposure?** Chronic damage of skin from the sun will lead to skin laxity and facial rhytids. However, alone it should not cause retraction of the eyelid if the septum and conjunctiva are unaffected.

- **Was there a history of trauma?** Cicatricial ectropion occurs following trauma (including surgery) to the lower eyelid. This may include iatrogenic trauma following blepharoplasty or repair of orbital fractures through periorbital incisions. Here, the outward rotation of the eyelid is caused by excess resection of skin comprising the anterior lamella or scarring of the septum in the middle lamella. The risk of cicatricial ectropion is greater with a transcutaneous approach to blepharoplasty than with a transconjunctival approach.

- **When the problem occur?** The time course is also important since early recognition of retraction may be treated with upward traction on the lid for a week or two rather than surgical correction which is required in more chronic settings.

- **Does the patient have excessive tearing of the eyes?** Poor drainage of normal tear production occurs if the superior and inferior puncta are pulled away from the surface of the globe as occurs with lid retraction.

- **Does the patient have an antecedent history of nerve problems?** Paralytic ectropion occurs with conditions of facial nerve paralysis, such as caused by trauma or infection (Bell's palsy). Spastic ectropion is seen in the setting of exophthalmos as a result of the pull of the orbicularis oculi muscle.

- **Was there a developmental problem of the eyelids for birth?** Congenital ectropion is usually caused by a deficiency in the anterior lamella, such as with a coloboma.

- **Does the patient take any medications?** Specific agents that predispose to bleeding such as aspirin, ibuprofen, Plavix, or Coumadin should be discontinued at least 2 weeks prior to surgery.

- **Does the patient smoke?** Smoking tobacco-related products causes the skin to age faster than normal and impairs blood supply to any flaps that may be necessary for repair.

2. Physical examination should include a basic ophthalmologic examination as well as identify the possible etiology of the retraction or ectropion. It should determine whether the problem is a retraction of the lower lid, which may be adequately addressed with canthal suspension, or a true ectropion, in which there is lid eversion and requires a more extensive repair. In doing so, the involved structures/lamellae of the lid must be identified.

- **Is there scleral show?** This is perhaps the most telling signal of lid malposition. The amount of scleral show in the normal population is variable but too much exposure is often related to a problem with the eyelid.

- **Is there rounding of the lateral canthus?** Lid eversion and laxity may be because of malposition of the lateral canthal tendon. The tendon normally inserts just inside the lateral wall of the orbit approximately 2 mm above the level of insertion of the medial canthal tendon. With dehiscence, the lid may pull away from the globe and produce an ectropion.

- **Is there conjunctival exposure?** Chronic exposure of the conjunctiva may lead to metaplastic change of the epithelium to a keratinized squamous epithelium, causing persistent irritation.

- **Is the lid tense when pulled on?** Upward traction on the lower lid will identify which structures are insufficient. A tense lid with skin laxity indicates contraction of the septum in the middle lamella, which initial tension on the skin indicates deficiency of the skin in the anterior lamella.

- **Does the lid snap back to the globe when released?** Poor tone in the orbicularis oculi muscle is seen with senile ectropion and other disorders of the muscle.

- **Are there scars on either the external eyelid or within the conjunctiva indicating prior surgery?** Even if the patient does not offer a history of recent trauma or surgery, the incisions for exposure should be visible.

- **Are there bony step-offs?** Trauma to the bony orbit may be associated with trauma to the eyelid.

- **Is the eye able to move through all six visual axes?** A basic ophthalmologic examination should note function of each of the eye muscles.

Table 1: Function and innervation of the six extraocular muscles.

Medial rectus	Medial rotation	Oculomotor (CN III)
Lateral rectus	Lateral rotation	Abducens (CN VI)
Superior rectus	Superior rotation	Oculomotor (CN III)
Inferior rectus	Inferior rotation	Oculomotor (CN III)
Superior oblique	Downward and outward rotation	Trochlear (CN IV)
Inferior oblique	Upward and outward rotation	Oculomotor (CN III)

- **Are the pupils equal and reactive?** Pupillary response to light may be indicative of optic nerve injury. Normally, light shone in one eye causes constriction of the pupil in both the ipsilateral and contralateral eyes. With partial injury to the optic nerve, there may be paradoxical dilatation of the pupil rather than constriction. This is referred to as a "Marcus Gunn" pupil. Its presence should warrant further investigation as to the cause.

- **Is there vision in each eye?** A baseline examination of visual acuity is important with any problems related to the eyes or periorbital structures.

- **Is the anterior chamber clear?** Blood in the anterior chamber occurs with trauma. Shining a light across the anterior portion of the globe and noting a blood-fluid level will identify the presence of a hyphema.

- **Do all branches of the facial nerve function normally?** Evaluation of facial nerve is important to determine if the findings are related to paralytic condition.

3. There are no specific studies to obtain prior to treatment. Of course, a plain film of the head and neck may be helpful in cases following reduction and fixation of fractures around the orbits. The plates and screws may need to be removed at the time of reconstruction. A CT scan will provide further information regarding any prior fracture but is similarly not critical.

4. A formal **ophthalmology** consultation should be obtained in addition to the basic ophthalmologic examination. This will include dilation of the pupils and examination of the posterior chamber by funduscopy.

- Tests for dry eyes should have preceded initial blepharoplasty and are often deferred to the consulting ophthalmologist.

   — With the **Schirmer test**, a small strip of filter paper folded on one side is placed inside the lower eyelid. The eyes are closed for 5 minutes and the amount of moisture measured. Sometimes a topical anesthetic in placed into the eye before the filter paper to prevent tearing because of the irritation from the paper. Of note, several clinical studies have shown that it may not be sensitive enough to identify all patients with dry eyes.

   — A newer test of **lactoferrin** may be more closely related to tear production.

5. The treatment options will differ greatly depending on how recent was the inciting event or how long the problems has persisted. Prior to any management, a discussion should address the patient's expectations, the anticipated results, and potential problems that might occur.

- The treatment of early lid retraction is very different from that which presents in a delayed fashion. Early cases may be managed with tape or sutures through the lower lid and suspended to the brow for a period of 7 to 10 days.

- Patients who present later but within 6 months following blepharoplasty may require division of scar tissue and resuspension of the eyelid. This may be performed under local anesthesia through a lateral canthotomy to expose the orbital rim and lateral canthus.
  - With **tarsal strip canthopexy**, the eyelid is elevated laterally and superiorly so that it rests at the desired position over the inferior limbus and a mark is made along the eyelid at the junction of the lid with the upper portion of the lateral canthus. The lid is then sectioned sagittally into anterior and posterior components up to the mark. A strip of posterior eyelid is preserved while the conjunctival lining the remainder is scraped with a scalpel blade to prevent the development of inclusion cysts. The strip of tissue is then pulled laterally and sutured to the periosteum of the lateral orbital rim and/or superior limb of the lateral canthal tendon. Next, the lateral portion of the orbicularis muscle is dissected from the overlying skin and fixed at the desired level to the periosteum over the frontal process of the zygoma. The temporal margins of the upper and lower eyelid are reapproximated to reconstruct the lateral canthal angle. Finally, a brow suspension suture may be used to provide temporary postoperative support to the lower eyelid.
  - A **midface lift** may be performed with the above technique in older patients to simultaneously resuspend the malar soft tissues into a more youthful position.
  - **Kuhnt-Szymanowski procedure** may also be performed. A triangular area of skin is excised lateral to the lateral canthus. A similar triangular area of conjunctiva and lid margin is excised laterally. The medial extent of the cut lower lid is sutured to the lateral edge of the upper lid at the canthus. The lower lid flap is sutured to the area of skin excised lateral to the canthus.
- Cases of late lid retraction are less common but are often more severe. These frequently require tissue in the posterior lamellar to fill space and compensate for secondary shortening of this layer. Options for the spacer grafts include a hard palate and an ear cartilage. The recipient bed is created after the tarsal strip procedure as described above. The palatal graft is taken from one side of the roof of the mouth after adequate injection of local anesthesia with epinephrine. The width of the graft is determined by the amount of preoperative shortening. The recipient site tends to bleed easily but may be left open since it will heal by secondary intention in a short period of time. A graft of auricular cartilage may be also be harvested via a posterior incision and used as a posterior lamella spacer.

A second resuspension procedure may be required after complete healing of the graft to the surrounding tissues.

- Treatment of ectropion requires more than simple canthal suspension.
  - Replacement of deficient skin from the anterior lamella is achieved with a full thickness skin graft harvested from either the contralateral upper eyelid (if sufficient) or the retroauricular sulcus. Unlike a split thickness graft, this has a diminished tendency for secondary contracture. The graft is inset into a defect created 1 to 2 mm below the lash line with the more superior lid suspended by traction sutures affixed to the brow. A subcutaneous dissection is performed to the level of the orbital rim and any scar tissue is released. The graft is inset to the surrounding skin and a tie-over bolster dressing is fabricated for gentle compression.
  - Middle or posterior shortening is best addressed with addition of a rigid mucosal graft. Mucosa from the lateral hard palate may be harvested and placed into a horizontal defect created just below the level of the lower eyelid tarsal plate. It is sutured into place with fine buried chromic sutures to avoid corneal irritation.

6. Lid retraction and ectropion are frequently complications of prior intervention and therefore all attempts should be made to minimize further complication. The more common complications include the following.

- Inaccurate diagnosis and treatment may cause **persistent deformity**.
- **Injury to the globe** should be rare and may be minimized with lubrication of the cornea and use of a corneal shield while operating around the globe. Of course, visualization of the limbus and the position of the lid in relation to the limbus will be necessary at some point during repair.
- **Skin graft failure** occurs most commonly because of either a poorly vascularized wound bed, fluid collection beneath the graft, or shearing of the graft. Graft failure may be managed secondarily by repeat grafting.
- Dissection within the lower eyelid and floor of the orbit may result in **injury to the inferior oblique muscle**. The patient will present with a postoperative complaint of vertical dystopia. Corrective extraocular muscle surgery may be necessary but should be delayed for a judicious period of time in hopes that the problem will resolve with time.
- **Postoperative bleeding** can be a devastating complication and should be considered in all cases involving the orbit. Like the head, the orbit has a limited volume and rigid walls. Bleeding within the orbit is thus not tolerated well and should be addressed rapidly. Avoidance begins before with adequate management of a patient's hypertension and coexisting medical conditions. During surgery, controlled anesthesia and a calm environment will lessen anxiety and acute

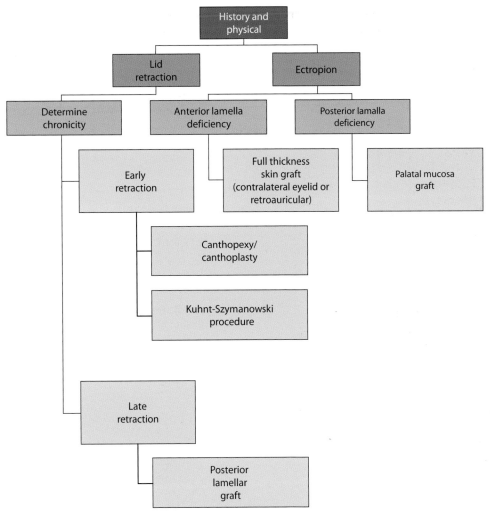

Algorithm 7-1 Algorithm for management of patients with problems related to position of the lower eyelid.

1. Augmentation of the posterior lamella with a hard palate graft will be more likely if more than 6 months have passed, the patient has prominent eyes or severe retraction, or prior attempts with resuspension alone have failed to fix the problem.

2. Local hemostasis is best achieved with 2% lidocaine with epinephrine and hyaluronidase. The medication should be given 15 minutes to take effect before proceeding to minimize bleeding, maximize visualization, and avoid complication.

3. When harvesting a skin graft for replacement of deficient skin, primary contraction is managed by harvesting 30% to 40% more skin than is thought to be needed and trimming any excess.

4. Since the lateral canthal tendon arises from the inner surface of the lateral orbit, all attempts to resuspend the canthus to a point similarly within the orbit should be made.

5. Attachment of a lateral canthal tendon or a strip of tarsus is best performed with a 6-0 double-armed polypropylene suture to maximize fixation during healing.

elevations in blood pressure. Careful hemostasis is of paramount importance. In the recovery area, patients should be well monitored and kept with their head elevated. Any complaint of pain should be addressed seriously. Serious pain and bulging of the eyes warrants immediate release of any sutures (including the lateral canthoplasty which may be restrictive) and a return to the operating room to identify potential sources of bleeding. An osmotic agent such as mannitol and a carbonic anhydrase inhibitor such as acetazolamide should be administered to reduce the intraocular pressure. The final intervention is osteotomy of one or more orbital walls.

References

1. Knize DM. The superficial lateral canthal tendon: Anatomic study and clinical application to lateral canthopexy. *Plast Reconstr Surg.* 2002;109(3):1149-1157.

2. Patipa M. The evaluation and management of lower eyelid retraction following cosmetic surgery. *Plast Reconstr Surg.* 2000;106(2):438-453.

3. Jelks GW, Jelks EB. Repair of lower lid deformities. *Clin Plast Surg.* 1993;20:417-425.

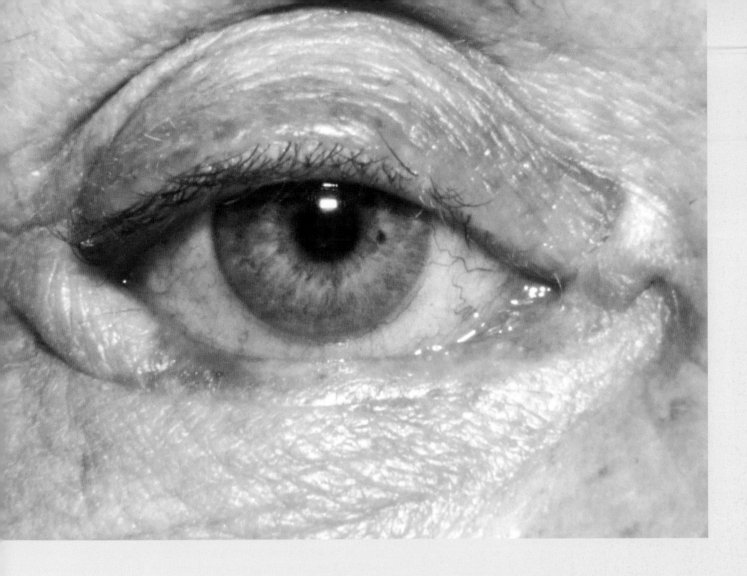

A local ophthalmologist asked you to evaluate and treat this patient with a pigmented lesion of the lower eyelid.

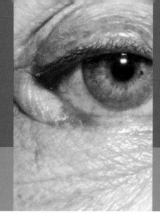
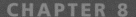

CHAPTER 8

Lower Eyelid Lesion

Malcolm A. Lesavoy and Mark Gelfand

1. The lesion in question is located along the lower eyelid and appears to have a pigmented color. Irrespective of the area, it is important to establish a diagnosis of any skin lesion of questionable behavior. A directed patient history is critical to determine the nature of the lesion.

   - **How long has the lesion been present?** Long-standing lesions that have not changed of late are of lesser concern than those that demonstrate some recent change in size of character. Chronic wounds tend to be of greater concern than acute ones since they may predispose to the development of squamous cell carcinoma.

   - **How has the lesion changed?** Rapid growth in a previously small, stable lesion or the development of areas of ulceration or bleeding can signal malignant degeneration.

   - **Is the patient older than 60 years of age and fair skinned?** These are two of the strongest risk factors for the development of malignant skin lassions, especially basal cell carcinoma.

   - **Does the patient have a history of chronic or repeated sun exposure, or trauma?** Malignant lesions of the skin including basal cell, squamous cell, and melanoma are directly related to a history of chronic sun exposure.

   - **Is there a history of radiation to the orbital region?** Similar to ionizing radiation from the sun, radiation to the skin as part of treatment for other malignant conditions can be related to the development of secondary malignancy.

   - **Does the patient have visual problems?** With any lesions or trauma to the periorbita, a history of visual symptoms is important. They may be unrelated to the lesion in question or symptoms of more extensive involvement.

   - **Does the patient have a history of skin malignancy?** The presence of malignant skin lesions elsewhere should increase the concern for the presence of malignancy in the eyelid lesion.

2. A directed physical examination should be performed.

   - **Where is the lesion located?** Malignant lesions of the periorbita are more likely to affect the lower eyelid and medial canthus than elsewhere. Only approximately 10% of malignant tumors occur on the upper lid. The position of the lesion on the lid can also affect the reconstructive options.

   - **Is the lesion fixed or freely mobile?** A rigidly fixed lesion can imply involvement of the underlying orbital rim or deeper orbital cavity. Excision would thus require a more extensive resection.

   - **Is there any ulceration or bleeding?** As stated, these symptoms may imply the presence of malignancy.

   - **Are there any visual changes?** Problems with extraocular movement or visual disturbance may also imply the presence of malignancy because of the extension of the lesion into the deeper soft tissue structures within the orbit.

   - **Is there any palpable adenopathy in the head and neck?** As opposed to basal cell tumors, which rarely metastasize, squamous cell tumors and melanomas can metastasize to lymph nodes of the face and neck area, including the parotid gland and cervical lymph node chain.

3. Pathologic diagnosis is the most important step in the management of a questionable lesion. A tissue sample can be obtained either with an incisional or excisional biopsy. An excisional biopsy is appropriate for small lesions in which the edges of the defect may be closed primarily and is adequate treatment for benign tumors of the eyelid, such as epidermal inclusion cyst, seborrheic keratosis, chalazion, and apocrine hydrocystoma. Similarly, excision to clear margins is sufficient treatment for premalignant lesions, such as actinic keratosis, Bowen's disease, and keratoacanthoma. If the lesion proves to be malignant, then further studies should be performed to stage the tumor. Malignant lesions of lower eyelid are rare.

   - The most common malignant tumor seen is **basal cell carcinoma**. Several subtypes exist; the most common being localized or nodular. These lesions usually have pearly margins that surround a translucent papule. Ulceration may occur, leading to bleeding. The sclerosing type may have no distinct margins. Such tumors are extremely rare but may invade the orbit or metastasize to local lymph nodes. Recurrent basal cell carcinoma usually is an aggressive tumor and has a high recurrence rate even after repeat excision.

- **Squamous cell carcinoma** is much less common, with a reported frequency of less than 2% to 10% of all eyelid tumors. It originates in the spindle cell layer of the epidermis and extends into the dermis. Risk is associated with sun exposure, radiation, chronic wounds, chemical exposure (especially cytotoxic drugs), actinic keratosis, and Bowen's disease. These tumors tend to spread into the orbit or cranium and to metastasize into regional lymph nodes.

  - Sebaceous gland adenocarcinoma can arise from meibomian glands or Zeis glands. These rare tumors are frequently misdiagnosed as benign lesions.

  - Malignant melanoma rarely occurs in eyelids, accounting for less than 1% of all eyelid tumors. Different subtypes with variable aggressiveness include superficial spreading, nodular and lentigo maligna exist. These lesions are usually elevated, bluish in color, hyperpigmented, and have irregular borders. Bleeding and ulceration are poor prognostic signs. Involvement of regional lymph nodes must be ascertained on initial physical examination.

4. Patients with malignant lesions will greatly benefit from a multidisciplinary team approach to their care. Input from a pathologist, oncologist, radiation therapy specialist, as well ophthalmologist and head and neck surgeon should be sought. Complicated cases should be presented to a local tumor board.

5. Prior to embarking on reconstruction, a surgeon must ensure that all of the cancer has been resected with negative margins appropriate for the given type of pathology. For basal or squamous cell skin cancers, these can be achieved either with Mohs' micrographic surgery or excision with frozen section control of the margins. An adequate margin should not be compromised for the sake of easier reconstruction, as tumor recurrence is often catastrophic for the patient both emotionally and physically. Recurrences tend to be much more aggressive than the original tumors. Defects of the lower eyelid may be partial or full thickness. The three lamella of the lower eyelid include skin and orbicularis oculi muscle, the tarsal plate for support, and the conjunctival lining. The type of reconstruction will vary depending on the thickness of the defect and the tissues involved. The goals of reconstruction are the closure of defect and provision of a stable lid margin, supporting the eyelid in opposition with the globe.

- In general, if the eyelid margin is involved, then full-thickness lid excision and primary closure should be performed. The shape of the excision should be perpendicular to the eyelid and then converge to a point in the midline similar to the shape of home plate to preserve vertical height.

- **Superficial partial-thickness** defects may be closed by primary approximation if there is enough adjacent eyelid skin, usually not more than 3 to 4 mm. Vertical closure is preferred since horizontal closure may result in ectropion.

  — If such defects are not amenable to closure then conversion to a full-thickness defect can allow for primary closure of up to 30% of a horizontal dimension.

  — If primary closure is not possible, a skin graft may be used for partial thickness defects. It is usually better to use full-thickness grafts for the lower lid when indicated because of their minimal contract and good color match. The skin of both upper lids in the supratarsal fold can be used as donor sites, and each can often provide sufficient graft. Another excellent source for donor full-thickness skin is the postauricular area, which can provide up to 5 to 6 cm of full-thickness skin with usually excellent color match. These grafts heal with some stiffness, which tends to lend additional support when they are used as grafts to the lower lid. With large defects of the lower lid, fixation of the medial and lateral margins of the graft beyond the medial and lateral palpebral fissures tends to lend support to the lower lid area by a sling-like effect.

  — Local flaps are the next option, and include a bipedicled Tripier flap from the upper eyelid, Fricke flap, midline forehead flap, superiorly based nasolabial fold flap, or a cheek flap.

- For **full-thickness defects**, excision of one-fourth to one-third of the lid can usually be closed primarily. The excision is again vertically oriented at the lid margin so the shape of the defect is a modified pentagon.

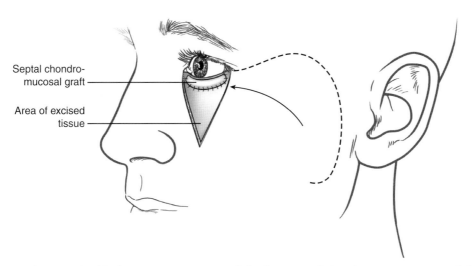

Figure 8-1 Schematic drawing highlighting reconstruction of the lower eyelid with a composite graft for internal lining and medial structure and a rotational cheek flap for external coverage.

Approximation of the vertical cut edges usually results in a straight lid margin without notching.

— If primary closure is not possible, a lateral canthotomy can be performed to allow medial advancement of the lid. If there is only 1 or 2 mm of gap before the canthotomy, closure should be possible. Lining is not a problem since the lateral conjunctiva of the fornix is attached to the lower lid when it moves medially for closure. If the lateral canthotomy does not allow closure undermining of the cheek for a few centimeters may be necessary.

— If there is still difficulty approximating the margins, a subcutaneous back-cut at the end of the lateral cheek incision, usually 4 to 5 cm lateral to the canthal tendon, should be done. The incision from the lateral canthus must be directed superiorly and laterally in an arch and then downward toward superior helix. Mobilization of the cheek flap is similar to a Mustarde flap. A septal cartilage-mucosal composite graft may be used to lend support to the reconstructed lateral canthal area. Sagittally splitting the graft with a No. 10 blade allows for slight convex curvature of the cartilage side of the graft while the concave mucosal side conforms to the curved globe. The deep dermis of the cheek flap is sutured to the lateral orbital rim periosteum. Advancement of this flap along with advancement of the conjunctiva then generally allows closure of these defects, in some cases up to nearly three-quarters of the lower lid. If needed, a lateral mucosal defect may be managed with a small graft from the nasal septum.

● Special circumstances:

— For total or near-total loss of the lower lid, a larger cheek flap is indicated along with a composite septal mucosa-cartilage graft for lining if conjunctiva is insufficient. The conjunctival defect is again estimated using a paper pattern, which is placed on the cocainized septal mucosa, and the composite graft is excised. The vertical dimension of the cartilage graft must be made larger than the area of the defect in order to overcorrect. This allows good support over time for the newly reconstructed lower lid. The initial anchoring of the cheek flap must be at the deep lateral canthal area approximating the dermis of the flap to the lateral canthal tendon or periosteum of Whitnall's tubercle.

— For small, full-thickness defects of the medial canthus and lower lid area combined, a small medially based musculocutaneous supratarsal flap from the upper lid can be used in association with a small cartilage graft. In this case, a lateral canthotomy or cheek advancement is not necessary. A composite mucosa-cartilage graft, however, may be required to fill the inner two layers of the defect.

— For a small, lateral horizontal defect that cannot be closed primarily, a flap of skin and orbicularis muscle from the upper eyelid can be used in a similar manner to cover a small composite mucosal cartilage graft. The donor area can be closed primarily in the supratarsal fold and good healing is generally ensured.

— For a horizontal defect of the entire width of the lid, a composite graft can be sutured beneath a bipedicled skin and muscle flap from the upper lid. If the defect involves the inferior lacrimal punctum, the lacrimal canaliculus can sometimes be mobilized and redirected medially. If this step is necessary, a 1 mm Silastic tube (Jones tube) should be placed in the lumen to maintain patency until healing is complete. An alternate method, the Hughes tarsoconjunctival flap, is used for reconstruction of the lower lid defect using a turn down "book" flap of conjunctiva and tarsus from the upper lid in association with a full-thickness skin graft for cutaneous coverage. The eye must remain closed for several weeks after the procedure to allow for

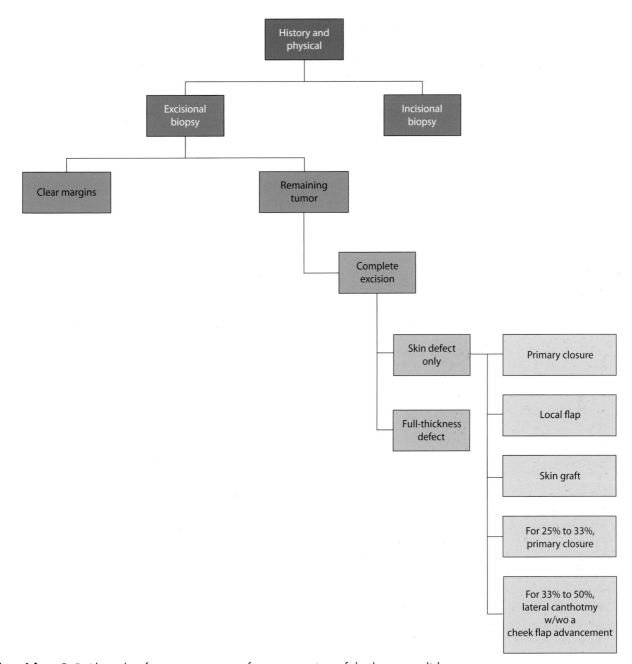

Algorithm 8-1 Algorithm for management of reconstruction of the lower eyelid.

1. It is always important to confirm clear margins following resection prior to reconstruction.

2. Defects of one-quarter to one-third of the width of the lower eyelid as a general rule can be closed primarily.

3. For reconstruction of large full-thickness defects, a mucocartilaginous graft from the nasal septum can provide inner lining and stability, while a cheek flap can provide surface coverage and a vascular bed for the graft.

4. When using a cheek flap, it should be firmly attached to the lateral orbital periosteum to prevent ectropion.

5. Temporary Frost sutures or a tarsorrhaphy should be used to minimize the development of an ectropion.

revascularization until it is time to detach the lower lid from the upper lid.

6. Potential complications following eyelid reconstruction should be considered before they occur so that specific steps to avoid them are carried out.

- **Corneal injury** should be avoided by using an ophthalmologic ointment early in the case and applied liberally to the inner surface of a corneal shield. Inadvertent injury would warrant an ophthalmology consult and possible antibiotic drops for several days.

- The development of postoperative eyelid eversion or **ectropion** may require a lid shortening or suspension procedure.

- Lid **entropion** can be corrected by excision of a horizontal tangential "V" wedge of tarsus.

References

1. Mustarde J. Reconstruction of the eyelids: The lower lid. In: Mustarde J. *Repair and Reconstruction in the Orbital Region—A Practical Guide.* 2nd ed. London, UK: Churchill & Livingstone; 1980: 92-129.

2. Cook B, Bartley G. Treatment options and future prospects for the management of eyelid malignancies—an evidence-based update. *Ophthalmology.* 2000;108(11):2088-2096.

3. Lesavoy M, Gimbel M. Correction of involutional entropion by horizontal tangential wedge excision of tarsus. *Ann Plast Surg.* 2006;56(3):330-335.

4. Miller T. Eyelid reconstruction. In: Lesavoy M. *Reconstruction of the Head and Neck.* Baltimore, MD: Williams & Wilkins; 1981:49-62.

5. Bernardini F. Management of malignant and benign eyelid lesions. *Curr Opin Ophthalmol.* 2006:17:480-484.

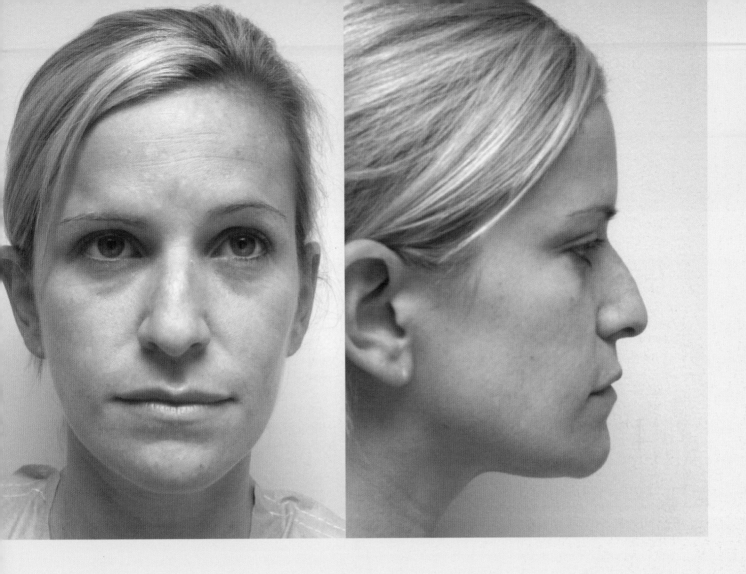

A 28-year-old woman presents to your office with concerns about the appearance of her nose.

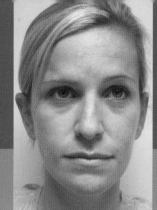

CHAPTER 9

Subjective Nasal Deformity

Sean G. Boutros

1. Evaluation of the patient who is unhappy with the appearance of nose and desiring rhinoplasty should be thorough and not be rushed. It should begin with a directed, but complete history, noting specific concerns. Functional complaints may be discussed first, followed by aesthetic goals. The latter should be precise, addressing specific, patient concerns regarding size, shape, contour, etc.

   - **How well does the patient breathe through nose?** Nasal breathing should be easy and unencumbered. In general, patients who complain about the quality of their nasal breathing will have some evidence of obstruction. Not all obstruction, however, can be corrected with surgery. Allergic symptoms and reactive airway disease may actually be worsened by inappropriate surgical intervention.

   - **What interventions have the patient tried (topical/ oral decongestants, breathe-right strips)?** Topical decongestants can improve breathing both in patients with functional obstruction and those with subjective nasal obstruction. The greatest benefit is generally seen in patients with allergic symptoms who note a symmetrical return of breathing. In patients with septal deviation, there will be improvement in breathing; however, more benefit will be noted on one side versus the other. Breathe-right strips, on the other hand, are often of benefit in patients with middle vault collapse and improvement in breathing with their use often points to underlying anatomical problems that can be surgically corrected though again, all patients will are some improvement with their application.

   - **Is there a cyclical pattern to the patient's breathing problems?** With the normal airway cycle, there is alternating increases and decreases in nasal airflow in each nostril. This is due to turbinate swelling and is part of the normal nasal function. It should be discussed discussed with patients preoperatively so that it is not a surprise in the postoperative period.

   - **Is there a history of trauma?** Traumatic injury may lead to problems with both nasal appearance and function. A history of trauma will help point to specific, correctable problems including nasal bone collapse and septal deviation.

   - **Is there a history of prior nasal surgery?** Patients undergoing secondary procedures should have special consideration. These patient's poor results are generally as a result of one of the four problems: (1) poor evaluation of the original problem by the primary surgeon, (2) poor execution of the surgical plan, (3) misguided surgical planning, or (4) patient misconception of the goal of rhinoplasty. Whatever the problem leading to a second procedure is, it must be identified prior to surgery if an acceptable result is to be obtained.

   - **What are the patient's aesthetic goals?** While the patient often will not understand the intricacies of the nose, they should describe their basic concerns and goals. This serves two functions. It allows patient to communicate the desired result, and allows the surgeon to evaluate the appropriateness of the patient for surgery.

2. Physical examination of the nose should focus on any deviation from the normal aesthetics, as well as functional structures. This should include evaluation of the chin and facial skeleton, as well as the nose.

   - **Examine the inside of the nose first without decongestant then again with decongestant.** In order to examine the nose, a strong light source and speculum in needed. It is important to note the appearance of the nasal mucosa. The surgeon should note if it is friable and bleeds easily. Topical decongestant should then be applied and the nose examined again. The surgeon should evaluate the size and position of the turbinates and, the position of the septum, noting any spurs along the maxillary crest. The septum should be inspected for position and the presence of any perforations. The septum may be deviated in an anteroposterior direction, a right to left direction, a cranial to caudal direction, or any combination of these. In secondary cases, a cotton tip applicator can be used to feel for residual septal cartilage. The area of the internal nasal valve should be inspected for signs of collapse or scarring.

   - **Examine the nose with breathing.** The surgeon should note changes in the nose with breathing. Attention should be paid to the middle vault and alar rims for signs of collapse. Feedback from the patient should also be elicited. When performing the Cottle maneuver, even asymptomatic patients will have improvement in airflow with lateral distraction of the cheek. However, patients with internal valve collapse will note a dramatic improvement in breathing.

- **Examine the dorsum and upper two-thirds of the nose.** The height of the dorsum of the nose is often either too high or too low. Specific attention should be given to the location of the radix as well. The surgeon should note any deviation of the nasal dorsum. Following the dorsal aesthetic lines is the most useful. They should be symmetric, starting at the brow and gently curving to the tip defining points. The width of the dorsum should be noted not only at the base of the nasal bones, but at the apex of the dorsum as well. A dorsum that is too narrow will often indicate collapse of the internal nasal valve. The length of the nose should also be evaluated at this stage. This is also evaluated along with the tip and lower third of the nose.

- **Examine the tip and lower one-third of the nose.** Projection describes the distance of the tip from the face on lateral view. An overprojected tip appears large in relation to the desired dorsal height, while an under-projected tip appears small. Rotation refers to the position of the tip to the lip and face. An overrotated tip will have a more obtuse columellar-labial angle and increased nostril show on the anterior view, while an underrotated tip will have a more acute columellar-labial angle, appearing droopy with an undesirable amount of nostril show. Tip support is difficult to quantify. It is the strength of the medial cura and their connection to septum. Support is evaluated by palpating the tip for ease of displacement. It is important to note that some noses with strong projection may have minimal support. The classic example is the tension nose. In this case, the tip support is actually reliant on the dorsal height and is transmitted through the skin. If the dorsum is lowered, the tip will become ptotic and collapse.

- **Is there one or more tip-defining points?** The symmetry of the tip is formed by the paired lower lateral cartilages. Asymmetry will result from deviation of these cartilages. Superiorly, the tip may be boxy with poor tip definition, or pinched with a narrow angle

at the domes. The alar base may be wide with flaring of the nostrils, although this may also be at the nasal sill.

- **How thick or thin is the skin over the nose?** The skin of the nose should be examined for its thickness. Caution is taken in skin that is excessively thin as any irregularities will be obvious post. Furthermore, patients with very thick skin, especially patients with rhinophyma, will be better served with skin treatments than with rhinoplasty.

3. As part of the patient's preparation for surgery, a standard set of photographs from eight views is important to document the preoperative appearance and assist in planning the surgery. These views include frontal, lateral, oblique, lateral smiling, and worm's eye. It is always prudent to document the surgical plan and the specific maneuvers that will be performed to address the problems identified in the history and physical. These should then be used in discussing the proposed procedure with the patient on one or more occasions. These points are general guidelines as rhinoplasty can in many ways be exploratory surgery. Even the most experienced surgeon will need to modify the surgical plans intraoperatively to achieve the desired effect on the nose.

4. No specific consultations are required prior to proceeding with cosmetic or functional rhinoplasty.

5. Numerous surgical interventions may be performed to effect the changes highlighted in the preoperative evaluation.

- The first decision in rhinoplasty is whether to perform it via the open or closed approach. In general, the open approach should be used for cases where the tip projection is insufficient and a columellar strut is required. It is also helpful on secondary cases in order to define the anatomy. Spreader grafts can be placed and secured via the closed approach, although it is easier to place via the open exposure. Overall, the surgeon must determine if the visibility required by the open approach justifies the loss of tip support and increased swelling that can occur with the open approach. Furthermore, if the closed approach is chosen, it should be converted to the open technique if intraoperative finding necessitate.

- Local anesthesia is important to provide hemostasis as well as anesthesia. The major nerves supplying the external nose arise from the supratrochlear (V_2) and infraorbital (V_1) nerves. Externally, the glabella is supplied by nasal branches of supraorbital nerve (off frontal off V_1). The tip is supplied by an external branch of the anterior ethmoidal nerve (off nasociliary off V_1). The alar base is supplied by the infraorbital nerve (off V_2) and the columella by nasal branches of the infraorbital nerve (V_2). The internal lateral mucosa is supplied by the anterior ethmoidal branch of the ophthalmic nerve, the internal nasal branch of the infraorbital nerve (off V_2), the anterior superior alveolar branch of the maxillary nerve (V_2) via the inferior conchae, and the posterior nasal branch of the maxillary nerve (V_2) via the sphenopalatine foramen. The internal medial mucosa of the superior septum is innervated by the posterior ethmoidal nerve (off nasociliary off V_1). The inferior septum is innervated by the infraorbital nerve (V_2). The anterior and posterior septum are innervated by the anterior ethmoidal nerve (off nasociliary off V_1) and the nasopalatine nerve (V_2), respectively. The external vascular supply arises from the superior labial artery (off facial artery, off maxillary artery). The internal vascular supply to the septum arises superiorly from the posterior ethmoidal artery (off ophthalmic off the internal carotid) and inferiorly off the greater palatine artery (off descending palatine artery). The anterior septum is supplied by the anterior ethmoidal artery (off the ophthalmic off the internal carotid) and superior labial artery (off facial artery, off maxillary artery). The posterior septum is supplied by the posterior septal artery. Injection of dilute lidocaine and epinephrine, usually ½% lidocaine with 1:200,000 epinephrine, provides adequate anesthesia and hemostasis. A total of 3 to 5 mm is all that is necessary over the skin of the nose with another three to five over the septum. Packing the nose with pledgets soaked in 4% cocaine is used for cases performed under sedation. Oxymetazoline hydrochloride 0.05% may be preferable in cases performed under general anesthesia.

- The dorsum is often addressed first in cases where it must be lowered. The bony dorsum is more commonly reduced with a rasp, but may be taken down with an osteotome in cases requiring greater reduction. It is sequentially palpated until the desired bony height is achieved. The cartilaginous dorsum is reduced next. The septum is reduced along with the paired upper lateral cartilages. It is important to perform this sequentially. The surgeon must take into consideration that with superior retraction of the nasal skin, the upper lateral cartilages are pulled up as well. If they are trimmed to the proper septal height, they will be too low when the skin envelope is relaxed.

- The septum is addressed after the dorsum is reduced. This order is important for two reasons. If the dorsum is reduced after the septum is resected, there may be insufficient dorsal cartilage left. Also, if the dorsum is rasped after the septum is resected, the septal cartilage may be dislocated from the perpendicular plate resulting is loss of dorsal support. The submucoperichondrial plane is obtained and dissection is carried to the vomer and the perpendicular plate. A long nose will require resection of the caudal septum and this is performed prior to the harvest of the posterior septum. While only a 1 cm L strut is necessary for nasal support, it is prudent to leave more except in cases requiring extensive grafting. Enough cartilage can usually be obtained if posterior septum is harvested properly. The harvest should include a portion of the bony vomer and the perpendicular plate, as this will ensure harvest of the entire useable cartilaginous portion of the septum. Once the cartilaginous portion is harvested in one piece, any deviation of the bony septum is addressed to fully open the airway.

- For cases requiring dorsal augmentation, septal cartilage is the best option. The edges should be gently crushed with a morselizer. If multiple layers are needed, the deep layers are not crushed and the most superficial is crushed more extensively to give a smooth natural contour. In secondary cases, auricular or rib cartilage can be used as well.

- After septal harvest is complete, the septum will often appear straight. In cases in which the caudal septum remains deviated, it will need to be released from the maxilla and then secured in the midline after the maxillary crest has been reduced.

- Spreader grafts may be fabricated from the thick, firm septal cartilage in the shape of a matchstick and be sutured along the superior edge of the upper lateral cartilages next to the septum, outside the mucosal envelope. They serve to open the internal nasal valve and allow for improved airflow. They are also useful to provide aesthetically pleasing dorsal aesthetic lines. Furthermore, they can be used to camouflage any nasal deviation. Asymmetric placement (i.e., two on one side, one on the other) or unilateral placement can be useful in cases of septal deviation to provide a straight appearance to the nose.

- Osteotomies are performed next. The three most common approaches are a direct intranasal approach to the piriform aperture, a gingivobuccal sulcus approach, and a transcutaneous approach. The internal approach is perhaps the simplest and leaves no external scar. The osteotome is started along the piriform aperture and directed cephalad. Significant attention has been placed on the starting and ending points of the osteotomy, which may be somewhat confusing. It is best to feel the nasal bones and to make the osteotomy in a location where there will be a smooth transition from the face of the maxilla to the nose. A transverse medial

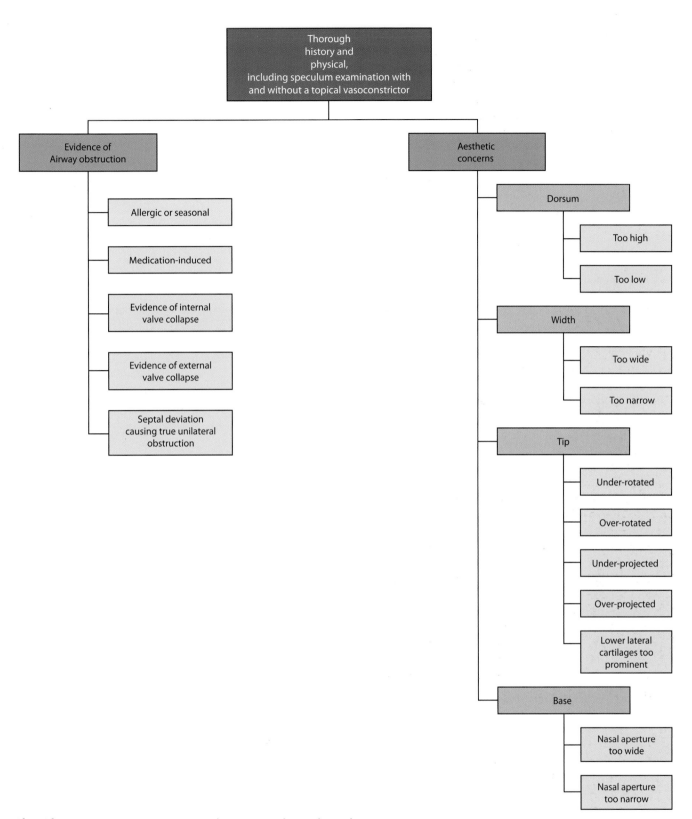

Algorithm 9-1 Managing a patient desiring aesthetic rhinoplasty.

osteotomy is not usually necessary if the bony dorsum was reduced, as the rasp weakens the bone and allows for fracture in the proper location. Once the osteotomy is created, gentle pressure is used to mobilize the bone medially. The displacement should not be a violent maneuver. It is gentle and precise. If performed in this manner, there will be less postoperative swelling and bruising. For surgeons not as comfortable with osteotomies, they can be delayed until the last portion of the case to prevent edema from obscuring the anatomy.

- Manipulation of the shape of the tip is perhaps the most written about in the literature. It usually involves techniques to narrow and refine the external appearance. Basic maneuvers include trimming the cephalic border of the lower lateral cartilages and placing sutures into the middle crura to better define the nasal tip. In general, the manipulation of the tip cartilages requires experience.

- To increase tip projection, a strut of cartilage is placed within the columella between the lower lateral cartilages that pushes on the underlying maxilla. The lower laterals are supported on this strut. This can also be used to rotate the tip. Rotation can also be increased by resection of the caudal septum, resection of the cephalic scrolls, tip sutures, and resection of the lateral cura. The rotation can be decreased by extended spread grafts which are sutured to the medial cura. The tip can be deprojected by division of the medial and lateral cura.

- Changing the position of the ala is usually performed to decrease the circumference of the nasal aperture. The simplest and most effective way to judge what should be reduced is to ask, "What is the most objectionable portion of the nostril?" It can be the nasal sill, the ala, the internal nostril, the external nostril, or any combination of these.

6. Complications

- With edema formation during the procedure, there is a risk of **overresection of the dorsum.** Should this occur, a secondary cartilage graft may be required to augment the area of deficiency.

- The **crooked dorsum** may also result from an inability to accurately judge its straightness during the procedure. To minimize the chance of the dorsum shifting in the postoperative period, the nose is packed with Vaseline gauze for a day or two and covered with a plaster or Thermaplast splint for a week or two. An established deviation requires repeat osteotomy.

- **Collapse of the external valve** on inspiration results from insufficient support to the nasal rim. It may occur following overresection of the lower lateral cartilage. In this case, a cartilage graft will need to be returned to the alar rim to provide support.

- **Obstruction of airflow through the internal nasal valve** results from scarring at the valve angle. Spreader grafts may be used primarily to ameliorate the risk or secondarily to manage the complication.

PRACTICAL PEARLS

1. Know the normal or ideal nose both aesthetically and anatomically. This includes performing anatomic dissections on cadavers.

2. Operate on the right patients and refuse to operate on the unrealistic or problem patient.

3. Formulate an operative plan in advance of the date of surgery, but remain flexible intraoperatively.

4. Resection in rhinoplasty serves an important purpose, but reconstruction should include support with grafts and sutures.

References

1. Howard BK, Rohrich RJ. Understanding the nasal airway: Principles and practice. *Plast Reconstr Surg.* 2002 Mar;109(3):1128-1146.

2. Behmand RA, Ghavami A, Guyuron B. Nasal tip sutures part I: The evolution. *Plast Reconstr Surg.* 2003 Sep 15;112(4):1125-1129.

3. Rohrich RJ, Griffin JR, Ansari M, Beran SJ, Potter JK. Nasal reconstruction—beyond aesthetic subunits: A 15-year review of 1334 cases. *Plast Reconstr Surg* 2004 Nov;114(6):1405-1416.

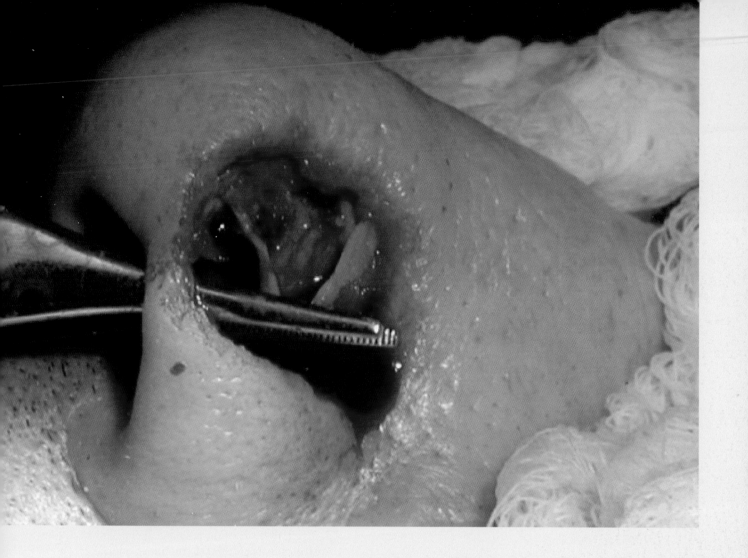

A dermatologist refers you a patient who earlier in the day underwent excision of a lesion of the nose.

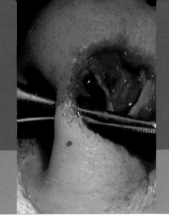

CHAPTER 10

Nasal Reconstruction

Donald R. Mackay

1. Lesions of the nose are fairly common on account of its anterior position on the face and almost inevitable sun exposure. Patients with skin lesions on and around the nose may present prior to/or following excision of the lesion by another physician. In cases where the lesion has not been removed or biopsied, a directed patient history is of invaluable assistance in determining the etiology and appropriate management.

   - **Does the patient have a history of chronic or repeated sun exposure?** The nose is the most prominent feature of the face and as such, sun exposure is the first, second, and third most common risk factors for the development of malignancy.

   - **How long has the lesion been present?** Chronic wounds predispose to the development of squamous cell carcinoma (SCC). Frequently, these present with a history of cyclical healing followed by recurrence of ulceration and bleeding.

   - **Has the lesion changed of late?** A relatively static lesion is of less concern than one that has undergone a recent change in size or color, as these might be hallmarks for malignant degeneration.

   - **Does the patient have preexisting medical conditions?** Numerous patients have coexisting medical issues that might need to be addressed prior to diagnosis and treatment. Some conditions may affect which management options are preferable.

   - **Does the patient take medication that interferes with the coagulation cascade?** Medications that interfere with clotting should be avoided perioperatively, if possible. Often, the patient's primary care or specialty physician is wary about temporarily discontinuing such medications and alternative strategies may be required.

2. A directed physical examination of the nose and potential sites for lymph node drainage should be performed. Here, the histologic and anatomic components of the nose should be evaluated individually.

   - **Where on the nose is the lesion located?** It is important to catalog the component parts of any defect. Those involving the nose may include the overlying skin, the cartilaginous or bony framework, or the internal lining. There are also nine anatomic subunits and two different skin types of the nose. The skin may be thick and glabrous or thin and waxy. The subunits include:
     — Dorsum (thin skin).
     — Left and right nasal side wall (thin).
     — Tip (thick).
     — Left and right ala (thick).
     — Left and right soft triangle (thick).
     — Columella (thick).

   Loss of more than half of any subunit may require excision and restoration of the entire subunit.

   - **Are there any facial scars?** Scars may interfere with using certain flaps for reconstruction.

   - **Is there laxity of the surrounding tissues?** Key areas where local skin and soft tissue might be recruited for reconstruction should be inspected. Elderly patients often have laxity of the malar, glabellar, and nasal skin that is valuable for reconstruction. Common locations to inspect include the nasolabial crease and the central forehead.

   - **Is there any palpable adenopathy in the head and neck?** As opposed to basal cell tumors, squamous cell tumors are noted to metastasize to regional lymph nodes. Nodes in the preauricular and cervical areas must be carefully palpated for evidence of dissemination.

3. It is most important to know whether any lesion on the nose is benign or malignant. Specimens sent for permanent sectioning are more reliable in demonstrating histopathologic cell types and detail at the borders of a lesion than are specimens examined after frozen sectioning.

   - The **biopsy** of a lesion may be excisional or incisional. An excisional biopsy is preferred when the lesion is relatively small and the defect can be closed primarily. When doubt exists about the diagnosis or in difficult anatomical areas, an incisional biopsy is preferable to identify the nature of the lesion. A small sample of the lesion is removed either with a 2-mm punch biopsy tool or with a knife. The margins are closed with a simple suture pending further complete excision of the lesion.

     — Melanomas and Merkel cell tumors need management that includes histologic measurement of the depth of the lesion, a metastatic workup, wide resection, and sentinel node biopsy for lesions more than 0.75 mm in depth.

— Mohs' surgery is a technique that repeatedly provides a small amount of skin for diagnosis while excising the tumor cells to the margin of uninvolved tissue. It is an effective and reliable technique for BCC and SCC but controversial for melanoma and Merkel cell carcinoma where it should not be used.

● The extent of disease may be determined locally by directed physical examination and with appropriate imaging such as CT/MRI as well as examining for regional or distant spread in cases with extensive disease.

4. In preparation for excision and reconstruction, a preoperative evaluation of the patient's health status should be performed.

● The presence of hypertension, diabetes, and other comorbidities should be noted and controlled.

● The need for chemotherapy or radiation therapy should be discussed with an oncologist based on physical and diagnostic findings.

5. For large, full-thickness defects, there is little role for nonsurgical management. In cases where further operative intervention is contraindicated, such as for medical reasons, fabrication of a partial or complete prosthesis may be preferable. A mirror image of the contralateral side composed of silicone and held in place with adhesive usually produces a better aesthetic appearance than multistaged procedures. The surgical steps should include obtaining negative margins by histologic examination, subsequent reconstruction of all necessary components involved, and possible adjuvant therapy.

● Negative excision margins, including underlying cartilage and mucosa, must be obtained before beginning any reconstructive effort.

— Standard nodular basal cell with translucent pearly borders can be removed by surgical excision with 2 mm margin with a 5-year cure rate of 90% to 95%. Radiation therapy, cryosurgery, or curettage yield similar results.

— Recurrent and morpheaform basal cell carcinoma (BCC) needs to be treated more aggressively and monitored by careful pathologic evaluation to ensure adequate excision. These are cases that are good indications for Mohs' surgery.

— SCC should be resected with a 1 cm margin.

— The resection margin for melanoma is based on the depth of the lesion.

  a. In situ lesions: 5 mm margin.

  b. Up to 1 mm: 1 cm margin.

  c. 1 to 2 mm: 1 or 2 cm margins.

  d. >2 mm: 2 cm margins.

— These margins are sometimes modified when strict adherence to the surgical margins are too mutilating; for example, a nasal sidewall lesion that with a 2 cm margin would require an ocular enucleation.

● Final **reconstruction** should be delayed until after the final margins are known. Defects following Mohs' surgery for basal cell and squamous cell tumors may be safely reconstructed immediately following the resection. The choice of surgical technique will depend on the extent of the defect. Full-thickness defects will require lining, support, and coverage.

● **Nasal lining** is often the most difficult to create. It may be provided by uni- or bilateral nasolabial turn-in flaps, pedicled septal mucoperichondrial flaps, or bipedicled mucosal flaps from above the site of the defect. Prefabrication of a forehead flap with split thickness skin graft on the undersurface of the flap can also provide lining. In each case, postoperative stenting may be helpful to prevent collapse of the nares from contracture.

● The **supporting framework** may be reconstructed either with bone, provided from available sites in the calvarium, ilium, or rib, or by cartilage, harvested from the ears or ribs. Bone is frequently used for dorsal and columellar reconstruction where tip support is needed. Cartilage is more commonly used along the alar rim for support of the external nasal valve.

● There is a plethora of options for **skin coverage**. The selection is based on the principles of the reconstructive ladder with the proviso that the option that will provide the best functional and aesthetic result is selected. The size and shape of the necessary donor tissue may be planned using a foil template. Another

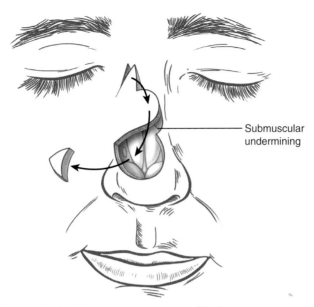

Figure 10-1 Schematic drawing highlighting reconstruction of the nose with a bilobed flap for external coverage.

principle is to reconstruct an entire aesthetic subunit where the defect is more than 50% of the subunit. This may require excision of uninvolved tissue. The principle is more important in young patients where scars are not as easily camouflaged as they are in older individuals. The options with increasing size defects and levels of complexity are:

— **Primary closure** of the wound margins should be considered first if possible. Significant tension or deformity as a result of primary closure would be an indication to consider alternative options.

— **Healing by secondary intention** may be a plausible option, especially for lesions in difficult anatomic areas, such as the inner canthus.

— **Skin grafting** should match the type of skin being replaced. Full and partial thickness skin grafts are available for use. Preauricular skin (followed by postauricular and supraclavicular) has adequate color match for the nose.

— **Local rotation flaps** are better for thicker areas, but the surgeon must be cognizant of the arc of rotation of each flap.

   a   For the dorsum and tip, a rotational flap from adjacent tissue (banner flap), a Limberg flap based on angles of 120 degrees/60 degrees or 150 degrees/30 degrees, a bilobed flap, or a dorsal advancement flap are all viable options.

   b   For the rim, a Kazanjian bipedicle flap, a Z-plasty, a perialar transposition flap, a lateral dorsal advancement flap, or a nasolabial flap may be used. The **nasolabial flap** is an axial pattern flap that may be based superiorly (angular branch of the anterior facial artery, as well as branches from the internal maxillary artery, transverse facial artery, labial artery) or inferiorly. It is drained by tributaries of the angular vein. Its thickness makes it a better option for lower nasal defects. The donor site scar is preferred for adults since the medial incision placed in the nasolabial crease. It should be avoided if crossing a concavity. An **auricular composite graft** may also be used for small defects of the nasal rim. For the columella, the options include a nasolabial flap,

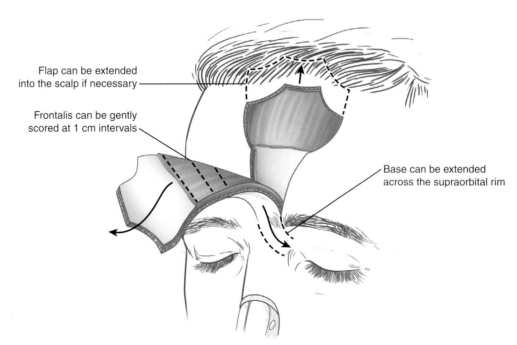

Figure 10-2 Schematic drawing highlighting reconstruction of nose with a paramedian forehead flap for external coverage.

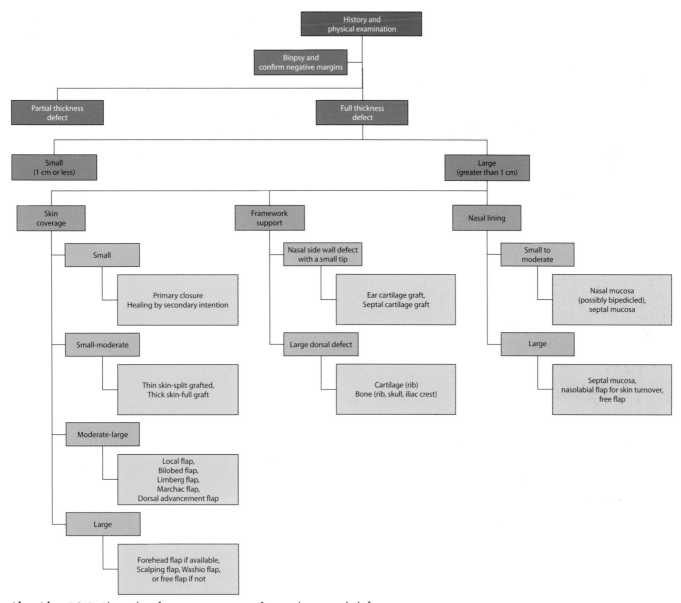

Algorithm 10-1 Algorithm for management of complex nasal defects.

which is commonly used in adults. The Washio flap, on the other hand, may be preferred for pediatric cases. A composite graft from the helical rim is another option for defects of less than 1 cm in otherwise healthy patients.

— The most widely used regional flap for coverage of the nose is the **paramedian forehead flap**. It is an axial flap based on supratrochlear vessels. It may be prefabricated prior to rotation with cartilage and/or skin for structure and lining. Most of donor site may be closed primarily with the rest left open to heal by secondary intention. The flap may be thinned in an intervening stage before flap division.

— Where the forehead flap is not an option a **scalping flap**, which is based on superficial temporal vessels and borrows tissue from behind the hairline to advance into the defect temporarily and is then replaced after 3 to 4 weeks may be considered. A full-thickness skin graft is required for the donor site. This may be better for a longer defect. Alternatively, a Washio flap, which is a **tempororetroauricular flap** based on posterior branch of superficial temporal artery may be used. It can be folded on itself for lining.

6. The potential for **scarring** and **distortion** of the reconstructed tissues should be discussed with all patients preoperatively. Patients should be warned that multiple stages and revisions are commonly needed before the best result is achieved. Truer complications include:

- **Bleeding** should be a rare complication with attention to hemostasis following excision and prior to closure. Collection of blood beneath a reconstruction noted postoperatively should be evacuated to minimize further distortion and potential for secondary infection.

- **Infection** in the head and neck is less commonly seen than in other areas of the body on account of its healthy blood supply and minimal hypovascular soft tissue.

- **Flap loss** is usually caused by ischemia and less commonly infection. Ischemia is more commonly seen in smokers. It may be minimized by carefully designing flaps to maximize vascularity. A fallback plan should always be considered.

PRACTICAL PEARLS

1. Make certain that the diagnosis is known and that the margins are clear in malignant cases prior to proceeding with reconstruction.

2. Think in terms of (1) lining, (2) support, and (3) coverage when planning the reconstruction. The skin coverage should incorporate the concept of the aesthetic subunits.

3. Plan the skin coverage so that the flap sits within the defect with absolutely no tension.

4. The nasolabial flap is normally raised with 2 to 3 mm of subcutaneous tissue but should be left thick in smokers or diabetics. The lateral incision is placed 2 to 3 cm lateral to the medial one.

5. Distally, the forehead flap is kept thin and raised in a subcutaneous plane. More proximally, it is raised in a submuscular (frontalis) plane to preserve vascularity.

References

1. Burget GC. Aesthetic reconstruction of the nose. In: Mathes SJ, ed. *Plastic Surgery*. London, UK: Elsevier; 2005;573-648.

2. Menick FJ. A 10-year experience in nasal reconstruction with the three-stage forehead flap. *Plast Reconstr Surg*. 2002;109:1839-1861.

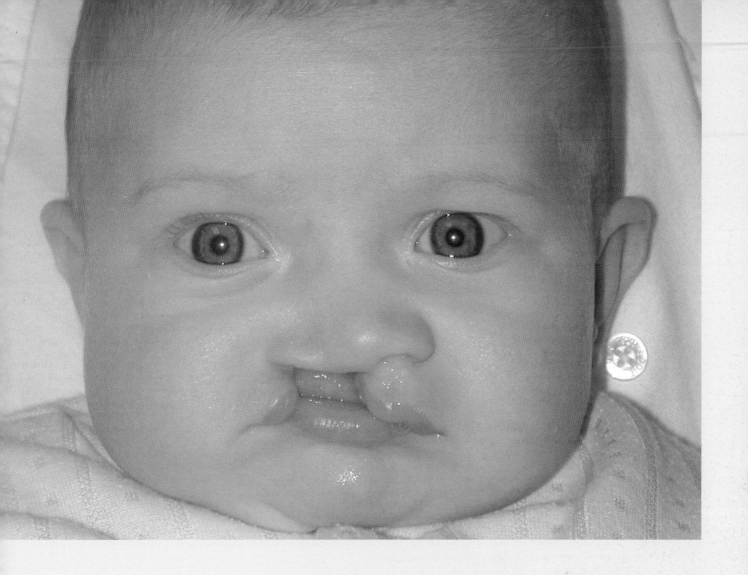

A 2-month-old infant presents to
the plastic surgery clinic with
the deformity of the upper lip.

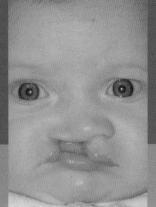

CHAPTER 11

Unilateral Cleft Lip

Jeffrey Weinzweig

1. Patients with a cleft of the lip are usually seen as infants, often in the setting of a craniofacial team conference and rarely, as adults. When such a patient is seen for consultation, several concerns are paramount to understanding the etiopathogenesis of the anomaly and providing optimal treatment.

   - **Were any prenatal problems identified that might be related to the development of the cleft?** While the molecular mechanism of cleft lip remains elusive, and multiple theories have been postulated. Currently, the multifactorial etiology of clefting is well accepted. Numerous agents have been directly associated with clefting, including smoking and the use of a myriad of drugs, during the critical period in gestation when fusion of the lip elements occurs.

   - **How old is the child and does the cleft interfere with either breathing or feeding?** Infants with a cleft lip but an intact palate should be able to generate enough suction pressure to feed adequately. When associated with a cleft of the palate, management strategies must accommodate issues that arise related to feeding and airway protection.

   - **Is there any family history of clefting or congenital anomalies?** A genetic predisposition for clefting has been well established. Although the genetics of orofacial clefting are only partially understood, such information is of great importance in counseling families of affected children. The overall incidence of clefting is higher in whites (1 in 700) and lower in African Americans (1 in 1300). The incidence of isolated cleft palate in whites is 0.5 in 1000. The incidence of a cleft lip (with or without an associated cleft of the palate) is higher in males, while the incidence of an isolated cleft palate is higher in females. For unclefted parents with one child with a cleft lip/palate, the risk of having a second child with a cleft is approximately 4%. This risk increases to 9% when there are two affected children. If one parent and one sibling have a cleft, the risk is 17%. As the degree of familial relationship increases, the recurrence risk decreases; first-, second-, and third-degree relatives have 4%, 0.7%, and 0.3% risk, respectively. Further, recurrence risk increases with the severity of the cleft.

   - **Are there any other known congenital anomalies?** While there are more than 250 documented syndromes associated with orofacial clefting, most cases occur as an isolated abnormality—"nonsyndromic" cleft lip/palate. Patients with a cleft lip, irrespective of palate involvement, less commonly present as part of larger syndromes than do patients with an isolated cleft palate.

2. A meticulous physical examination is paramount to discerning anatomic subtleties that make each patient unique and will contribute to the development of a specific surgical strategy that will address each of those anatomic variations. The examination should focus on the lip, nose, alveolus, and posterior palate with special attention paid to the specific details of the anatomy of the lip, which will be utilized in the repair.

   - **What portion of the lip is involved?** The entire lip, including the Cupid's bow, philtral columns, philtral tubercle, vermilion, white roll, mucosa, nasal sill, columella, and orbicularis oris muscles may be involved (*complete cleft*), or simply portions of these components can be involved (*incomplete cleft*). A cleft in which the skin and mucosa are intact but the muscles are aberrant is referred to as a *forme fruste* cleft lip. A *microform cleft* is characterized by a furrow extending the vertical length of the lip, a vermilion notch, imperfections of the white roll, and varying degrees of lip shortness. If the nostril sill is intact, much of the structure of the nose is preserved. An *incomplete cleft* is characterized by varying degrees of vertical separation of the lip but they all have an intact nasal sill, or Simonart's band.

   - **Is the palate involved? If so, does that adversely affect the lip?** A complete cleft of the palate will generally distort the lip more than an isolated cleft of the lip alone owing to the malpositioning of the alveolar arches and inherent maxillary hypoplasia which, invariably, have an impact on positioning and development of all structures related to the lip and nose.

   - **Is the nose distorted?** A complete cleft of the lip and palate usually causes distortion of the nose. The typical cleft nasal deformity has splaying of the lower lateral cartilage and buckling of the lateral crus. In addition, a cleft of the alveolus will produce asymmetry of the base as a result of a deficient platform at the alar-facial crease, the result of maxillary hypoplasia.

- **Are the dental arches aligned?** Clefts that do not involve the alveolus generally have well-aligned dental arches. Those that do involve the alveolus and portions of the palate will often demonstrate malaligned dental arches. When the arches are not well approximated, a nasoalveolar molding appliance may be fabricated from alginate impressions and used within the first weeks of life to mold the segments facilitating the ultimate repair.

3. There are no specific studies, either blood tests or radiographic images that are necessary to plan for treatment. Specific preparation for presurgical nasoalveolar molding should be discussed in conjunction with the cleft lip and palate team. This may delay initial lip repair by several weeks.

4. The input of a multidisciplinary team of specialists that evaluates and manages children with clefts and possibly other craniofacial anomalies is critical for optimizing and individualizing each child's treatment plan. Such a team ideally includes plastic surgeons, orthodontists, otolaryngologists, speech pathologists, audiologists, geneticists, social workers, child psychologists, and ophthalmologists.

- Initial problems with feeding may be addressed by the cleft team's **speech and swallowing specialist**. Maneuvers to improve swallowing include upright feeding and use of a wider-bore nipple to improve the flow of milk or formula. It is rare for a child to require prolonged nasoenteral feeds or even placement of a gastrostomy tube.

- Consultation with the cleft team's **pediatric dentist** or orthodontist should occur as soon as possible. The dentist should evaluate the feasibility and necessity of preoperative nasoalveolar molding prior to cleft lip repair. In addition, the molding device may assist with molding the cartilages within the nasal alar rim to facilitate primary cleft rhinoplasty and improve the initial appearance of the nose.

- Associated anomalies, occurrence in other family members, and possible etiopathogeneis are topics of discussion with the team's **geneticist**.

- Evaluation of the child's postnatal audiogram and examination of the external ear canal, tympanic membrane, and middle ear should be done by the team's pediatric otolaryngologist. The pediatric otolaryngologist should evaluate the need for myringotomy tubes either before or at the time of lip and/or palate repair.

5. Cleft lip repair is often performed at approximately 3 months of age (or according to the "rule of 10's": 10 kg, 10 g of hemoglobin, and 10 weeks of age), when the risk of anesthetic complications diminishes. This may be delayed, however, if the patient has undergone a lip adhesion or is undergoing presurgical nasoalveolar molding.

- Particularly wide, complete clefts can be converted to incomplete clefts by a preliminary lip adhesion procedure that preserves all natural landmarks and tissue necessary for the definitive repair while contributing to the alignment of the maxillary components. With the advent and prevalence of presurgical orthopedics, lip adhesions are performed less frequently but should still remain within the armamentarium of the cleft surgeon who may be called upon to perform a wide cheiloplasty without the benefit of presurgical orthopedics. The advantages of performing a lip adhesion include: (1) narrowing of the cleft, (2) decreased tension across the maxilla, (3) easier correction of the nasal deformity caused by the resultant improved bony framework, (4) elongation of a short lip prior to definitive repair, and (5) fewer secondary revisions.

  — Standard markings and measurements for an adhesion are similar to those of the complete unilateral repair. Care is taken to avoid violation of vital landmarks including the philtral columns and the vermilion medial to the base of the cleft-side philtral column. Two rectangular flaps are raised from the cleft margins away from the definitive lip repair incision markings. One rectangular flap is based on the mucosal side and one on the skin side. The flaps are raised deep enough to expose the orbicularis muscle so one or two removable muscle-approximating, tension sutures can be placed and maintained for 10 to 14 days.

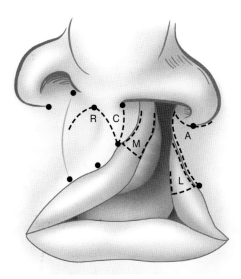

Figure 11-1 Schematic drawing highlighting reconstruction of a unilateral cleft lip by the rotation-advancement repair.

- The primary objective of presurgical orthopedics is to correct the skeletal deformities of the cleft maxilla before surgery, facilitating primary repair of the lip, and decreasing the need for secondary revisions. Presurgical orthopedic management is indicated in children with wide clefts or in cases where a gingivoperiosteoplasty may be desired. Millard was a strong proponent of the use of the Latham appliance for the presurgical alignment of the alveolar segments and maxilla into an edge-to-edge or "touch" position, facilitating cleft repair without tension or the need for a lip adhesion.

- Alveolar and nasoalveolar molding are performed increasingly more commonly in an effort to reposition the maxillary segments into proper alignment as well as to reposition and mold the elements of the nasal cartilages of the tip and nostril. Multiple methods have developed that range from external taping to apply pressure and approximate the separated alveolar segments, simulating a nonsurgical lip adhesion procedure, to modifications that involve the use of a molding bulb attached to a dental plate as an outrigger to mold the nose in conjunction with the external taping of the lip. The combination of force from the taping and counterforce from the molding bulb provide the force necessary to bring the alveolar segments into proper alignment. These molding techniques are usually started within the first 2 weeks after birth; careful monitoring is required every 1 to 2 weeks for a period of 3 to 6 months to produce the desired result.

- The specific goals of cleft lip repair are:
  — Reconstruct the normal lip contour (Cupid's bow).
  — Restore the vertical height of the lip along the philtral ridge. This includes creation of a natural appearing philtral tubercle.

- Realign the fibers of the orbicularis oris muscle. The major muscle within the lip is a sphincter that normally encircles the mouth and inserts onto itself. In the patient with a cleft of the lip, the muscular ring remains open with the ends aberrantly inserting onto the maxilla along the posterior edge of the cleft.

- Minimize the appearance of scars on the lip.

- With the aforementioned goals in mind, a myriad of repair techniques have been described over the past half century to reconstruct clefts of the lip. The most widely used technique, currently performed by the majority of plastic surgeons worldwide is the *rotation-advancement* technique first described by Millard in 1957 and refined by him many times over subsequent decades.

- A spectrum of techniques has evolved over decades, largely to improve the placement and appearance of scars on the lip while optimizing lip length. These techniques typically encompass some variation of a Z-plasty of the upper or lower aspect of the lip, or both. Straight-line and quadrangular designs have also been described with similar goals. Selected techniques are listed below for historical purposes.
  — Straight line repair (Rose-Thompson).
  — Lower Z-plasty repair (Randall-Tennison and LeMesurier).
  — Upper Z-plasty repair (Millard).
  — Upper and lower Z-plasty repair (Trauner and Skoog).
  — Quadrangular repair (LeMesurier).

- Prior to commencing with the actual lip repair (cheiloplasty), several anatomic landmarks should be identified and tattooed in the dermis to facilitate the repair:
  — High point of Cupid's bow on the noncleft side of the major lip element.
  — Low point of Cupid's bow with the philtral dimple of the major lip element.
  — High point of Cupid's bow opposite the cleft on the major lip element.
  — High point of Cupid's bow opposite the cleft on the minor lip element.
  — Commissures.
  — Alar bases.
  — Columellar midpoint.

- With the rotation-advancement technique, several flaps are elevated and transposed to close the cleft defect, while the incisions on the lip are largely confined to the philtral column and alar-facial groove to minimize scarring.
  — A **rotation flap** is created opposite the cleft on the major lip element. The medial incision begins at the high point of Cupid's bow opposite the cleft on

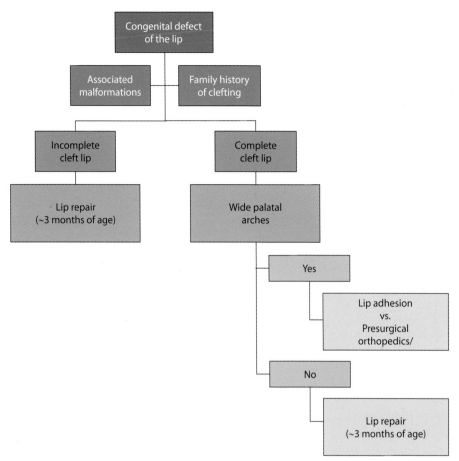

Algorithm 11-1 Algorithm for management of patients with a cleft of the lip and/or palate.

the major lip element, sweeps toward the margin of the cleft, and extends to the base of the columella. From there, a back-cut, one that extends as much as two-third the width of the philtrum, approaching the philtral column in parallel but never crossing it, allows rotation of the flap and length to be gained for the repair. A Mohler variation extends the rotation flap a couple millimeters onto the columella to borrow tissue and facilitate columellar lengthening.

— An **advancement flap** is created on the cleft side. The medial edge is designed along the white roll of the lip to match the length of the philtral column on the noncleft side.

— A **columellar flap** (C flap) is created at the base of the columella medial to the incision for the rotation flap on the major lip element. It is used to fill in the defect in the upper portion of the lip left by the rotation flap.

— A **lining flap** (L flap) is created within the vermilion on the cleft side. It is used in clefts with nasal involvement to augment the surface area of the nasal lining. An incision with the base of the nasal sidewall is created to accept the flap and allow medial rotation of the alar base.

— A **mucosal flap** (M flap) is created within the vermilion on the opposite side of the lining flap. It is used to fill in any gaps left after an incision is made within the gingivobuccal sulcus to advance the major lip element toward the defect.

● Edge-to-edge alignment of the alveolar segments also facilitates the performance of a gingivoperiosteoplasty, a procedure introduced by Skoog in 1967. Gingivoperiosteoplasty is thought to promote bony union of the alveolus and, thus, stabilize the arch, providing a platform for reconstruction of the lip and nose. This procedure remains controversial as a result of reports of resultant facial growth disturbances.

6. The cleft surgeon must understand the complications that may occur with cleft lip repair and how to best manage them.

● **Bleeding**, which can occur with any procedure, can certainly occur following cleft lip repair. It is generally the result of the subdermal plexus oozing and self-limited. More vigorous bleeding from the muscle can readily be controlled by gentle compression of the labial vessels laterally (*away from the actual repair*), if necessary.

● **Infection** is, fortunately, rare because of the abundant blood supply to the lip and the use of sterile technique. The rare occurrence is easily treated with antibiotics.

● **Wound dehiscence** occurs uncommonly and should be managed with local wound care and antibiotics until the edges have sufficiently healed. Anytime thereafter, a secondary closure may be performed if indicated.

● **Hypertrophic scarring** may be managed with frequent massage and application of local steroids. This may be administered via injection or topically.

PRACTICAL PEARLS

1. Although generally repaired at 3 months of age, cleft lip repair is not an emergency procedure. *Be certain* that the repair has been optimized either by performing presurgical orthopedics or a lip adhesion, when indicated, and the child has no other comorbidities that require attention prior to lip repair.

2. For wide clefts or those with significant alveolar segment malalignment, presurgical orthopedics and nasoalveolar molding optimize the ultimate result and are strongly advocated. When using a molding bulb to mold the nose, *be certain* the child is monitored closely to avoid excessive pressure being applied to the nasal cartilages or skin, a potentially disastrous situation that can result in tissue necrosis.

3. In the absence of presurgical orthopedics, there is no reason to not perform a lip adhesion as the first stage of a two-stage cheiloplasty in the case of a particularly wide cleft. *Be certain* to mark and preserve anatomic landmarks that will be used for the definitive repair.

4. Each surgeon should select the technique with which they are most comfortable and with which they obtain the most reliable, predictable, and reproducible results. While the Millard repair is the most commonly used technique, some feel it is not ideal for repair of especially wide clefts. If a lip is short on the operating table, it will be short down the road. *Be certain* that you have achieved adequate lip length intraoperatively, extending the back-cut as necessary to accomplish this but never crossing the philtral column.

References

1. Millard DR. The unilateral deformity. In: Millard DR, ed. *Cleft Craft—The Evolution of It's Surgery,* Vol I. The Unilateral Deformity. Boston, MA: Little, Brown; 1976.

2. Millard DR. Refinements in the rotation-advancement cleft lip technique. *Plast Reconstr Surg.* 1964;33:26-38.

3. Mulliken JB, Pensler JM, Kozakewich HP. The anatomy of Cupid's bow in normal and cleft lip. *Plast Reconstr Surg.* 1993;92:395-403.

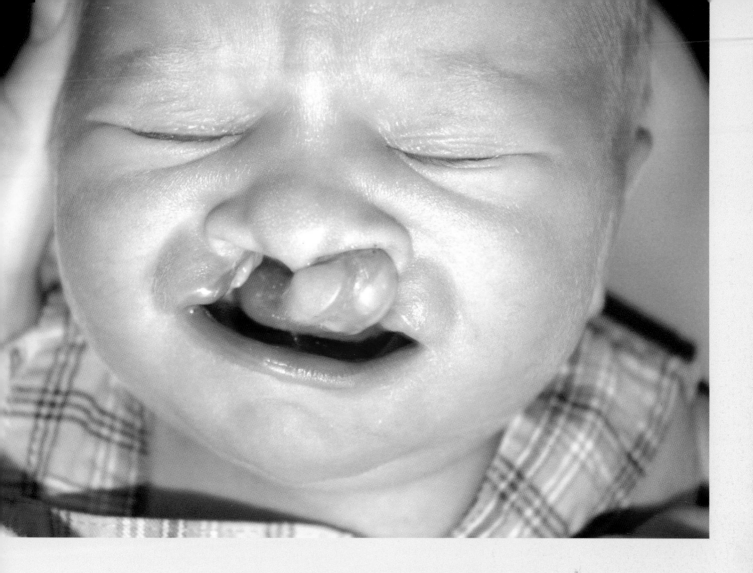

The neonatal intensive care unit requests

your consultation on the infant

shown above.

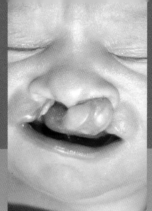

CHAPTER 12

Bilateral Cleft Lip

Joseph E. Losee

1. The patient in question appears to have a cleft of the lip with or without extension into the palate on both sides of the face. The general management of patients with a bilateral cleft lip is similar to that of a unilateral cleft lip. Many families come to the surgeon and cleft–craniofacial team for prenatal consultation and greatly benefit from this antenatal meeting. Patients are seen soon after birth; and depending upon the severity of the deformity, may require intervention prior to definitive lip repair. During the initial consultation with the infant and family, several questions are paramount.

   - **Is there a family history of clefting or other congenital anomalies?** A thorough history should be obtained with particular attention paid to any relatives with clefting or congenital anomalies, as well as any prenatal conditions that might be related to orofacial clefting. The general incidence of clefting found in Caucasians (1 in 500) and Asians (1 in 400) is higher than that of African Americans (1 in 1300). The incidence of cleft lip (with or without cleft palate) is higher in males; while the incidence of an isolated cleft palate is higher in females. The increased risk of having a second child with a cleft is 4%; and this risk increases to 9% when there are two affected children in the family. If a parent and single sibling have a cleft, the risk for another child with orofacial clefting increases to 17%.

   - **Are there associated congenital anomalies?** Infants with cleft lip (with or without cleft palate) have associated medical conditions up to 30% of the time. Cleft lip (with or without cleft palate) is less likely to present as part of a larger syndrome, when compared to isolated clefts of the palate. Infants with cleft palate alone have nearly a 10% risk of carrying the 22q. 11 deletion of Velocardiofacial syndrome, as well as an increased risk for Pierre Robin sequence and Stickler syndrome.

   - **Is the infant eating and gaining weight?** Children with orofacial clefts may have initial feeding difficulties, requiring extra time and attention; however, it is unusual for them to not ultimately do well. Those infants with complete clefts of the lip and palate are unable to generate a seal and create negative pressure necessary for successful sucking. Infants with clefts need to have liquid "dispensed" into their mouths, often with the use of a specialized bottle, while they go through the motions of suckling. Infants, with isolated clefts of the lip with intact palates, are often able to generate enough negative pressure to feed normally.

   - **Is the infant having respiratory or breathing difficulties?** More frequently associated with isolated cleft palate, breathing difficulties can occur in children with micro-retrognathia and Pierre Robin sequence. Infants with cleft lip (with or without cleft palate) usually do not have associated breathing difficulties.

2. A complete physical examination should be performed to determine whether associated congenital anomalies (i.e., heart disease) exist. Particular attention should be paid to the craniofacial examination; and the full extent of the cleft and its involvement of the lip, alveolus, and palate determined. Clefts of the lip can be classified as complete (affecting the entire lip), incomplete (affecting a portion of the lip with an intact Simonart's band in the nostril sill), or forme fruste (affecting the orbicularis oris with intact skin).

   - **Is it a complete cleft?** If a complete bilateral cleft of the lip exists, the lateral alveolar segments are often widely separated, and the premaxilla is anteriorly displaced resulting in a "fly away" premaxilla. A "fly-away premaxilla" exists when the midline prolabium (lip tissue anterior to the bony premaxilla) and premaxilla protrude anteriorly on a stem of the vomer, as they have no connections to the more posterior lateral palatal shelves. Primary surgical setback of the premaxilla, practiced historically, is no longer advocated since it has been shown to affect midface development. In addition, a complete cleft of the lip and nose results in a flat nose lacking projection, a short or nonexisting columella, and flared alar bases tethered to widely displaced pyriform rims. Within the nasal tip, the lower lateral cartilages are also widely displaced. Generally, complete clefts of the lip, nose, and palate require presurgical infant orthopedics (i.e., nasoalveolar molding) prior to definitive repair. Nasoalveolar molding realigns the premaxilla and alveolar segments, as well as elongating the columella and approximating the lip segments, facilitating the definitive lip and nose repair. If presurgical infant orthopedics is not available or able to be obtained, a preliminary surgical "lip adhesion" may be performed, converting the wide complete cleft into an incomplete cleft.

- **Is it an incomplete cleft?** If a child is born with an incomplete bilateral cleft of the lip and/or palate, the deformity is less severe. This deformity can be repaired primarily at approximately 3 months of age without the need for presurgical infant orthopedics.

- **Is the nose distorted?** A bilateral complete cleft of the lip and palate will almost always cause distortion of the nose since the premaxilla onto which the columella and septum rest is anteriorly displaced.

- **Are the dental arches well aligned?** A bilateral complete cleft of the lip and palate will also usually result in malalignment of the dental arches. In these cases, an appliance may be created to mold the segments and within the first weeks as a means of facilitating the ultimate repair.

3. No particular studies are required prior to surgery, provided the complete physical examination has not raised any concern about any comorbidity (i.e., heart disease).

- A thorough examination by a pediatrician must "clear" the infant for surgery. Prior to the elective lip and nose repair, the child should be eating well, gaining weight, and growing normally. If an associated syndrome is suspected, further studies are often required (i.e., renal ultrasound, echocardiogram, ophthalmologic evaluation). Most cleft surgeons perform the definitive primary cleft lip and nose repair around 3 to 6 months of age (for the full-term infant) when the risk of anesthetic complications diminishes. However, the time of surgery may be delayed, particularly if the infant is undergoing presurgical infant orthopedics. The "rule of 10's" has been offered as a guide or prerequisite for surgery: 10 kg, 10 g of hemoglobin, and 10 weeks of age.

4. The current standard of care dictates that infants born with orofacial clefts benefit from evaluation in the setting of a cleft and/or craniofacial team. The input of the team's professionals, with experience in managing the complex care of these unique patients, is important.

- Often, infants born with complete clefts experience initial problems with feeding, and these issues may be addressed by the cleft team's **speech and swallowing specialist**. Maneuvers to improve swallowing include upright feeding and use of a wider-bore nipple to improve the flow of milk or formula. Fluids are "dispensed" in the infant's mouth as they make the suckling motions. It is exceedingly rare for a child with a cleft to require prolonged nasoenteric feeds or placement of a gastrostomy tube.

- For those infants with complete clefts, consultation with the cleft team's **pediatric dentist or orthodontist** should occur as soon as possible. The pediatric dentist or the orthodontist will evaluate the feasibility of presurgical infant orthopaedics (i.e., nasoalveolar molding) prior to cleft lip repair. Nasoalveolar molding repositions the "fly away" premaxilla, aligns the maxillary segments, and molds the nasal cartilages while elongating the columella. This will greatly facilitate the definitive cleft lip and nose repair. If presurgical infant orthopaedics is not available or possible, consideration is given to a preliminary surgical "lip adhesion," converting the complete cleft into an incomplete cleft, prior to definitive cleft lip and nose reconstruction.

- If the history or physical examination identifies any associated anomalies, a consultation with the cleft–craniofacial team's **medical geneticist** is necessary. Further evaluation and testing may be appropriate (i.e., ophthalmological assessment for suspected Stickler syndrome in a child with Pierre Robin sequence, and routine screening for the 22q.11 deletion of Velocardiofacial syndrome in all isolated cleft palates).

5. The concept of a "reconstructive ladder" has little implication in cleft surgery, and the goals of cleft lip and nose repair are quite specific. Cleft lip and nose repair can be conceptualized as "philtral subunit reconstruction," reconstructing a symmetric Cupid's bow. The deformities unique to complete bilateral clefts include: (1) splayed lower lateral cartilages, (2) a deficient columella and poor tip projection, (3) splayed alar bases tethered to wide pyriform rims, (4) loss of a philtrum, (5) anteriorly displaced premaxilla and displaced lateral maxillary segments, and (6) orbicularis oris muscle discontinuity. Therefore, the goals specific to bilateral cleft lip and nose reconstruction include: (1) nasal tip reconstruction, (2) creation of a columella from nasal tissue, (3) release and repositioning (overcorrection) of the alar bases,

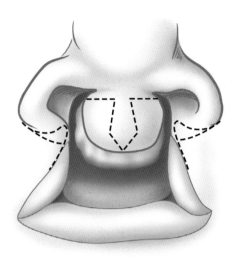

Figure 12-1 Schematic drawing highlighting reconstruction of a bilateral cleft lip.

(4) creation of a philtrum from prolabial tissue, placing the scars along the normal philtral ridges, (5) creation of a Cupid's bow, and central lip tubercle from lateral lip tissue, and (6) reestablishment of a muscular sphincter.

- **Nasal reconstruction.** The alar bases, which are stretched across a wide pyriform rim, need to be completely released and radically mobilized from the facial skeleton. They are overcorrected with a narrowing cinch suture using permanent material such as nylon or Prolene. Bilateral rim incisions allow for dissection of the lower lateral cartilages, removal of the fibrofatty tissue interposed between them, and intradomal sutures bringing the alar domes together. The soft triangles are judiciously excised and columellar shaping stitches are placed.

- **Philtral reconstruction.** The new "tie shaped" philtrum is designed from the prolabial tissues. The lateral long edges of the philtrum bow inward slightly. Postoperatively, the philtrum will stretch in both the horizontal and vertical dimensions, and is thus created narrow with future growth in mind. The philtrum is marked 2- to 3-mm wide at the columellar-philtrum junction superiorly. The philtrum is made 6 to 8 mm in height. The low point of Cupid's bow is marked inferiorly, and the height of Cupid's bow marked 2 mm on either side, for a total width of Cupid's bow being 4 mm on the new philtrum. The remaining skin of the prolabium may be discarded.

- **Lateral lip elements.** The corresponding high points of Cupid's bow, on the lateral lip elements, are determined where the lateral lip vermilion "begin to lose their fullness." The white roll of the new Cupid's bow is obtained from the lateral lip elements, 2 mm on either side. Extra mucosa is harvested from the lateral lip elements to create a "pouting tubercle" for the central lip. The lateral lip advancement flaps are created 1 to 2 mm longer than the length of the philtral "tie flap." The lateral lip elements are cut and buccal sulcus incisions allow for radical mobilization and advancement to the midline.

- **Muscle reconstruction.** The orbicularis oris muscle is freed from the overlying skin and underlying mucosa bilaterally. Following repair of the mucosa, the muscle is approximated in the middle, on top of the premaxilla and beneath the neophiltrum. It is sutured to the nasal spine.

- **Skin repair.** The lateral lip elements are advanced to the new philtrum and deep subcutaneous and cuticular sutures are placed. Great care is taken in placing these buried sutures so that the skin edges are perfectly coapted. This obviates the need for external cutaneous sutures.

6. The cleft surgeon must have a clear understanding of the potential postoperative complications of cleft lip, nose, and palate repair.

- Early postoperative complications include **bleeding** and **airway compromise** from tongue swelling and/or narrowing of the nasal airways. Persistent or significant postoperative **bleeding** should be explored in the operating room. Following cleft lip nasal reconstruction, **swelling** may temporarily decrease the nasal airways and affect the obligate nasal breather. Swelling affecting the tongue or nasal airways can be treated with racemic epinephrine, steroids, and close observation. Early wound complications (i.e., wound **dehiscence** or acute infection) are rare events. The treatment of minor wound separation is usually conservative. Significant breakdown can be treated conservatively or with immediate "re-repair" depending upon the etiology (i.e., trauma or infection). **Stitch abscesses** should be addressed immediately with suture removal to prevent a granulating "pimple" that will likely compromise the ultimate scar.

- Late postoperative complications include **hypertrophic scarring** which can be managed with frequent massage and application of local steroids. Should significant scarring occur, linear scar contraction might result in secondary deformities (i.e., whistle deformity) requiring revisional surgery.

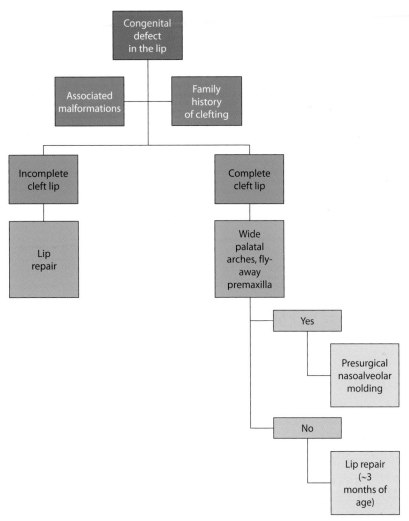

Algorithm 12-1 Algorithm for management of patients with bilateral clefts of the lip and/or palate.

PRACTICAL PEARLS

1. Presurgical infant orthopaedics (nasoalveolar molding) repositions the "fly away" premaxilla, aligns the neonatal maxillary segments, approximates the lateral lip segments, and stretches the columella, setting the stage for definitive lip and nose repair.

2. If presurgical infant orthopaedics are unable to be performed, a preliminary "lip adhesion" will convert the complete cleft into an incomplete cleft prior to definitive repair.

3. The bilateral cleft lip nasal deformity is reconstructed with: (1) radical release of the widely splayed alar bases and overcorrection with alar base cinch stitch, (2) infracartilaginous or rim incisions to dissect the fibro-fatty tissue from between the splayed lower lateral cartilages, (3) intradomal tip suture reconstruction, (4) soft triangle excision and columellar shaping sutures.

4. A narrow philtrum should be created from the central prolabial tissue cognizant that it will grow with time.

5. A natural-appearing Cupid's bow should be created from the white roll of the lateral lip elements.

6. A "pouting" central lip tubercle should be created from the lateral lip element vermilion.

7. Care should be directed toward accurate reconstruction of the orbicularis oris muscle beneath the neophiltrum

References

1. Mulliken JB, Wu JK, Padwa BL. Repair of bilateral cleft lip: Review, revision, and reflections. *J Craniofac Surg.* 2003;14(5):609-620.

2. Mulliken JB. Primary repair of bilaterel cleft lip and nasal deformity. *Plast Reconstr Surg.* 2001;108(1):181-194.

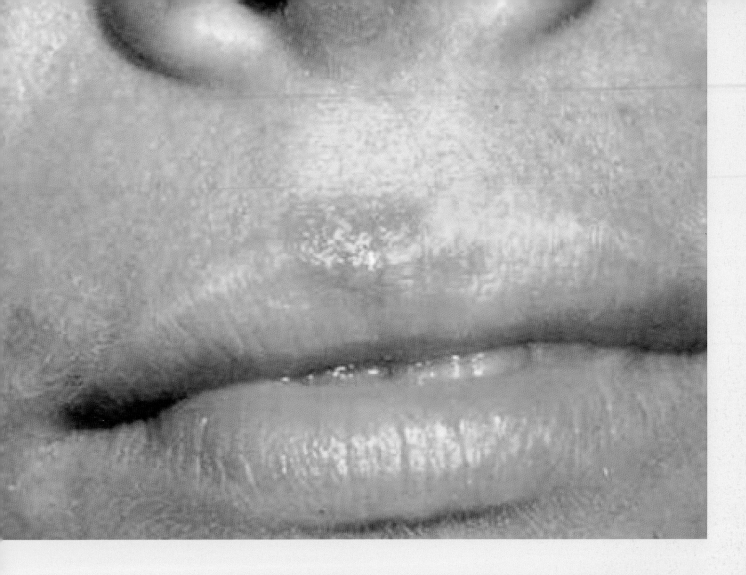

A 35-year-old man asks your opinion

regarding a lesion on the upper lip

that has not improved after several

weeks of observation.

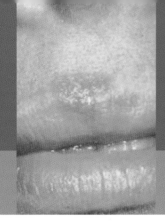

CHAPTER 13

Upper Lip Lesion

Stephen B. Baker

1. The presence of a nonhealing lesion in an area of chronic sun exposure, such as the upper lip that has not gone away with observation should warrant concern for malignancy. Skin cancer affecting the lip is a relatively common site among head and neck tumors, accounting for 25% of all oral cavity cancers. Most are squamous cell cancers with the remainder being basal cell carcinomas and melanomas. It is important to begin to establish a diagnosis of either benign or malignant disease with a directed patient history.

- **What is the patient's age and skin type?** Lip cancer is most common in patients with a fair complexion, such as those with Fitzpatrick I and II skin types. It is also more common in males, especially those older than 50 years of age who have a longer chronicity of sun exposure.

- **Is the patient male or female?** There is roughly a 6:1 male to female ratio for the development of squamous cell carcinoma of the lip.

- **Does the patient have a history of chronic or repeated sun exposure?** Sun exposure is perhaps the first, second, and third risk factors for the development of skin cancers. One-third of the patients either work outdoors or participate in avocations that are carried out outdoors. The highest rates of skin cancer are in Australia, Granada, and Spain, where exposure to intense UV rays is high. The lip is susceptible to metaplasia since it lacks a layer of pigmentation for protection. Cancers of the lip are also commonly seen in conjunction with other primary skin malignancies.

- **How did the lesion present?** Patients typically report the presence of an initial lesion that crusts over and subsequently bleeds with removal of the scab. Continued problems warrant more extensive examination which often reveals a nontender infiltrative ulcer with metaplastic changes of the lip.

- **How long has the lesion been present?** Long-standing lesions with little evidence of a change in character are less suspicious for carcinoma. Chronic wounds that fail to heal or recur over time predispose to the development of squamous cell carcinoma.

- **How has the lesion changed?** Changes in appearance might be a hallmark for malignant degeneration.

- **Does the patient have a history of skin cancers in the past?** Following an initial lesion, the presence of a separate, metachronous lesion is common.

- **Does the patient have any comorbidities or take any medication?** The presence of significant medical conditions, such as hypertension/cardiovascular disease, diabetes, or immunologic compromise, should be noted. Diabetic patients or those continuing to use tobacco must be advised to begin more appropriate blood-glucose management or quit smoking, respectively, as immediate improvements in either status facilitates likely surgical efforts. Many patients take blood thinners that may cause difficult bleeding and may or may not be able to be discontinued for the perioperative period.

2. A careful physical examination of the head and neck directed to the areas in and around the lips should be performed. This includes sites of possible spread in the oral cavity and draining lymphatic areas in the neck. Lymphatic drainage from the upper lip is mainly to the submental, submandibular, and parotid lymph nodes on the same side as the lesion. The submental nodes also secondarily drain to the submandibular nodes; and both the submandibular and parotid nodes secondarily drain to ipsilateral jugulodigastric lymph nodes. Midline lesions may have some cross-drainage to one or both sides of the neck.

- **Where on the lip is the lesion located?** It is important to catalog the component parts of any potential defect. Upper lip is composed of lateral and medial elements with the central portion called the philtral dimple, which is bound by two curvilinear philtral columns. Lesions involving the lip may also involve the skin, wet/dry vermilion, muscle and/or mucosal lining.

- **Is the lesion mobile or does it feel fixed to underlying structures?** Most tumors remain localized and grow slowly for an extended period of time, while some rapidly infiltrate and invade, deeper structures such as periosteum or bone. They can involve the mandible by direct extension, perineural invasion, or lymphatic spread.

- **Are there any local scars?** Scars around the face may indicate damage to available flaps useful for reconstruction.

- **Is there palpable adenopathy in the lymph nodes that drain the upper lip?** As opposed to basal cell tumors, squamous cell tumors can metastasize to lymph nodes of the face and neck area.

3. It is most important to know whether the lesion is benign or malignant. Most malignant neoplasms of the upper lip are basal cell carcinomas, whereas most malignancies of the lower lip are squamous cell carcinomas. The nature of the tumor plays a role in overall therapy. Basal cell carcinomas of the upper lip do not require as large an excisional margin as the lower lip tumors, which are usually squamous cell carcinomas.

   - Specimens sent for permanent section will more clearly show histopathologic detail at the borders of a lesion than frozen section specimens, and therefore are more heavily relied on.

   - A tissue **biopsy** may be excisional or incisional. An excisional biopsy is preferred, when the resultant defect is able to be closed primarily with little tension. In areas of difficult anatomy, such as the medial canthus of the eye, an incisional biopsy is preferable to identify the nature of the lesion. A small sample of the lesion is removed and the margins closed primarily knowing that the bulk of the lesion was left behind.

   - **Mohs' surgery** is a technique that repeatedly provides a small amount of skin for diagnosis while excising the tumor cells to the margin of uninvolved tissue. Many believe it is not indicated for melanoma since the depth of the lesion is not able to be ascertained.

   - The extent of disease may be determined locally by directed physical examination and regionally/distantly by **CT scan** and/or MRI.

   - The entire upper lip may be anesthetized by bilateral infraorbital nerve blocks. A 25-gauge needle is passed transcutaneously or transmucosally. The infraorbital foramen faces downward and is located approximately 7 mm from the infraorbital rim. The foramen can be accurately located by tracing an imaginary line downward from the medial limbus.

4. In preparation for excision and reconstruction, a preoperative evaluation of the patient's health status should be performed.

   - The presence of hypertension and diabetes should be noted and be well controlled.

   - The need for chemotherapy should be discussed with an oncologist based on the physical and diagnostic findings.

   - The following stages are used for nonmelanoma skin cancer:
     — Stage 0: Carcinoma in situ.
     — Stage I: Tumor is 2 cm or smaller.
     — Stage II: T is larger than 2 cm.
     — Stage III: Tumor has spread below the skin to underlying structures such as lymph nodes, cartilage, muscle, and/or bone, but not to other parts of the body.
     — Stage IV: Tumor has spread to distant sites in the body.

   - The following stages are used for melanomas:
     — Stage I: Lesion up to 1.5 mm with no lymphadenopathy.
     — Stage II: > Lesion 1.5 mm with no lymphadenopathy.
     — Stage III: Lymphadenopathy present.
     — Stage IV: Metastatic disease present.

5. Treatment of lesions of the upper lip involves making a histologic diagnosis, resecting the lesion with tissue-specific margins (as outlined below), and reconstruction to achieve a lip that provides sensate tissue, a functional sphincter, adequate opening for food and dental care, and an aesthetic appearance.

   - Prior to reconstruction, excision of the lesion with margins appropriate for the histologic type of tumor, including underlying muscle, if necessary, must be performed.
     — Standard nodular, basal cell carcinoma with translucent pearly borders can be removed by surgical excision with 2 mm margin and yield a 5-year cure rate of 90% to 95%. Radiation therapy, cryosurgery, or curettage yield similar results.
     — Recurrent, basal cell carcinoma is treated more aggressively and monitored by careful pathologic evaluation to ensure adequate excision.

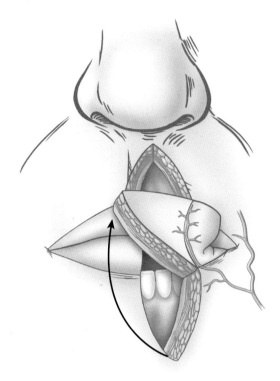

Figure 13-1 Schematic drawing highlighting reconstruction of an upper lip defect by an Abbe flap from the lower lip.

—Squamous cell carcinoma should be resected with a more aggressive margin, usually 1 to 2 cm, if possible.

—The resection margin for melanoma is based on the depth of the lesion:

   a. In situ lesions: 5 mm margin.

   b. Up to 1 mm: 1 cm margin.

   c. 1 to 2 mm: 1 or 2 cm margins.

   d. 2 to 4 mm: 2 cm margins.

   e. >4 mm: >2 cm margins.

- The goals in upper lip reconstruction are a sensate lip, a functional sphincter, good apposition of lower vermilion to upper vermilion, a watertight seal, adequate opening for food and dental care, and an aesthetic appearance. Unfortunately, in subtotal and total resections, not all these criteria can be satisfied. Frequently, the closure results in a tight, inverted lower lip that disappears beneath the curtain of the upper lip. Postoperative microstomia may require a regimen of lip stretching by appliances and dentures designed to collapse during insertion or removal. The dentulous patient must be able to open his mouth sufficiently to provide access for dental manipulation. Lip surgery should have little long-term effect on speech.

- The final **reconstruction** should be delayed until after the final margins are known. If the lesion is located on the **vermilion** and excision of the white roll becomes necessary, the surgeon should mark it prior to injecting local anesthesia and make all incisions

perpendicular to the vermilion skin junction. Occasionally, a small V-Y advancement flap may be effective.

- Up to one-quarter of the upper lip may be resected and closed primarily. In older patients who have lax skin, as much as one-third of the upper lip can be closed, although philtral distortion may occur particularly in the case of a more central wedge excision.

- If the lesion extends across the mucocutaneous border, partial or full-thickness wedge excision and primary performed, with excellent results. Accurate repair must include correct alignment of the vermilion and the white roll, and reapproximation of the orbicularis oris muscle.

   — Defects that remove the philtrum may leave the lip without a Cupid's bow. In males, the defect may be concealed with a mustache. In females, however, primary closure gives the lip a flattened appearance. In this instance, an Abbe flap, full-thickness skin graft, or composite graft should be adequate.

- If the lower lip is to be used for reconstruction of the upper lip, it is essential that it be of sufficient volume to serve as a donor. Following transfer, cross-lip flaps are typically left attached for 14 to 21 days before division with the timing dependent upon the size of the flap, the size of the mucosal attachment, and maintenance of the axial vessel.

- For defects **between one- and two-thirds of the upper lip**, primary closure may result in a tight oral stoma. Numerous options exist that make use of more extensive flaps of neighboring tissue. Local tissue from the cheeks may be advanced with or without compensatory excisions of healthy skin and subcutaneous tissue. Most will require revision.

   — The **Abbe flap** is useful to reconstruct full-thickness defects up to one-half of the upper lip. The flap transfers lower lip tissue pedicled on the labial artery to the upper lip defect (**figure**).

   — The **Reverse Estlander flap** is based on the lateral elements of the lower lip which are rotated into the lateral upper lip. It may cause distortion of the commissure (**figure**).

   — The **Webster flap** was described as a **combination procedure** in which vermilion is advanced from the edges of the defect to reconstruct the mucosa while a flap of lower lip skin and muscle is rotated upward to reconstruct the remainder of the lip.

   — **Bilateral nasolabial flaps** are superiorly based and may borrow tissue from beneath the nasal sill, if available. Similarly, a superiorly based flap of the entire cheek may be advanced into the upper lip with the donor site in the lateral cheek closed with a skin graft.

   — **Bilateral lower cheeks flaps** are the inferiorly based counterparts of the nasolabial flap as described by Kazanjian and Converse.

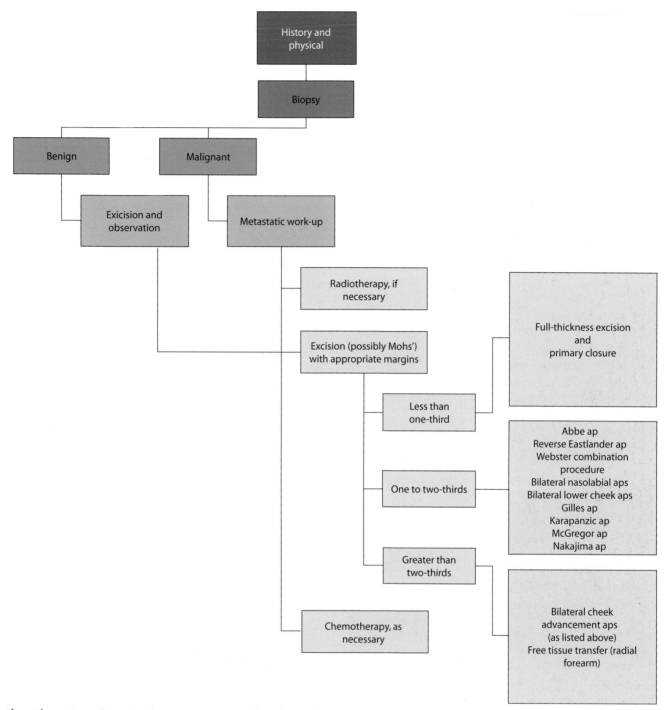

Algorithm 13-1 Algorithm for management of lesions of the upper lip.

— The **Reverse Gilles fan flap** rotates lip tissue lateral to the defect and compensates the donor site, by placing a Z-plasty at the base of the rotation lateral to the lower lip and closing the donor site at the tip of the flap in a V Y fashion at the alar base (**figure**). With better options listed, it is rarely used.

— The **Reverse Karapandzic flap** creates a circumoral incision of the remaining upper and lower lip, dividing the skin, muscle, and mucosa while leaving the facial nerve branches and vessels intact to preserve the functional elements of the lip (**figure**). Disadvantages of the technique are the extensive circumoral incisions and resultant microstomia.

— The **McGregor flap** incises full-thickness lateral cheek tissue which is then rotated around a fixed commissure. The lateral edge of the defect becomes the new vermilion edge and the donor site is closed primarily (**figure**). The **Nakajima flap** involves the same rotation and closure but, like the Karapanzic flap, attempts to spare the vessels and nerves traversing the incision (**figure**).

- **Upper lip defects greater than two-thirds** may require microvascular free tissue transfer.

  — A composite radial forearm palmaris longus free flaps may be used for reconstructing large upper lip defects as well as total lower lip and perioral reconstruction. Secondary commissuroplasty in these instances is often required.

6. Surgical reconstruction may leave the lips with reduced sensation and elasticity. Reconstructive techniques that use full-thickness nasolabial tissue may also denervate the upper lip muscle to a great degree.

- Patients who have **anesthesia of lip**, in addition to **poor sulcus depth**, have a tendency to drool. Reduction in sensation, to a degree significant to cause this problem, occurs more often after lower lip reconstruction than after upper lip reconstruction. Deepening of the vestibular trough, repositioning of the frenum, and broadening of the zone of attached gingiva may be required.

- **Infection** is possible but less likely around the oral cavity. Meticulous technique should be stressed when handling the remaining tissues.

- **Flap loss** results from leaving an inadequate vascular supply to the flap. Following the general principles of plastic surgery, including early recognition of the vascular supply to either a random or axial flap, avoidance of scar tissue as a base for the flap, avoidance of tension and gentle handling of tissues will minimize flap loss.

- When loss of both vermilion and muscle occur, local tissue reconstruction is best. Slight whistle or notching defects may be corrected by local flaps from either or both sides of the defect, mucomuscular advancement flaps, or simple V-Y advancement of the upper lip buccal mucosa. When larger areas of vermilion and muscle are required, unipedicle flaps from the lower lip, tongue flaps, and modified Abbe flaps may be used.

PRACTICAL PEARLS

1. The upper lip generally tolerates large excisions well.

2. When a deep laceration passes through the orbicularis, muscle closure is mandatory.

3. Suture placement into the white roll should be avoided because the redness associated with healing has the potential for creating an indistinguishable mucocutaneous junction.

4. Do not underestimate the need for mucosal lining.

5. When dissecting an Abbe flap, the full-length incision on one side of the flap serves as an excellent anatomical map for the contralateral side. Since the artery is seen and divided on the side of complete division, its exact location may be known.

6. Avoid the lower lip as a donor source if there is insufficient bulk to avoid microstomia.

References

1. Lesavoy MA, Smith AD. Lower third face and lip reconstruction. In: Mathes SJ, Hentz VR, eds. *Plastic Surgery*. 2nd Edition. Philadelphia, PA: Saunders Elsevier; 2006.

2. Langstein H, Robb GL. Lip and perioral reconstruction. *Clinics in Plastic Surgery*. 2005; 32(3):431-445.

3. Erol OO, Pence M, Agaoglu G. The Abbe island flap for the reconstruction of severe secondary cleft lip deformities. *J Craniofac Surgery*. 2007;18(4):766-772.

4. Burget GC and Menick FJ. Aesthetic restoration of one-half of the upper lip. *Plast Reconstr Surg*. 1986;78:583.

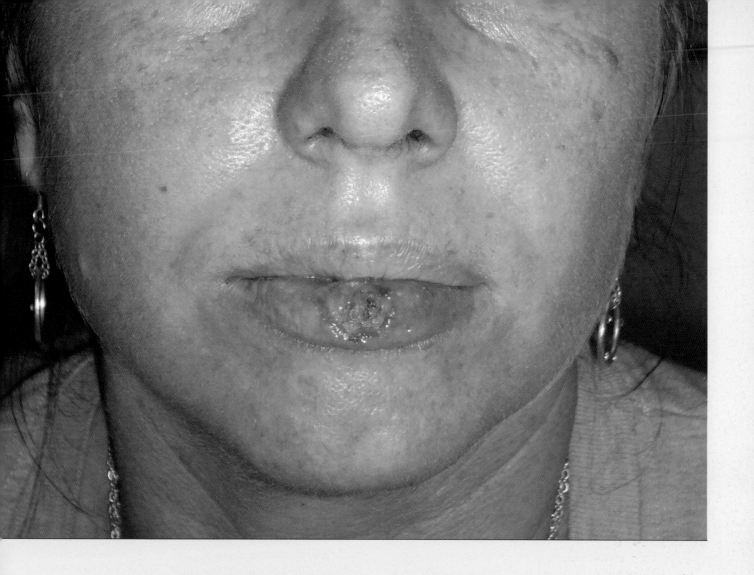

A dermatologist requests your opinion regarding a patient with a questionable lesion in the lower lip.

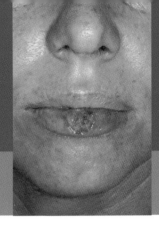

CHAPTER 14

Lower Lip Reconstruction

Jack C. Yu

1. The patient in the photograph has lesion of the lower lip of questionable behavior. Like cancer of the upper lip, cancer of the lower lip is relatively common among those affecting the head and neck. Approximately 3500 new cases are diagnosed in the United States each year and the incidence is approximately 2 per 100,000 persons. Ninety percent are squamous cell cancers with the rest made up of basal cell carcinomas, salivary gland carcinomas, and melanomas. Unlike the upper lip which has characteristic philtral columns, the lower lip has no definitive central structure and therefore may sustain greater loss without distortion. This also permits the lower lip to donate larger amounts of tissue for upper lip reconstruction. As with all lesions, it is important to start with establishing a diagnosis. This is first performed with a directed patient history.

- **What is the patient's age and skin type?** Lip cancer is most common in fair-complexioned white males in their sixth decade of life.

- **Is the patient male or female?** There is roughly a 6:1 male to female ratio for the development of squamous cell carcinoma of the lip.

- **Does the patient have a history of chronic or repeated sun exposure?** Sun exposure is perhaps the first, second, and third risk factors for the development of skin cancers. One-third of all the patients have outdoor occupations or outdoor pastimes. The lip is susceptible to metaplasia since it lacks the pigmented layer for protection. As such, cancers of the lip are commonly seen with other primary skin malignancies.

- **How did the lesion present?** Patients typically report a history of crusting that bleeds with removal of the scab.

- **How long has the lesion been present?** Long-standing lesions with little evidence of a change in character are less suspicious for carcinoma. Chronic wounds that fail to heal or recur over time predispose to the development of squamous cell carcinoma.

- **How has the lesion changed?** In addition to failure to heal over a sufficient period of time, recent increases in growth or changes in color, consistency, or mobility may indicate malignant degeneration.

2. A physical examination directed to the areas in and around the lips should be performed. This includes sites of possible spread in the oral cavity and draining lymphatic areas in the neck. Lymphatic drainage from the lower lip is largely into several primary trunks that lead to bilateral submental nodes if the lesion is located in is the central portion of the lip and to ipsilateral submandibular lymph nodes if the lesion is in the more lateral portion of the lip.

- **Where on the lip is the lesion located?** It is important to catalog the component parts of any potential defect. Those involving the lip may include skin, wet/dry vermilion, muscle, and mucosal lining. As noted above, this is also relevant for the site of lymphatic drainage.

- **Is the lesion mobile or does it feel fixed to underlying structures?** Most tumors remain localized and grow slowly for an extended period of time, while some rapidly infiltrate and invade tissues. Perineural spread may be along the course of the mental nerve into the body of the mandible.

- **Are there any local scars?** Local scars may compromise the use of flaps for eventual reconstruction.

- **Is there any palpable adenopathy in the head and neck?** As opposed to basal cell tumors, squamous cell tumors can metastasize to lymph nodes of the face and neck area. As noted, these are primarily to the submental and submandibular lymph nodes.

3. It is most important to ascertain is whether the lesion is benign or malignant. Unlike the upper lip, in which most malignancies are basal cell carcinomas, those of the lower lip are more commonly squamous cell carcinomas. The nature of the tumor plays a role in overall therapy.

- **Biopsy** of the lesion may be excisional or incisional. An excisional biopsy is preferred when the resultant defect is able to be closed primarily with little tension. In areas of difficult anatomy, such as the medial canthus of the eye, an incisional biopsy is preferable to identify the nature of the lesion. A small sample of the lesion is removed and the margins closed primarily knowing that the bulk of the lesion was left behind. Specimens sent for permanent sections will more clearly show histopathologic detail at the borders of a lesion than frozen section specimens, and therefore are more heavily relied on.

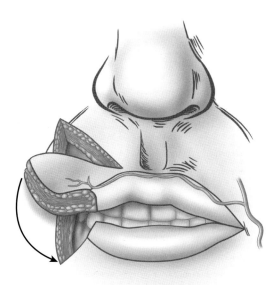

Figure 14-1 Schematic drawing highlighting reconstruction of a lower lip defect by Estlander flap from the upper lip.

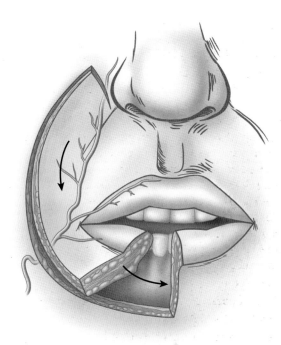

Figure 14-2 Gilles flap for repair of a lower lip defect.

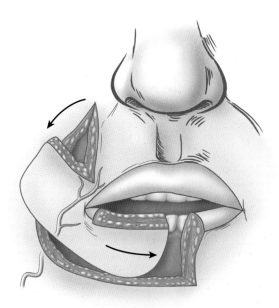

Figure 14-3 Nakajima (McGregor) flap for repair of a lower lip defect depending if the neurovascular pedicle is (or is not) preserved.

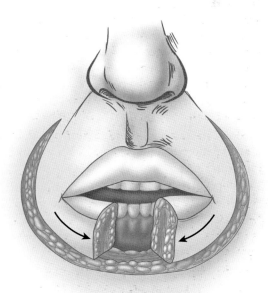

Figure 14-4 Bilateral Karapanzic flaps for repair of a central lower lip defect.

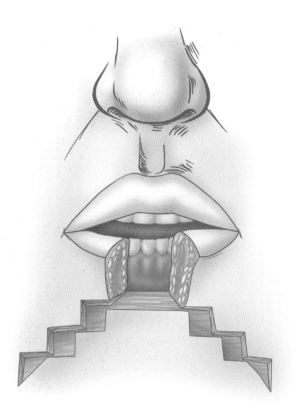

Figure 14-5 Step reconstruction of a central lower lip defect. The length of each step should approximate half the width of the defect.

- **Mohs' surgery** is a technique that repeatedly provides a small amount of skin for diagnosis while excising the tumor cells to the margin of uninvolved tissue. Many believe, it is not indicated for melanoma since depth is not able to be ascertained.

- The extent of disease may be determined locally by directed physical examination and regionally/distantly by **CT scan** and/or MRI. A **panorex** is indicated when the tumor is felt to be fixed to the mandible, extends over the gingiva into a tooth root, when the dentition is loose, or with hypesthesia of the mental nerve. Further intervention is not indicated since less than 2% of patients have distant metastasis at time of workup.

4. In preparation for excision and reconstruction, a preoperative evaluation of the patient's health status should be performed. The need for chemotherapy should be discussed with an **oncologist** based on physical and diagnostic findings. The presence of hypertension and diabetes should be noted and be well controlled.

- The following stages are used for nonmelanoma skin cancer:
  — Stage 0: Carcinoma in situ.
  — Stage I: Tumor is 2 cm or smaller.
  — Stage II: Tumor is larger than 2 cm.
  — Stage III: Tumor has spread below the skin to underlying structures such as lymph nodes, cartilage,

muscle, and/or bone, but not to other parts of the body.
  — Stage IV: Tumor has spread to distant sites in the body.

- The following stages are used for melanomas:
  — Stage I: Up to 1.5 mm with no lymphadenopathy.
  — Stage II: >1.5 mm with no lymphadenopathy.
  — Stage III: Lymphadenopathy.
  — Stage IV: Metastatic disease.

5. Proper management of the malignant lesion of the lower lip (as with those elsewhere) involves excision of the lesion while sparing the surrounding uninvolved structures.

- Radiation and surgery are the primary modalities employed in the treatment of lip cancer. Both appear to be equally effective in controlling early stage lesions. Five-year survival rates for lesions less than 3 cm average 90%. Radiation is advantageous in that it is noninvasive and may be the only option for candidates who cannot undergo surgery. It does, however, prolong the treatment time and may result in local tissue destruction, hindering later reconstruction.

- Surgical excision of any lesion must yield negative margins, including underlying muscle.

  — **Basal cell carcinomas** of the upper lip do not require as large an excisional margin as the lower lip tumors, which are usually squamous cell carcinomas. Standard nodular basal cell carcinoma with translucent pearly borders can be removed by surgical excision with 2 mm margin with a 5-year cure rate of 90% to 95%. Radiation therapy, cryosurgery, or curettage yield similar results. Recurrent basal cell carcinoma is treated more aggressively and monitored by careful pathologic evaluation to ensure adequate excision.

  — **Squamous cell carcinoma** should be resected with a more aggressive margin. Lower lip lesions measuring 1 to 1.5 cm should be excised with a margin of 7 to 10 mm. Patients with SCC of the lower lip commonly have actinic changes of the remaining lip. As the incidence of carcinoma in situ is typically approximately 12% in this setting, performing a lip shave in conjunction with a full-thickness wedge excision is usually recommended in patients with actinic changes of the vermilion. Alternatively, carbon dioxide laser can also be used.

  — The resection margin for **melanoma** is based on the depth of the lesion:
    a. In situ lesions: 5 mm margin.
    b. Up to 1 mm: 1 cm margin.
    c. 1 to 2 mm: 1 or 2 cm margins.
    d. 2 to 4 mm: 2 cm margins.
    e. >4 mm: >2 cm margins.

- Definitive **reconstruction** should be delayed until after the final margins are known. Similar to the upper lip, the goals in lip reconstruction should be a sensate lip with a functional sphincter mechanism that allows for adequate opening for food and dental care, and appears natural. Unfortunately, in subtotal and total resections, not all these criteria can be satisfied. Lip surgery should also have little long-term effect on speech. Reconstruction following surgery may then involve local or regional tissue and must address mucosal lining as well as superficial skin coverage. Defects of up to one-third of the lip can be closed primarily. Larger defects may require tissue transfer, and the preferred donor site is the adjacent cheek or upper lip.

— Anesthesia may be provided by bilateral mental nerve blocks and local infiltration. The mental nerves may be located by rolling the lower lip outward and stretching the mucosa away from the canine root. Mucosal infiltration about 1 cm lateral to the canines into the lower buccal sulcus should provide ample anesthesia.

— Resection is usually approached with a full-thickness excision and primary closure. If excising the white roll becomes necessary, the surgeon should mark it prior to injecting local anesthesia and make all incisions perpendicular to the vermilion skin junction. Occasionally, a small V-Y advancement flap may be effective.

— A lip shave procedure is typically performed for premalignant lesions such as severe actinic cheilitis, leukoplakia with atypia, widespread carcinoma in situ, and in combination with full-thickness excision for lip carcinoma. The defect may be closed with a bipedicle mucosal flap with an incisional release at the depth of the labial sulcus or a tongue or adjacent buccal mucosa flap.

• Reconstruction of defects <30% may be managed with shield-shaped excision extending to, but not crossing the labiomental fold, to avoid hypertrophic scar formation. When incisions do cross the labiomental fold, a Z-plasty should be used. With larger lesions, the flared W-plasty or the barrel-shaped excision yield a more aesthetic result.

• For defects involving 30% to 65% of the lower lip, borrowing upper lip tissue will usually yield an excellent result. Alternatives include the lip switch flap, cheek advancement flap, oral circumference advancement, or an innervated composite flap.

— An **Abbe flap** transfers upper lip tissue pedicled on the labial artery. The central portion of the upper lip should never be used for donor tissue, as the philtral columns and dimple are irreplaceable. A flap from the junction of the middle and lateral thirds of the upper lip is preferable. Although the procedure requires two stages, the second step is relatively minor. The tissue is initially denervated, but in follow-up, sphincteric function returns. A third stage may be necessary to equilibrate the vermilion.

— In the **Bernard procedure**, the tumor/lesion is removed en bloc from the central lower lip and incisions are then extended outward from the commissures. In the original description, full-thickness triangles were removed lateral to the upper lip (in the nasolabial fold area), allowing advancement of bilateral lower cheek flaps. Multiple modifications of this concept now exist for the reconstruction of larger lower lip defects. The triangular excisions now only include skin to prevent upper lip denervation.

— The **Abbe-Estlander** flap employs a full-thickness, medially based, triangular upper lip flap, which is transferred to reconstruct defects that comprise one-third to two-thirds of the lower lateral lip mass, which involve the commissure. It is only the involvement of the commissure that makes it different from the standard Abbe flap.

— **The Gillies fan flap** is an extended version of the Estlander flap. It carries the commissure and lower lateral lip inward for the more medially located lower lip defects. Like the Estlander procedure, the resulting commissure is distorted and the lower lip is shortened.

— The **McGregor flap** further modified the Estlander technique with the inclusion of vermilionectomy. According to McGregor, the other techniques do not rid the patient of the malignant potential of the remaining lower lip vermilion.

• **For defects of greater than 65% of the lower lip,** bilateral cheek advancement, bilateral oral circumference advancement, or bilateral innervated composite flaps are more suitable. The method chosen must be based on the availability of local donor tissue. If local tissue is not available, distant flaps, or microvascular free tissue transfer (fasciocutaneous radial artery flap) may be the only options.

6. Complications related to reconstruction of lower lip defects may be functional as well as visual. Both should be taken into account during preoperative planning and postoperative follow-up.

• Frequently, the procedure results in a tight, inverted lower lip that disappears beneath the curtain of the upper lip. Postoperative **microstomia** may require considerable postoperative lip stretching by appliances and dentures that have been constructed especially to collapse during insertion or removal. Surgical reconstruction may leave the lips with reduced sensation and elasticity. Reconstructive techniques that use full-thickness nasolabial tissue may also denervate the upper lip muscle to a great degree.

• Patients who have reduction of lip sensation in addition to poor sulcus depth have a tendency to **drool**. **Reduction in sensation**, to a degree significant to cause this problem, occurs more often after lower lip reconstruction than after the repair of upper lip defects. Deepening of the vestibular trough, repositioning of the frenulem, and broadening of the zone of attached gingiva may be required.

- Because of the rich blood supply in this area, lip reconstruction enjoys a low frequency of **infection**. However, if not properly designed or executed, tissue ischemia can occur. Devitalized tissue in the presence of heavy bacterial load will lead to infection postoperatively.

- It is important to not exceed the length to width ratio of any flap. Even though the region of the lower lip has a robust blood supply with rich collateral vessels, exceeding 2:1 ratio in random skin flaps is associated with more frequent **distal flap necrosis**. This is particularly problematic in smokers.

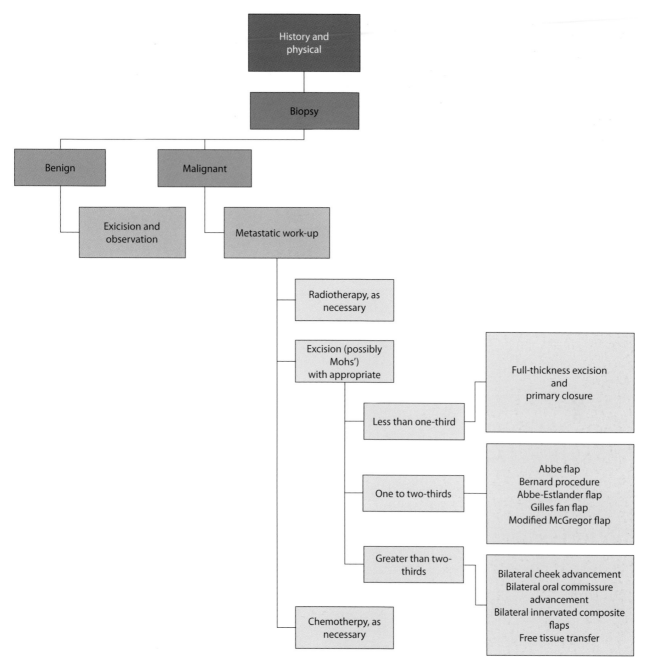

Algorithm 14-1 Algorithm for management of lesions of the lower lip.

PRACTICAL PEARLS

1. Ample use of tagging sutures to stabilize the lip.

2. Labial artery can be controlled transiently by holding the lip with thumb and index finger of the nondominant hand permitting more definitive measure to be deployed.

3. Always cut across the white roll at right angles whenever possible. Identify this with two closely placed dots on each side so that the resection will not completely remove the previously marked areas.

4. Make a pattern of the defect if a flap is to be used. This can be done with metal foil from a suture package, glove paper, or flat, cotton gauze.

5. Allow vasoconstrictor 5 to 7 minutes to work before incision.

References

1. Jackson IT. Local flaps in head and neck reconstruction. St. Louis, MO: Mosby; 1985.

2. Lesavoy MA, Smith AD. Lower third face and lip reconstruction. In: Mathes SJ, Hentz VR, eds. *Plastic Surgery*. 2nd ed. Philadelphia, PA: Saunders Elsevier; 2006.

3. Stark RB, ed. *Plastic Surgery of the Head and Neck*. New York, NY: Churchill Livingstone; 1987.

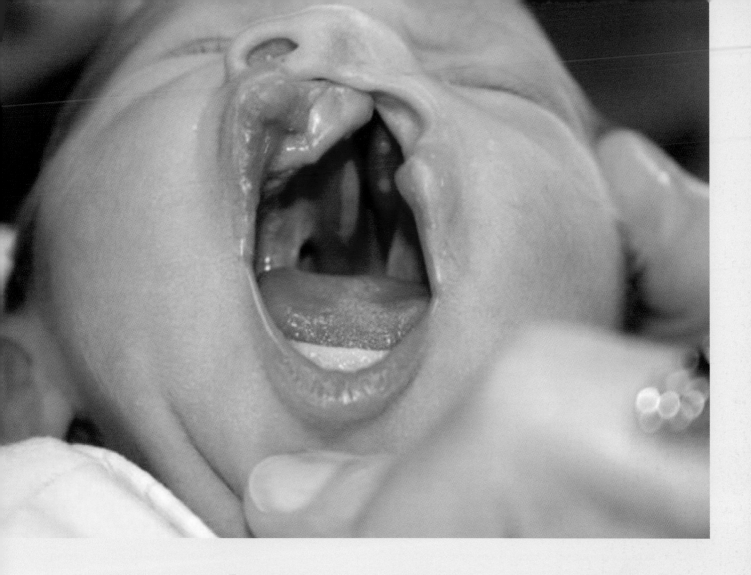

The neonatal intensive care unit asks you to consult on a newborn with difficulty feeding and congenital deformity shown above.

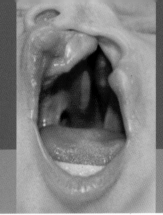

CHAPTER 15

Cleft Palate

William Y. Hoffman

1. The patient in question appears to have a unilateral complete cleft lip and palate. Patients with a cleft palate are often seen as infants in the setting of a craniofacial center. In less developed countries, lip repair is performed for cosmetic concerns and palate repair is deferred if the family cannot afford the cost of the procedure. In such cases, patients may present as adults with speech disturbances that are difficult to correct. When a patient with a cleft palate is seen for consultation, several concerns are paramount.

- **How old is the patient and does the cleft interfere with either breathing or feeding?** Clefts of the palate are associated with difficulty creating suction, as there is no seal of the posterior pharynx. Thus, breast feeding is usually difficult and specialized nipples and bottles are used to ensure adequate nutrition. Swallowing difficulties may reflect other problems (neurological, gastroenterology (GI)).

- **Are there any associated congenital anomalies?** Approximately 30% of cleft patient have an associated genetic syndrome. A cleft palate may be seen in infants with other craniofacial anomalies, including Apert syndrome, Treacher Collins syndrome, or with genetic syndromes such as van der Woude syndrome, Stickler syndrome, and velocardiofacial syndrome (22q), among others.

- **Did the patient pass his newborn hearing screen?** Since the incidence of fluid in the middle ear is higher in cleft patients, the results of the mandatory postdischarge hearing test should be obtained.

- **Is there a history of fluid within the middle ear or recurrent infections?** During the first year of life, infants are susceptible to otitis media, because of the shorter and more horizontal position of the Eustachian tube. The tensor veli palatini muscle is also positioned abnormally and its ability to open the distal portion of the Eustachian tube is altered. Serous fluid accumulation even without infection will produce hearing loss, which will have a negative effect on speech development. Chronic infection may lead to tympanic membrane perforation, hearing loss, or formation of a cholesteatoma.

2. At the time of consultation, a thorough physical examination should examine the entire head and face looking for associated craniofacial malformations.

- **What portion of the cleft is involved?** The palate is defined from the lip anteriorly to the uvula posteriorly. It is lined on both sides by mucosa and composed of bone in the anterior portion and muscle in the posterior portion. The primary palate includes the premaxilla, in which the anterior four teeth (central and lateral incisors) develop, and the hard palate back to the incisive foramen. The hard palate posterior to the incisive foramen and the soft palate together comprise the secondary palate.

— The muscles in the soft palate include the **tensor veli palatine** and the **levator veli palatine**, which function to pull the palate superiorly and posteriorly. The levator forms a transverse sling in the normal palate; in the cleft, the levator fibers are oriented more longitudinally, parallel to the margins of the cleft. The **palatoglossus** and **palatopharyngeus** muscles are interdigitated with the levator and extend down the tonsillar pillars, serving to pull the palate inferiorly and posteriorly. The **uvulus** shortens the uvula and moves it anteriorly. All the palatal muscles are innervated by the pharyngeal branch of the vagus nerve (CN X) except for the tensor, which is innervated by a branch of the mandibular nerve (V3).

— The blood supply to the palate arises from the **greater and lesser palatine arteries**, branches of the descending palatine artery off the third part of the maxillary artery. The greater palatine arises through a foramen at the posterior aspect of the hard palate; the lesser arises slightly more posterior, within the soft palate. The nasopalatine artery arises anteriorly via the incisive foramen. The greater palatine artery is critical for blood supply to the anterior mucoperiosteal flaps that are elevated during palate repair.

- **Are the dental arches well aligned?** If there is a complete cleft lip and palate, the pull of the orbicularis oris muscle contributes to the separation and displacement of the alveolar processes. When the arches are not well aligned, a molding plate may be fabricated and used within the first weeks of life to guide the segments into better position and thus facilitate repair. Newer modalities for managing children with cleft palate include the use of presurgical nasoalveolar molding, which adds an extension to shape the nose as well as moving the alveolar segments. Simple taping across the cleft may be helpful as well. The lip is closed around 3 months of age, and the repair of the orbicularis muscle will exert a great effect on the alveolus, providing further molding.

- **Does the patient have a normal lower jaw?** Pierre Robin sequence refers to an association of clefts with the classical triad of micrognathia, posterior displacement of the tongue and respiratory obstruction.

- **Is there fluid within the middle ear?** As noted, the presence of fluid within the middle ear may predispose the patient to hearing loss and recurrent infections, as well as more serious sequelae.

- **Are there any other congenital anomalies not previously noted?** A thorough examination of the remainder of the head and neck as well as the axial skeleton should be performed. The heart should be auscultated to appreciate any murmurs. The abdomen should be palpated to identify any masses and the perineum inspected for evidence of congenital anomalies of the genitourinary system.

3. No formal imaging studies are required prior to beginning treatment of the cleft lip and palate.

4. A cleft team should see all children with clefts; the minimum requirement for a team is a plastic surgeon, orthodontist, and speech pathologist although most teams also have genetics, otolaryngology, nursing, pediatrics, and other members. The team can coordinate care and minimize the number of interventions and office visits needed.

- Early consultation with a nurse/feeding specialist is important to be sure that nutritional intake and weight gain are appropriate. Genetics evaluation is obtained for every child with a cleft; this may alert you to other abnormalities including potential developmental delay, and will also inform parents regarding the chances of having another child with a cleft. **Pediatric otolaryngology** consultation is obtained for audiology and likely placement of ventilating tubes at the time of palate repair.

- Prior to formal palatal repair, the **pediatric dentist** or orthodontist on the cleft team can facilitate palatal movement by molding the arches with an intraoral appliance. These devices are either active ones that are fixed to each half of the maxilla and pull the edges into opposition or passive devices that act like orthodontic retainers to push the edges closer together. Added components can assist to reshape the malleable cartilaginous framework of the nose to improve its appearance.

5. The next issue that needs to be addressed is the timing of the repair. The lip, if involved, is generally closed first, followed by the palate, and then by the alveolus, which requires bone grafting. There has been debate concerning the optimal time for cleft palate repair. The issues that must be weighed include speech and language development versus midfacial growth. Earlier repair favors speech development, while later repair is thought to favor development of the maxilla. For this reason, some surgeons have favored staged repair of the soft palate followed by the hard palate. However, this technique has generally been associated with poorer speech outcomes and there has not been a demonstrable improvement in maxillary growth. Most centers repair the palate around 10 to 12 months of age, and there is increasing evidence that earlier repair is associated with improved speech outcomes.

- Several types of repair have been developed to reconstruct the hard palate:

  — The **von Langenbeck** repair utilizes bilateral, bipedicle flaps which are advanced to the midline. The technique was originally described for clefts of the secondary palate.

  — Bardach described the two-flap palatoplasty, which extends the Langenbeck incisions to the cleft margin behind the alveolus to complete the elevation of anterior flaps based on the greater palatine vessels. By shifting the larger flap (in a unilateral cleft) over the nasal closure, the anterior fistula rate is markedly reduced.

  — The **Veau-Wardill-Kilner** repair creates two mucoperiosteal flaps from either side of the hard palate. These are closed in a V-Y fashion (hence the term

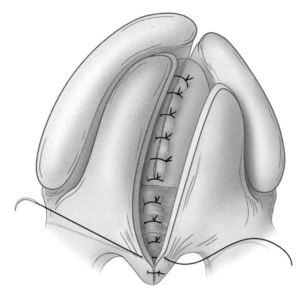

Figure 15-1 Schematic drawing highlighting reconstruction of a cleft palate with bilateral mucoperiosteal flaps and intravelar veloplasty.

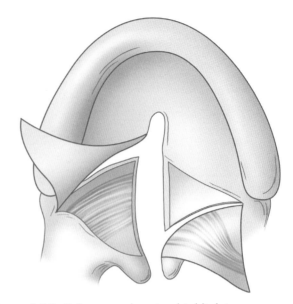

Figure 15-2 Schematic drawing highlighting reconstruction of a posterior cleft of the soft palate with double opposing Z-plasties.

pushback repair); the anterior portion of a complete cleft only has nasal closure, which is facilitated by elevation of uni- or bilateral, superiorly based flaps of nasal mucosa off the midline vomer. The incidence of fistula formation is more common with this repair than with the two-flap technique.

- There are essentially two main types of soft palate closure.

— The **intravelar veloplasty** is a straight-line closure that removes the mucosa at the medical edge of each hemipalate and separates the tissue into nasal mucosa, muscle, and oral mucosa. In doing so, the attachment of the levator palatini muscle needs to be taken down off the posterior aspect of the hard palate and rotated into the midline. Some surgeons recommend release of the tensor veli palatini tendon to permit greater rotation of the levator muscle into a posterior transverse position.

— The **Furlow double opposing Z-plasty** repair has gained increasing popularity, as it has been associated with low fistula rates and good speech outcomes. The cleft margins are the central limb of two Z-plasties that are designed in opposite directions on the oral and nasal side. The posteriorly based flaps on each side are developed together with the levator palatini muscle, while the opposite anteriorly based flaps are mucosa only. Transposition of these flaps creates overlapping levator muscles and recreates the normal transverse sling, while narrowing the width of the posterior pharynx and lengthening the soft palate.

- In areas where the nasal mucosa cannot be approximated, some surgeons have placed a thin sheet of acellular dermis. Long-term results with this technique are not available at present.

- Postoperatively, either a suture through the anterior tongue or a soft nasopharyngeal tube is placed and removed in the morning to protect the airway in the event of undue swelling. In the absence of complications, patients may be discharged home on the first postoperative day. Feeding is usually kept to full liquids or soft meals and arm restraints may be recommended if the child tends to place hard objects in the mouth.

6. Finally, the cleft surgeon needs to understand the complications that may occur with palatal repair and how to best manage them. The early complications include bleeding and airway compromise.

- Prevention of **hemorrhage** is addressed in several ways. Prior to the repair, the palate should be infiltrated with an appropriate amount of anesthetic with epinephrine and the solution should be given adequate time (7 to 10 minutes) to take effect. A thorough search to achieve hemostasis should be performed either with a monopolar or bipolar electrocautery. Minor bleeding can be addressed with Surgicel or Gelfoam in the raw lateral areas of the palate and gentle pressure over the mucoperiosteal flaps. Postoperatively, ice packs to the back of the neck will diminish bleeding considerably. Significant late hemorrhage may warrant a return to the operating room and search for the offending vessel.

- **Airway compromise** after surgery may have multiple etiologies. Infants are obligate nasal breathers, but this usually is corrected by 6 months of age. Isolated swelling of the palate should not give rise to airway compromise, but the closure of the palate does redirect airflow and also narrows the posterior pharyngeal airway. Furthermore, swelling of the tongue occurs with placement of the mouth gag for extended periods of time (greater than 90 to 120 minutes).

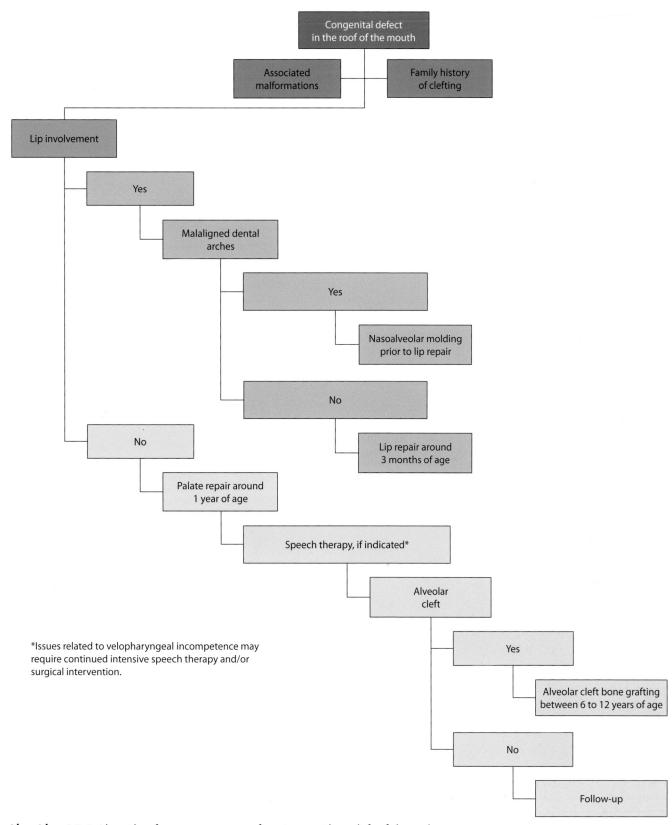

Algorithm 15-1 Algorithm for management of patients with a cleft of the palate.

*Issues related to velopharyngeal incompetence may require continued intensive speech therapy and/or surgical intervention.

- **Fistulas** form in areas of tension, notably at the junction of the hard and soft palates. Anterior fistulas are more common with the V-Y pushback technique, and are difficult to close. The rate of fistula formation is approximately 5% to 10% in many series, and higher in patients older than 2 years of age. Speech should be evaluated first since simple obturation may be temporarily effective. Small fistulas may not require any treatment. If necessary, surgical interventions include repeat elevation and closure, mucosal flap, facial artery myomucosal flap, tongue flap, and rarely free tissue transfer.

- **Incompetence of the velopharyngeal mechanism** is not truly a complication of palatal repair, but rather a result of either the scarring that occurs postoperatively or an innate problem with the muscles or the surrounding anatomy. Nasal air loss with positive pressure consonants is the hallmark of this problem. Specific causes include:
  - Neuromuscular insufficiency (may be associated with syndromes and developmental problems).
  - Disproportion between the depth of the pharynx and the length of the palate (either preexisting or because of a short palate after repair).
  - Scar formation in either the palate and/or the pharynx.
  - Regression of the adenoid pad.
  - Advancement of the maxilla, which may pull the soft palate forward and convert a borderline situation into one of overt nasal speech.
  - Workup includes evaluation by a skilled speech and language pathologist, as well as examination of the soft palate by either nasoendoscopy or videofluoroscopy. Treatment includes speech therapy at first; if there is inadequate length of the palate, surgical treatment may consist of lengthening with a Furlow Z-plasty or creation of a partial obstruction with either sphincter pharyngoplasty or pharyngeal flap. Augmentation of the posterior pharyngeal wall with a variety of materials has been proposed but has had mixed results. Non-surgical candidates may be treated with a speech bulb prosthesis, which creates bulk in the posterior pharynx.

PRACTICAL PEARLS

1. Initial evaluation by a complete cleft team facilitates care by multiple specialties and decreases the number of surgical interventions.

2. The diagnosis of syndromes is important for prognosis and outcomes.

3. Proper treatment of middle ear pathology is critical for good speech outcomes.

4. Repair of the levator palatini muscle is the key to soft palate repair.

5. Poor speech outcomes are more difficult to correct than maxillary growth problems.

References

1. Mount D, Hoffman WY. Cleft palate. In: Mathes SJ, ed. *Plastic Surgery*. London, UK: Elsevier; 2005.

2. Furlow LT Jr. Cleft palate repair by double opposing Z-plasty. *Plastic Reconstructive Surgery*. 1986;78:724-738.

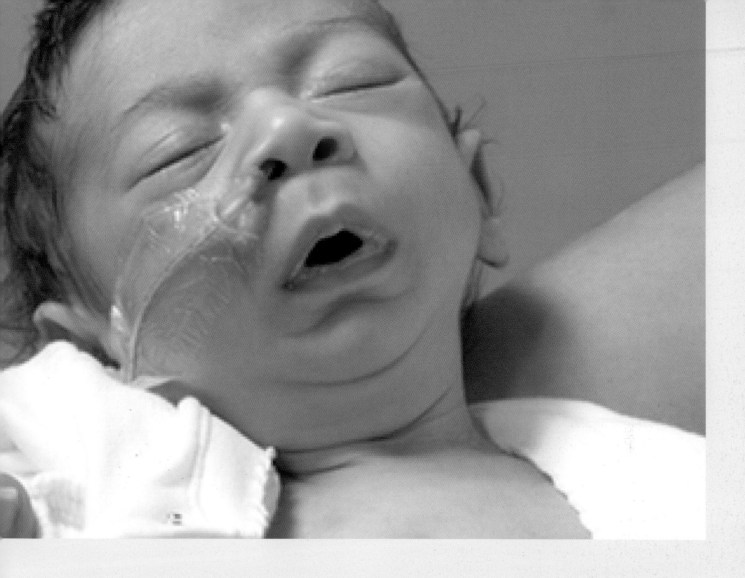

The neonatal intensive care unit asks you to see

a 2-week-old infant with failure to thrive.

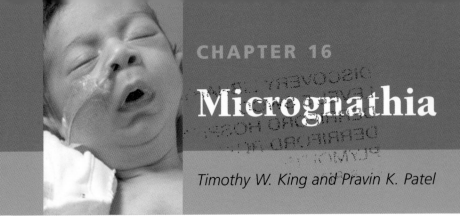

CHAPTER 16

Micrognathia

Timothy W. King and Pravin K. Patel

1. The patient in the photograph presents with the classic triad of Pierre Robin sequence (PRS) initially described in 1934, which includes micrognathia associated with paroxysmal respiratory obstruction caused by glossoptosis. In approximately one-quarter to one-third of these patients, a cleft of the secondary palate is also noted. In this definition of PRS, the cleft palate often cited as part of the triad is not considered essential. However, it is recognized that the definition of the Pierre Robin sequence has varied in the literature. Important questions to ask of the neonatal intensive care unit (NICU) staff and the family include the following.

   • **Is the patient having difficulty breathing?** In the neonate with PRS, respiratory compromise the primary concern. The posterior position of the tongue obstructs the airway and causes respiratory distress. With microretrognathia there is lack of structural support of the tongue and the tongue falls downward and backward (glossoptosis) into the posterior pharyngeal space, obstructing the epiglottis. In this position, the tongue acts as a "ball valve" allowing egress of air, but hampering inspiration. Thus, energy expenditure is diverted from normal growth and development (weight gain) to the work of inspiratory effort (sternal retractions). Labored breathing becomes more apparent with supine position. Chronic airway obstruction may lead to hypoxia, failure to thrive, and cor pulmonale. Mortality rates as high as 30% have been reported.

   • **Does the patient have any feeding difficulty?** Feeding problems in the infant with PRS are thought to be because of the abnormal anatomic position and the inadequate neuromuscular control of the tongue. Furthermore, a cleft of the palate when present with PRS further compounds the ability of the child to feed with the inability to generate adequate suction. In such situations, feeding should be upright with a specialized cleft palate nipple/bottle that does not require suction. The patient's weight should be followed closely to insure that they are gaining weight appropriately. If the infant is unable to gain appropriate weight in spite of these interventions, a feeding tube should be considered. Moreover, when severe airway obstruction is present energy expenditure is diverted from normal growth reflected by a lack in weight gain, surgical intervention should be considered.

   • **Is there a family history of craniofacial anomalies?** While not the norm, some patients may have relatives with similar findings. In such cases, consultation with a geneticist may be advisable.

   • **Does the patient have any coexistent medical conditions or congenital anomalies?** Numerous craniofacial conditions coexist with anomalies of the cardiovascular or genitourinary systems that may need to be addressed prior to proceeding with surgery, if indicated.

2. The single initiating cause is the hypoplastic development of the mandible with consequential posterior positioning of the tongue base that occurs between the seventh and eleventh weeks of gestation. The posterior position of the tongue impairs the retroglossal airway space and closure of the posterior palatal shelves that may result in a cleft of the secondary palate. Beyond the isolated sequence, PRS may occur in approximately 25% to 35% within the context of a formal syndromic condition such as Sticker, Treacher Collins, Nager Syndrome, and a multitude of others. In contrast to relative occurrence of 1 in 800 live births of the typical facial clefts of the lip and palate and 1 in 2000 births of the isolated cleft palate, the prevalence of PRS is of approximately 1 per 8500 live births with equal male-to-female predominance. Physical findings that are important to identify include the following.

   • **What is the size of the mandible?** Without a significant normal reference, it is often difficult for the inexperienced examiner to determine the severvity of the retromicrognathia. However, in patients with PRS the mandible is hypoplastic and symmetrically receded. Typically, the mandibular dental arch is *at least* 10 mm behind the maxillary arch. This can be easily assessed at the bedside and documented with a ruler.

   • **Does the tongue appear to be large or protrusive?** Glossoptosis is an essential finding. The tongue remains posterior and thrusts vertically above the palatal shelves into the nasopharynx resulting in complete obstruction of the oral and nasal airway.

- **Is there evidence of respiratory distress?** Respiratory signs, frequently aggravated by supine positioning, include labored breathing (stridor), inspiratory effort, sternal retractions, and periods of cyanotic attacks.

- **Is there an associated cleft palate?** Cleft palate, if present, may range from a submucous cleft to an overt cleft that may extend from the isolated soft palate to involvement of the secondary hard palate. In contrast to the typical "V-shaped" morphology of most palatal clefts, the cleft pattern is characteristically "U-shaped" and larger in width in PRS. However, the typical "V-shaped" cleft pattern has been reported and does not exclude PRS. A cleft of the lip may be present but is not specifically associated with PRS.

- **Does the child have fluid in the middle ear?** Fluid, or frank otitis media, occurs in concert with the palatal cleft.

- **Does the child have other congenital anomalies?** The presence of other facial anomalies, ocular findings, auricular anomalies, and/or anomalies of the extremeties or audible cardiac murmurs may be encountered in the setting of associated syndromic conditions.

3. A number of noninvasive diagnostic studies are important in the diagnosis and eventual management of these patients.

- Transcutaneous **pulse oximetry** is used routinely to monitor periods of the oxygen desaturation and determine the need for intervention.

- **Polysomnography** may document significant hypoxia in the absence of obvious clinical signs of obstruction and is useful to identify those infants who may be at risk following discharge. Additionally, obstructive versus central patterns of sleep apnea should be identified to guide future management.

- Complete assessment of the airway with **laryngoscopy/bronchoscopy** is paramount to discerning the site(s) of airway obstruction. The infant with PRS may not only have a tongue base obstruction, but also glottic/infraglottic obstruction, as with tracheomalacia or laryngomalacia. In such patients, the treatment requires a tracheostomy. Simply addressing the airway above this level will not alleviate the need for tracheostomy. In patients with tongue base obstruction in whom mandibular advancement is contemplated, an "Argamaso" maneuver can be performed in which mandibular advancement is simulated by a jaw thrust to assess whether this would relieve the airway obstruction.

- A **CT scan of the head and neck** with coronal, sagittal, and three-dimensional reconstructions should be performed to assess the anatomic size of the retroglossal airway, the mandibular anatomy, and aid in surgical planning. In PRS, the mandible is retrognathic relative to the maxilla and typically has a characteristic small body, obtuse gonial angle, and a posterior inclination of the condyle. Additionally, the airway space is significantly reduced volumetrically by the tongue base.

4. Because of the complexity of care required for these children, a multidisciplinary team approach should be utilized. The team should consist of craniofacial plastic surgery, pediatric otolaryngology, neonatology, sleep medicine, pediatric anesthesia, and when indicated by a comorbid syndrome, pediatric ophthalmology, pediatric cardiology, and genetics.

5. In the majority of the cases, conservative management will allow sufficient mandibular development to occur with resulting improvement in symptoms over the first several weeks of life. However, the initial management requires close monitoring in a neonatal intensive care setting.

- Initial therapeutic measures include prone positioning, feeding in an upright position, bypassing the lingual obstruction with the use of a nasogastric or feeding tube, or nasopharyngeal intubation. Most infants with PRS that can be successfully managed with progressive improvement are discharged by the second week of life generally with home pulse oximetry. However, a small subset of these patients cannot be managed conservatively and surgical intervention is required to ensure a stable airway.

- Considerable degree of judgment is required when to abandon conservative management and to proceed with operative intervention. The key question is "How much time does one allow for the mandible to exhibit "catch-up" growth for airway protection?" Among the considerations, continued inability to breathe easily while resting or sleeping, periods of cyanosis secondary to respiratory obstruction, and failure to gain weight are important. A useful "rule-of-thumb" as described by Parsons and Smith suggests that surgical intervention should be considered when progressive weight gain and control of tongue cannot be established within the first weeks of life or when endotracheal intubation is required.

- The surgical options for the infant with PRS include: tongue-lip adhesion, mandibular distraction, and tracheostomy. For the patient with PRS who has reached skeletal maturity and whose mandible failed to "catch up" would require conventional orthognathic surgery—that is, mandibular bilateral sagittal split osteotomy with advancement with or without an osseous genioplasty—to correct the class II dentofacial skeletal relation. Between infancy to adolescence, surgical treatment is guided by functional considerations.

  — With a **tongue-lip adhesion**, the mucosa on the inferior surface of the tongue, the floor of the mouth, the alveolus, and the lower lip are denuded. The most anterior portion of the tongue is sutured to the lower lip and the suture line is extended posteriorly and bilaterally to close the denuded areas together. This keeps the tongue in an anterior position and the airway open. The tongue is released and allowed to return to its normal position when the cleft palate repair is performed. However, some have suggested releasing the tongue earlier by 6 to 7 months of age if the maxillary-mandibular discrepancy becomes less than 3 mm. While tongue-lip adhesion remains part of the protocol in PRS management in a number of centers, mandibular distraction has increasingly replaced it in a growing number of institutions.

  — In severe cases of where either early mandibular distraction is not possible or the infant has comorbid condition of a glottic/infraglottic obstruction a **tracheostomy** is required. However, many patients who have a tracheostomy as an infant remain tracheostomy-dependent until mid-to-late childhood. Furthermore, decannulating becomes increasingly difficult because of dependence on the tracheostomy and a shift of the airflow pattern despite mandibular "catch-up" growth or surgical advancement. Thus, once an infant is identified with PRS and the obstruction isolated to the tongue base, early mandibular distraction is likely to alleviate the need for tracheostomy. Depending on circumstances, an acceptable alternative is to consider an early temporary tracheostomy followed by mandibular distraction and decannulation within the first year of life.

  — In infants with PRS, **mandibular distraction osteogenesis** will correct the airway obstruction and simultaneously have a beneficial effect on swallowing

and reflux. There are two basic approaches to mandibular distraction and is primarily directed by the type of mandibular distractor used: internal devices and external devices. Both have their merits and limitations. The internal distraction devices benefits include ease of use for the parents and closer proximity to the bone providing distraction force directly at the osteotomy site. The limitations of the internal distractors is that distraction is limited to a single vector, the maximal distraction distance is device dependent (typically, 25 to 30 mm) and the requirement for a second surgical procedure for its removal. However, for most cases of microretrognathia in the context of Pierre Robin, distraction lengths greater than 20 to 25 mm is rarely needed and a single vector is adequate. The need for a second surgical procedure may in time be eliminated with continued evolution of devices and the use of resorbable fixation.

To place internal distractors, symmetric submandibular incisions are made below the inferior-posterior border of the angle of the mandible. Typically either an inverted 'L' or a vertical ramal osteotomy is designed to minimize risk to the inferior alveolar nerve and developing tooth buds while maintaining adequate bone stock on either side of the osteotomy to allow for adequate footplate fixation. The distraction device is then temporarily fitted into the operative site on the basis of a predetermined vector, and its footplates are tailored to accommodate it. A counter incision is made in the postauricular area and the activating arm of the distractor is passed through this site. Once the position is verified the distractor is secured in place. The distractor is activated for approximately 1 to 2 mm and the corticotomy is converted to an osteotomy with the bone in tension using a thin interdental osteotome. To ensure that a complete osteotomy has been performed, the device is activated, revealing an osteotomy gap of several millimeters and is then returned to its original position.

The primary benefits of the external distraction devices are that the distraction can be guided in multiple planes, up to 40 mm of distraction in length can be achieved, and a second surgical procedure for removal of the device and pins is not required. The disadvantages are that they are bulky, more easily damaged/loosened/dislodged, and remain visible until consolidation. Furthermore, the distraction forces are not directly applied at the level of the mandible but at distance allowing the pins to bend. Thus, 2 mm/d at the device does not translate one-to-one at the level of the osteotomy. The placement of an external distractor, is similar to the placement of an internal distractor. However, rather than securing the distractor to the mandible directly, the distractor pins are passed transcutaneously and, under direct visualization, screwed into the distraction segments. With both approaches, the infant is then transferred to the neonatal unit. **Activation** of the device begins on the first postoperative day at a rate of 1.5 to 2.0 mm/day divided in three sessions. Serial plain radiographs are obtained to ensure proper lengthening is being achieved by monitoring the distance between the fixation footplates of the device. Clinically, the relative position of the mandibular to maxillary dental arches is observed. The mandibular advancement is overcorrected by 2 to 3 mm and any asymmetry in lengthening is adjusted at the termination of the activation phase. Experienced clinicians who prefer distraction for infants with PRS note a dramatic improvement in breathing by the end of the first week along with improving oral feeding. There is improvement in the tongue posture from a vertical to a horizontal position along the floor of the mouth.

At the end of the distraction period, a **consolidation** phase of a minimum of 6 weeks occurs to allow bone healing to occur. After this period of time, the distractors are removed and a laryngoscopy/bronchoscopy is performed. It should be noted that this minimum period of consolidation is not well defined and varies with the child's age.

- There is a subset of children with PRS whose mandibular growth remains deficient throughout childhood and into adolescence at time of skeletal maturity. In these cases, **conventional orthognathic surgery** is required to correct the Class II occlusal relationship and the maxillary-mandibular skeletal relation. Surgery is delayed until skeletal maturity unless functional considerations such as evidence of obstructive sleep apnea warrant earlier intervention. While typically these adolescents will require a mandibular advancement, bilateral ramal sagittal splitting approach with or without an osseous genioplasty, a number of them will also require simultaneous maxillary advancement to correct midfacial skeletal deficiency that may occur concomitantly.

6. Complications of surgical intervention for patients with PRS can and do occur, but must be weighed against the more imperative need for stabilizing the airway. The complications of lip-tongue adhesion include dehiscence, adjacent neural-vascular and salivary structures and interference with normal tongue function when adhesion is prolonged.

- Minor **pin site infection** with external devices or at the site of the activation arm with transcutaneous internal devices are not uncommon. Most may be managed conservatively with more aggressive pin site care to allow drainage and a short course of oral antibiotics. The typical picture is of cellulitis and rarely abscess collection that requires operative drainage. The pins should be cleaned meticulously with hydrogen peroxide to remove crusts followed by a topical antibiotic ointment. **Osteomyelitis** has been reported as a rare occurrence and would require prolonged intravenous antibiotics.

- In the infant, **dental injury** is a potential but rare complication. The risk is minimized by placing the mandibular osteotomy for the distraction as posterior as possible to avoid injury to the developing tooth buds. However, placement of the anchoring screws or pins for the anterior segment of the distractor may damage the tooth buds of the second and third molars. While every attempt is made to avoid dental injury, it may be inevitable given the anatomic limitations of distracting a diminutive mandible.

- **Injury to the inferior alveolar nerve** during surgery can be minimized by directing the osteotomy posterior to its entrance into the canal. However, there is a definite risk and its occurrence is unknown. It is likely that the nerve is injured in many instances and this should be openly discussed with the patient/family. It is a risk that may be inevitable given the anatomic limitations of a diminutive mandible and must be balanced against the need to improve airway.

- **Premature consolidation** and **malunion/nonunion** are a not a common complication if the distraction is performed correctly and the consolidation phase is allowed to occur prior to the removal of the distractor.

- There is a multitude of **device failures** that can occur with external devices such as loosening of pins, traumatic dislodgement, or problems with the complex worm gears of multidirectional distractors. Experience with internal devices has contrasted with elimination of such problems at the expense of a formal secondary operative procedure for removal of the submerged internal device.

PRACTICAL PEARLS

1. The primary components in a child with PRS is a microretrognathic mandible with airway compromise as result of glossoptosis. Cleft palate is not necessary to satisfy the definition and many infants with PRS occur within the context of other syndromic conditions.

2. The prognosis of mandibular catch-up growth correlates with the underlying cause of the primary event. All patients should be followed closely until skeletal maturity to guide intervention.

3. Most infants with PRS can be managed conservatively with prone positioning and feeding while the child is upright. However, infants must be closely monitored.

4. Surgical intervention should be considered early if there is clear evidence of continued airway compromise and failure to thrive within the first weeks of life.

5. Internal uniplanar mandibular distraction is a viable alternative to lip-tongue adhesion and will eliminate the need for tracheostomy when the obstruction is anatomically isolated to the retroglossal region (tongue base). It will not eliminate the need for tracheostomy, if the child has a glottic/infraglottic obstruction (tracheomalacia). Parents must be made aware of the need for tracheostomy despite mandibular distraction.

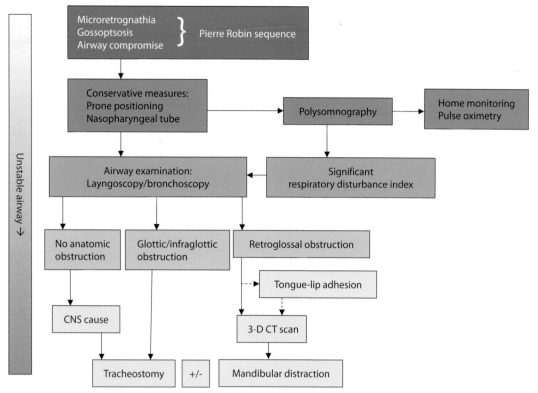

Algorithm 16-1 Algorithm for management of patients with Pierre Robin sequence that must be tailored to each institution.

References

1. Denny AD. Distraction osteogenesis in Pierre Robin neonates with airway obstruction. *Clin Plastic Surg*. 2004;31(2):221-229.

2. Izadi K, Yellon R, Mandell DL, et al. Correction of upper airway obstruction in the newborn with internal mandibular distraction osteogenesis. *J Craniofac Surg*. 2003;14(4):493-499.

3. Parsons RW, Smith DJ. Rule of thumb criteria for tongue-lip adhesion in Pierre Robinz Anomalad. *Plas Reconstr Surg*. 1982;70(2):210-212.

4. Patel PK, Novia MV. The surgical tools: The LeFort I, bilateral sagittal split osteotomy of the mandible and the osseous genioplasty. *Clin Plastic Surg*. 2007;34(3):447-475.

5. Pruzansky S. Not all dwarfed mandibles are alike. *Birth Defects Orig Artic Ser*. 1969;5:120-129.

6. Randall P, Krogman WM, Jahina S. Pierre Robin and the syndrome that bears his name. *Cleft Palate J*. 1965;2(3): 237-246.

7. Randall P. The Robin anomalad: Micrognathia and glossoptosis with airway obstruction. In: Converse JM, ed. *Reconstructive Plastic Surgery*. Vol 4. 2nd ed. Philadelphia, PA: Saunders; 1977:2235-2245.

8. Robin P. Glossoptosis due to atresia and hypotrophy of the mandible. *Am J Dis Child*. 1934;48:541-547.

9. Schaefer RB, Stadler JA, Gosain AK. To distract or not to distract: An algorithm for airway management in isolated Pierre Robin sequence. *Plast Reconstr Surg*. 2004;113(4): 1113-1125.

10. Shprintzen RJ. Pierre Robin, micrognathia and airway obstruction: The dependency of treatment on accurate diagnosis. *Int Anesthesiology Clin*. 1988;26(1):64-71.

11. Singhal VK, Hill ME. Craniofacial microsomia and craniofacial distraction. In: Bentz ML, Bauer BS, Zuker RM, eds. *Principles and Practice of Pediatric Plastic Surgery*. St. Louis, MO: Quality Medical Publishing; 2008:755-797.

12. Williams AJ, Williams MA, Walker CA, Bush PG. The Robin anomlad (Pierre Robin Syndrome)—a follow up study. *Arch Dis Childhealth*. 1981;56(9):663-668.

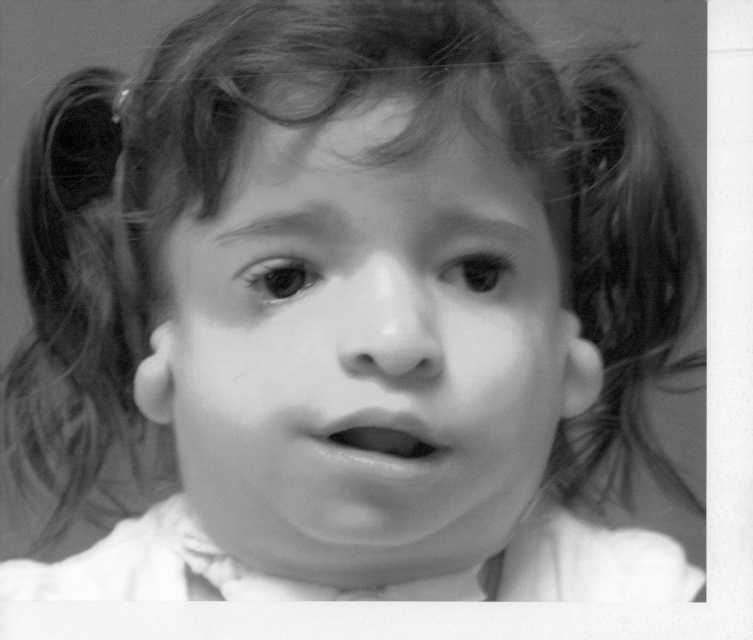

A child with several facial deformities

is referred to your office by a local

pediatrician.

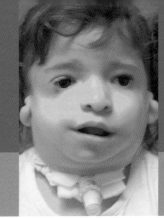

CHAPTER 17

Treacher Collins Syndrome

Davinder J. Singh

1. The appearance of the child suggests an anomaly affecting the midfacial structures, namely the eyes, cheeks, and ears. Since these structures all develop from the first and second branchial arches, one of the craniofacial syndromes, such as Treacher Collins, is likely. The first branchial arch ("mandibular arch") develops into the muscles of mastication (anterior belly of the digastric, mylohyoid, tensor tympani, tensor veli palatini), the maxilla and mandible, the incus and malleus, the trigeminal nerve (CN V) and the maxillary artery. The second branchial arch ("hyoid arch") develops into the muscles of facial expression (zygomaticus major and minor, orbicularis oculi and oris, buccinator, and platysma), stapedius, stylohyoid, and posterior belly of the digastric, the stapes, styloid process, lesser horn of the hyoid, and the facial nerve (CN VII). When interviewing the patient's family, several key points in the history should be obtained.

- **Are there any problems with breathing?** For patients seen at the time of birth, the primary emergent concern is the airway. In the neonate, difficulty with respiration warrants endotracheal intubation via an orotracheal route if possible or by tracheostomy. Potential sites of compromise include the choanae, which may be atretic, the mandible, which may be hypoplastic and force the tongue into the oropharynx, and the trachea, which may be underdeveloped. Tracheostomy is indicated if the patient has significant laryngo- or tracheomalacia. However, if respiratory problems are related to obstructive apnea, the patient may be appropriate for distraction osteogenesis of the mandible.

- **Are there any problems with feeding?** This is an equally pressing problem. Patients who have difficulty feeding require an orogastric tube as a short-term solution or a feeding gastrostomy tube as a more permanent solution.

- **Are there any drying or exposure concerns with the globe?** Without the ability to either close the eyes or roll the eyes upward at night (Bell's phenomenon), corneal drying will lead to visual compromise.

- **Does the patient have other ophthalmologic concerns?** Amblyopia (poor or indistinct vision in an eye that is otherwise normal) secondary to refractive errors, anisometropia (unequal refractive power, one eye may be more nearsighted and one more farsighted), strabismus (improper alignment of the eyes caused by lack of coordination between the extraocular muscles), and/or eyelid ptosis are all possible manifestations.

- **Has the child passed or failed a recent hearing test?** Early implementation of hearing aids should be arranged to greatly enhance speech and language development.

- **Does the patient have other developmental issues?** Mental deficiency is reported to occur in less than 5% of affected patients. Most children develop normally but should be followed for psychosocial concerns related to their physical appearance.

- **Is there any family history of similar findings?** Numerous craniofacial syndromes are transmitted in an autosomal dominant manner with variable penetrance. Those with autosomal transmission often fail to survive.

2. For patients with congenital anomalies of the head and neck, the diagnosis is often made by examining the constellation of findings. Here, the affected structures appear to be derived from the first and second branchial arches. Treacher Collins syndrome is generally symmetric with variable degrees of facial clefting in the No. 6 through No. 9 positions according to the Tessier classification system. The particular constellation of clinical manifestations in patients with Treacher Collins syndrome spans the craniofacial skeleton.

- **Does the skull appear normal?** The skull is usually normal other than constriction at the squamosal portion of the temporal bones. The skeletal deficiency encompasses the zygomatic bones with associated hypoplasia of the glenoid fossae, TMJ's, condyles, and mandibular rami.

- **Are the orbits fully formed?** The bony deficits affect the lateral and inferior orbital rims, which may be hypoplastic or totally absent. This produces a downward slope, or antimongoloid slant, to the palpebral fissures.

- **Are the eyelids fully formed?** Patients may present with one or more defects along the lower eyelid (epibulbar dermoid) or partial to total absence of the lower eyelashes. There may also be ptosis of the upper eyelid.

- **Are the eyes able to track objects in a coordinated fashion?** Inability of the eyes to follow objects would suggest the presence of anisometropia.
- **Is the mouth symmetrical?** Lateral facial clefts (Tessier No. 7), either unilateral or bilateral, may be present. This results in macrostomia and difficulty with feeding as adequate suction cannot be generated because of the splaying of the orbicularis oris.
- **Is the upper jaw fully formed?** The maxilla is often elongated anteriorly and shortened posteriorly, which produces a steep occlusal plane.
- **Is the lower jaw fully formed?** The occlusal plane is typically steep as a consequence of a short mandibular ramus on one or both sides.
- **What is the shape of the nose?** The nose often demonstrates a wide dorsum with a hump and a drooped tip.
- **Are the ears fully formed on each side of the head?** The external ears demonstrate variable degrees of microtia while the middle ear may also be underdeveloped.
- **Do all major branches of the facial nerve function appropriately?** The muscles that arise from either the first (mastication) or second (animation) branchial arch may be hypoplastic. Occasionally patients may have facial nerve weakness, although this is not typical.
- **Is there a cleft palate?** Failure to inspect the oral cavity and specifically the roof of the mouth will miss the presence of a cleft palate.
- **Are there other congenital anomalies?** While not common, patients with Treacher Collins may have one or more noncraniofacial anomalies, which should be sought. These include absence of the parotid gland, cryptorchidism, and/or congenital heart defects.

3. Several studies are important to obtain preoperatively to plan any surgical intervention. There are no specific perioperative laboratory studies to obtain.

- Patients with Treacher Collins syndrome have characteristic findings on AP and lateral **cephalograms.**
  - Decreased total facial height, as measured from nasion to menton (N-Me).

— Decreased mandibular projection, low SNB angle.
— Decreased AP length of the face.
— Decreased bitemporal width.
— Decreased posterior facial height.
— Obtuse angle between the sella-nasion line and the palate.
— Normal upper facial height, as measured from nasion to the anterior nasal spine (N-ANS).

- **Orthopantomogram** is a panoramic X-ray of the mandible.
- A thin-cut **CT scan of the head and facial bones,** which may be reformatted into a three-dimensional image is useful to identify the bony architecture. It should include the petrous portion of the temporal bones, which houses the middle ear structures.

4. In formulating a management plan, it is important to obtain appropriate consultations.

- **Genetics** consultation is important not only to ascertain the genetic nature of the syndrome but also to provide the parents with information regarding the risk in subsequent children. Treacher Collins has been mapped to chromosome 5q. Important syndromes in the differential diagnosis to rule out include:
  - **Treacher Collins syndrome** (mandibulofacial dysostosis) has been mapped to chromosome 5q. Frequent findings include lower lid colobomas, zygomatic hypoplasia, microtia, mandibular hypoplasia, and possible cleft palate.
  - Craniofacial microsomia presents with asymmetry of the face. The right side is likely to be affected twice as often as the left, with up to one-quarter of cases being bilateral. It is noticeable since the corner of the mouth on the affected side may be higher and the midpoint of the chin may not lie in the middle of the face. The ear may be microtia or absent (anotia) with a hemimandible that is flatter and shorter than the opposite side. The TM joint may be underdeveloped and some patients may have macrostomia or weakness of the ipsilateral facial muscles. Intelligence and development are normal.

— **Goldenhar syndrome** is a variant of craniofacial microsomia that presents with additional findings of epibulbar dermoids, cervical spinal fusions, and renal anomalies.

— **Nager syndrome** is an autosomal recessive variant of Treacher Collins that presents with hypoplasia of the soft palate and associated hand deformities.

- A **pediatric ophthalmology** consultation should be obtained at the first consult and prior to beginning any reconstruction around the eyes, including lid reconstruction and orbitozygomatic bone grafting.

- Consultation with the **pediatric otolaryngologist** is important since many patients will require bone conduction hearing aids for the development of normal speech and language. Later, they may undergo release of the ossicles if they are noted to be ankylotic. If the child has acute airway issues at birth, it is critical to have otolaryngology involved to assess for laryngo- or tracheomalacia, and also to have a sleep study performed to evaluate for central apnea, reflux, and obstructive apnea. These evaluations allow proper treatment for airway issues.

5. Prior to surgery, the extent of the reconstruction and the expectations should be discussed with the patient and his/her family. The "staged" nature of the surgical procedures and need for repeat surgeries depending on patient's growth should be stressed.

   - The earliest consideration is the airway. The base of the tongue can be displaced anteriorly to improve air exchange by prone positioning, tongue-lip adhesion, distraction osteogenesis of the mandible. Tracheostomy should also be considered.

   - Exposure of the eyes may be addressed with skin or skin/muscle flaps from the upper eyelid to replace missing tissue.

   - At 3 to 6 months, one may elect to repair the macrostomia component of the lateral facial cleft (Tessier No. 7 cleft) with superior and inferior vermilion flaps. It is important that the fibers of the orbicularis muscle from the upper and lower lips be identified and overlapped in the corner of the mouth to recreate the modiolus. The skin just lateral to the newly created corner is best closed with a straight line repair and the mucosa in a Z-plasty design.

   - Cleft palate repair may be performed approximately 10 to 12 months of age. Straight-line intravelar veloplasty or repair by double opposing Z-plasty (Furlow technique) may be used.

   - For severe mandibular hypoplasia, distraction osteogenesis may be considered after eruption of the first molars. The Pruzansky type III mandible with scant bone stock will require costochondral rib graft or iliac bone graft, which may then be distracted if further bone is required. A formal orthognathic procedure (sagittal split osteotomy and advancement of the mandible) is contemplated when skeletal growth is complete.

- Ear reconstruction with autogenous costochondral rib grafts or an alloplast should be offered in cases of complete microtia. Autogenous tissue reconstruction is begun around 6 to 8 years of age. This involves primary creation of a costochondral cartilage framework and secondary elevation of the framework from the temporal scalp with banked cartilage and split thickness skin graft and definition of the conchal bowl and tragus in two or more stages. Earlier reconstruction may be considered if alloplastic reconstruction is chosen. In this instance, a prefabricated alloplastic material is chosen in lieu of cartilage and is covered with a temporoparietal fascia flap and skin graft. Finally, some patients may opt for a prosthetic ear, which attaches to osseointegrated pins anchored into the temporal bone. If the mandible is severely hypoplastic, distraction is advised prior to ear reconstruction in order to better position the ear framework.

- Reconstruction of the zygoma, lateral orbit, and midface may also be performed around 7 to 8 years of age and timing may be integrated with ear reconstruction. This requires bone graft harvested from available sites including the outer table of the skull, ribs, or iliac crest.

- In early adolescence, orthodontia is initiated in anticipation of needed orthognathic surgery. In late adolescence, formal orthognathic surgery, including posterior lengthening and anterior shortening/impaction of the maxilla at the LeFort I level, bilateral sagittal split osteotomy to lengthen the rami and advance the mandible, and vertical reduction and advancement genioplasty of the chin.

- Formal rhinoplasty is best left until after any orthognathic procedure when the facial skeleton is set to improve cosmesis of the nose.

6. The potential complications from managing children with Treacher Collins syndrome as well as other craniofacial malformations can be life-threatening. In addition to the standard surgical risks such as bleeding, infection, poor scarring, and injury to surrounding structures (brain, meninges, globes) numerous complications at each stage of the reconstruction are possible.

   - With distraction of mandible, device failure, infection, and poor vector choice are all possible complications.

   - With ear reconstruction, postoperative **exposure** of the cartilage or alloplast is possible. In some instances, small local flaps may be designed to cover an area of exposure. In more severe cases, a temporoparietal fascial flap is required. This option is not possible if it has previously been used to cover an alloplastic implant.

   - With reconstruction of the midface using bone grafts, exposure, malposition, and resorption of the grafts are all potential complications.

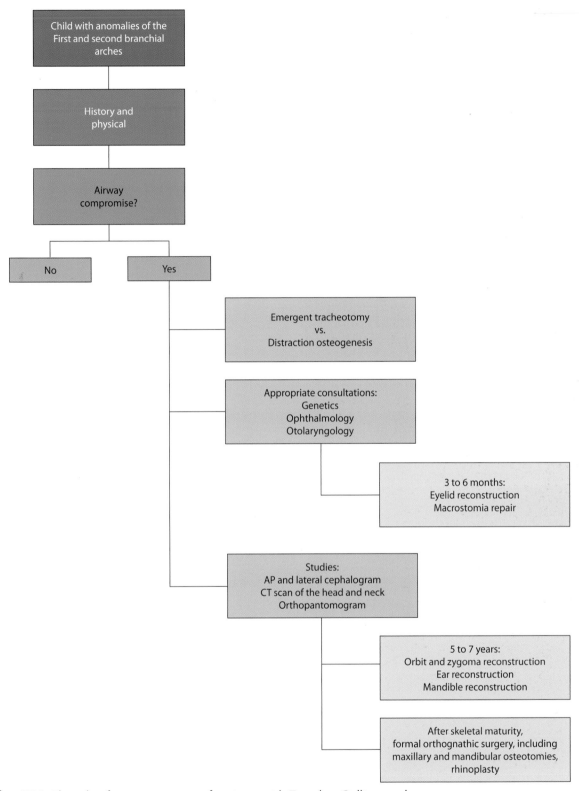

Algorithm 17-1 Algorithm for management of patients with Treacher Collins syndrome.

PRACTICAL PEARLS

1. The airway should always be assessed first. If there is any concern, the otolaryngologist should endoscope the proximal airway to document any narrowing and a sleep study should be obtained.

2. The upper eyelids should be spared as a donor site for skin since flaps of skin and muscle from the upper eyelid are used to reconstruct the lower eyelid.

3. Reconstruction of the lower eyelid and macrostomia should be repaired early (age 3 to 5 months), followed by the cleft palate around age 9 to 12 months.

4. The need for STAGED surgical procedures should be stressed to patient and family.

5. Appropriate imaging studies (three-dimensional CT, AP and lateral cephalogram, orthopantomogram) should be obtained to plan the skeletal surgical procedures.

References

1. Hunt JA and Hobar PG. Common craniofacial anomalies: The facial dysostoses. *Plast Reconstr Surg.* 2002;110(7):1714.

2. Gorlin RJ, Pindborg JJ, Cohen MM. *Syndromes of the Head and Neck.* 2nd ed. New York, NY: McGraw-Hill, 1976.

3. Pruzansky S. Not all dwarfed mandibles are alike. *Birth Defects.* 1969;5:120.

4. Jackson IT. Reconstruction of the lower eyelid defect in Treacher Collins syndrome. *Plast Reconstr Surg.* 1981;67:365.

5. Posnick JC. Treacher Collins syndrome. In: Aston S, ed. *Grabb and Smith's Plastic Surgery.* 5th ed. Philadelphia, PA: Lippincott Raven; 1997.

6. Freihofer HPM. Variations in the correction of Treacherr Collins Syndrome. *Plast Reconstr Surg.* 1997;99:657.

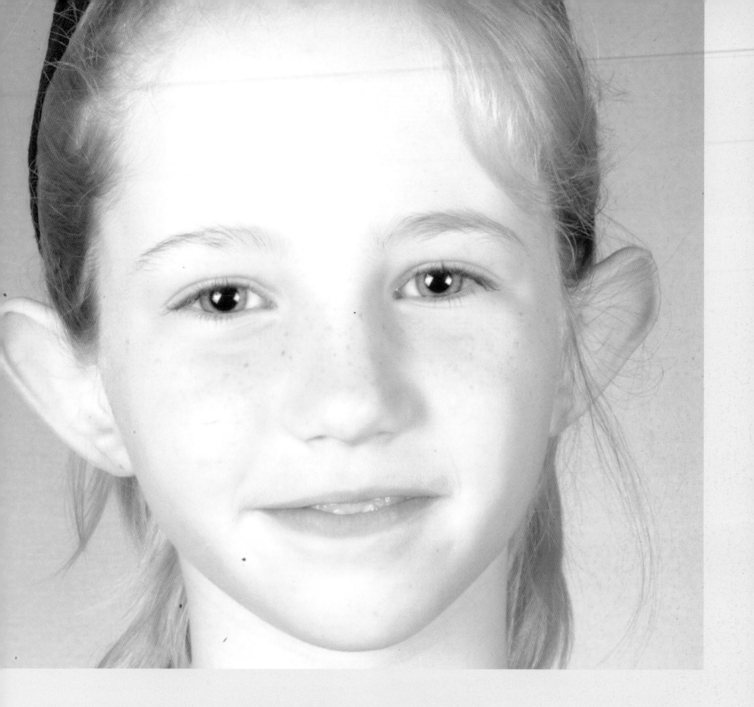

A 6-year-old girl is brought to your office

with concerns about the appearance

of her ears.

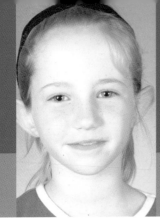

CHAPTER 18

Prominent Ear Deformity

Patrick Cole and Samuel Stal

1. Significant malformations of the ear are prevalent in today's society and affects more than 5% of the population. The child noted in the photograph has a prominent ear deformity, which may or may not present with the patient being self-consciousness about the appearance of the ears. Developmentally, the embryologic anterior hillocks form the helical root and tragus while the posterior hillocks form the helix, antitragus, triangular fossa, scapha, concha cymba, concha cavum, and lobule. The ear then develops rapidly over the first decade of life. By one year of age, approximately 90% of the eventual adult width is achieved. At 10 years, the ear is 97% to 99% of its expected adult width. Length develops at a slower rate. Throughout adulthood, the external length continues to grow at a slow rate primarily through lengthening of the fibrofatty lobule. At the first visit, a thorough history should be taken to determine the effect of the deformity and identify any other congenital anomalies.

- **Was the deformity present from birth?** Almost all cases have been present since infancy. If noted within 1 to 2 months of birth, high levels of residual circulating maternal estrogen may allow successful conservative ear restructuring. In this event, tape and dental compound may be used to effectively mold auricular framework. The auriculocephalic angle continues to increase from 16 degrees at one year of age to 22 degrees by 10 years. Although this angle slightly increases throughout the second decade of life, the auriculocephalic angle subtly retracts over the third decade before eventual plateau. Often the result of antihelix underdevelopment or an enlarged conchal bowl, the prominent ear necessitates thorough evaluation and a careful, rational approach to surgical correction.

- **Is there any associated hearing difficulty?** Difficulty with hearing is important to identify and manage early to allow normal speech and language development. Although the physiologic effects of ear deformity are negligible, the aesthetic and psychological impact on the patient can be profound.

- **Is the child teased at school?** While surgery is not performed for functional problems, the appearance of prominent ears may produce psychosocial concerns. Often teasing in school is the catalyst to proceed with correction. Interviewing the maturing child regarding his or her personal feelings on corrective surgery is imperative. While getting the pediatric patient "on board" with perioperative care is often incredibly useful, patient report of psychosocial stress resulting from ear prominence is always important to document and discuss before proceeding.

- **Are there any concomitant congenital anomalies?** Upon initial presentation, a thorough evaluation should be completed to determine if additional congenital anomalies may be present.

2. There are several causes for a prominent ear deformity. The presence or absence of each should be ascertained by careful physical examination. Prominent ear deformity may be caused by unfurling of the antihelical fold, deepening of the conchal bowl, an obtuse scaphomastoid angle, or a combination of findings. Because several factors may result in auricular prominence, successful evaluation and correction begins with a thorough knowledge of normal auricular anatomy. Although significant variation exists, objective measurements help define normal auricular dimension.

- **Are the ears fully formed?** The broad spectrum of ear projection makes it difficult to define normalcy based on absolute parameters. Although quantitative means can be defined for almost any dimension of the external ear, prominence must always be viewed in context of an individual's facial structure. Projection beyond an objective, average value can often be considered abnormal, but much of the final opinion should be derived from the patient's or family's perception as compared with a societal standard. By adulthood, ear length reaches 5.5 to 6.5 cm and width increases to approximately 50% to 60% of length (the height of the ear is approximately two times its width).

- **Where is the ear positioned on the side of the head?** The superior aspect of the ear typically corresponds to the brow, while the inferior border usually descends to the level of the columellar base. Various genetic syndromes affecting the craniofacial skeleton result in ears that are set lower than normal.

- **What is the vertical axis of the ear?** In profile, the vertical axis of the ear normally projects posterolaterally by 15 to 30 degrees.

- **Is the antihelical fold well defined?** The fold of the antihelix begins at the antitragus and continues in a smooth, uninterrupted anterior and superior to form the superior and inferior crura. The antihelical fold typically produces a conchoscaphal angle of 90 degrees or less. The acuity of this angle directly corresponds to the distance the helical rim is from the scalp. Obtuse angles are confirmed by flimsy antihelical development, as the auriculocephalic angle increases, the ear gains in prominence.

- **How deep is the conchal bowl?** Lateralization of the ear can also be enhanced by anterior rotation of the concha or deepening of the conchal bowl. In most cases, the hemispherical conchal bowl normally extends to a depth less than 1.5 cm, with a sharply defined rim.

- **By how much does the ear project off the side of the head?** The auriculocephalic angle, the measure of ear projection at the helical root, is approximately 23 degrees (21 degrees for females, 25 degrees for males) off the temporal scalp. An angle more than 25 degrees will appear prominent. Protrusion may also be measured along a hypothetical plane drawn from the helical margin to the scalp. From the scalp, the helical rim of the ear commonly projects laterally 10 to 12 mm at the superior pole, 16 to 18 mm at the midpoint, and 20 to 22 mm at the lobule. The helix should project beyond the antihelix in a smooth contour with an undistorted postauricular sulcus. In normal circumstances, the lobule does not project lateral to the upper two-thirds of the ear.

- **Are there secondary anomalies related to the prominent ear?** Secondary anomalies very often exist in this setting. These include an excessive helical root protrusion, an overprojected lobule, excessive protrusion of the antitragus, insufficient helical curling, a cup ear deformity, and macrotia.

- **Is the canal patent?** In almost all cases, the canal is patent and there are no underlying developmental issues related to the middle ear.

- The ear is supplied by the external carotid via posterior auricular and superficial temporal arteries. It is innervated by the auriculotemporal nerve on its anterior surface, the ear receives posterior surface sensation via greater auricular and lesser occipital nerves.

3. No specific radiologic studies are indicated prior to proceeding with correction of a prominent ear deformity.

4. No specific consultations are required in a child whose hearing has been normal.

5. Over the last century, numerous corrective maneuvers have been described that bend, suture, excise, score, and reposition the auricular cartilage. While the surgeon may enjoy the wide latitude that multiple corrective techniques offer, they are better off proceeding with specific techniques that are best suited to the specific auricular deformities present. By this approach, correction of the prominent ear can go beyond patient satisfaction to predictably maximize outcome in both form and symmetry.

- The timing and selection of intervention should balance the level patient maturity, appropriate ear development, psychosocial stress resulting from the deformity, and pliability of the auricular cartilage. Abnormalities in the dimension of the external ear typically reveal themselves at an early age. In order to minimize potential psychosocial stress, many surgeons advise correction prior to childhood socialization. Although abbreviating the negative social impact of deformity is always a primary stimulus for correction, the decision to operate must take into account additional factors. In many cases, waiting for the child to mature enough to become an active participant in his or her postoperative care is optimal. By 3 years of age, 90% of eventual ear growth is achieved; however, at 6 years, auricular cartilage begins to significantly harden. Following prominent ear correction in patients less than 6, Mustarde demonstrated a 1.8% recurrence rate at 10 years postprocedure. However, patients older than 6 years at the time of surgery experienced a 300% increase in relapse rate. Many surgeons take advantage of the 3 to 6-year-old age window to correct major ear constriction, before the start of school. In general, the goal of surgery is to produce a symmetrical result of perceivably normal form within 3 mm of variation from the contralateral ear. The more severely deformed ear should be addressed first; in time, the

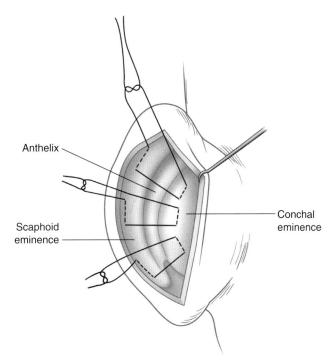

Figure 18-1 Schematic drawing highlighting the placement of posterior cartilage sutures to redefine the antihelical fold.

less-affected ear can be tailored to complement the contralateral correction.

- When presented with a series of anomalies, the concha should be addressed early on in order to minimize the need for excessive Mustarde suture tightening. For mild to moderate conchal depths of less than 2.5 cm, the Furnas technique of conchomastoid suturing is extremely effective.

- Prior to beginning, markings made on the anterior surface are transferred to the posterior surface with a 25-gauge needle dipped in methylene blue to stain the skin and underlying cartilage. These may include the superior rim of the triangular fossa, the upper border of the superior crus, and the junction of the scapha and helix. A vertical incision is made in the posterior conchal skin 2.5 cm lateral to the sulcus. Anterior and posterior skin flaps are then elevated for access to the helical rim, scapha, and mastoid fascia. Instead of excising a posterior ellipse of skin, soft tissue should be preserved to minimize the tension on the posterior sulcus, reinforce positioning of the mid-helix, and decrease the incidence of suture granuloma formation or bow-stringing over the Mustarde sutures. The postauricular muscle and ligament are divided downward until the ponticulus, the cartilaginous insertion, is identified (Elliott maneuver). Dissection is then directed toward the mastoid with soft tissue elevation for approximately 2 cm. The ear is then drawn directly backward with the use of nonabsorbable suture until the desired look is achieved. At this point, the contact areas between the conchal cartilage and the mastoid fascia are marked, and three to four 4-0 Merseline

mattress sutures are used to approximate these markings. On the conchal side, the sutures must contain both the anterior and posterior perichondrium, although great care must be taken to avoid inclusion of the anterior auricular skin. It is imperative to obtain secure bites of the mastoid fascia in order to minimize the incidence of suture pulling through the fascia. To minimize forward rotation or external auditory canal narrowing, place sutures in an anteroposterior direction. In the event substantial canal narrowing occurs following Furnas suture placement, the use of a Spira posterior conchal flap can effectively limit stenosis. By excising postauricular muscle and fibrofatty tissue, a deep mastoid pocket can be created to further accentuate the setback. Further enhancement can be accomplished by conchal cartilage thinning along the area adjacent to the mastoid prominence.

- In addition to cartilage-sparing techniques, a hypertrophied concha may require cartilaginous excision. Either an anterior or posterior incision can be used to expose underlying conchal cartilage. A curvilinear rim incision is then made in the cartilage followed by creation of posterior and anterior skin flaps. Excessive cartilage of the ascending conchal bowl is excised, and the remaining cartilaginous tissues reapproximated with 4-0 clear nylon suture. The anterior skin flap is allowed to redrape the newly created conchal bowl and closed in its new position.

- In the case of significant antihelical deformity, a new antihelix can be created through the use of scaphoconchal mattress sutures and anterior cartilage scoring. In order to create an antihelical rim, Mustarde advised placing four to five horizontal scaphoconchal mattress sutures (Figure 1). Prior to the placement of permanent sutures, temporary 4-0 nylon sutures placed at 4 mm. intervals are used to fold the scapha and evaluate the neoantihelix. Moderate-caliber mattress sutures are then placed through the base of the auricular cartilage with careful incorporation of the anterior and posterior perichondrium. Again, maximal care must be taken to avoid skin incorporation within the closure. Sutures should be placed obliquely at the mid-conchal region to facilitate a naturally anatomic, "C"-shaped curve. Symmetrical nonoblique sutures tied to an overly straight neohelix may produce a "game postdeformity." In addition to Mustarde sutures, anterior scoring is commonly required on the rigid cartilage of those older than 6 years of age. Although a variety of methods are effective in scoring the anterior auricular cartilage, our preference is to create a 2 mm anterior skin excision in the area of the inferior crus. Blunt dissection is then used to elevate the skin from along a path between the new antihelix and superior crus. The cartilage is further scored with a Dingman otobrader to facilitate pliability and increase scarring, thus leading to greater healing potential. The auricular cartilage is then repositioned, followed by careful reapproximation of the skin.

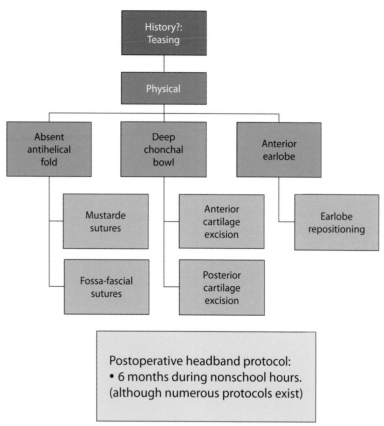

Algorithm 18-1 Algorithm for management of patients with prominent ear deformity.

- An enlarged earlobe is frequently associated with the protruding ear. Unfortunately, the application of the Mustarde technique to create a new antihelical fold often exacerbates this finding. Because of the significant elastic recoil and skin resiliency of the ear's lower third, substantial surgical latitude is allowed and many reduction methods have proven capable. Retroposing the helical tail effectively decreases the lobule's lateral angle from the scalp, and effectively retracts inferior tissues. With a recurrence rate of only 4%, suturing the helical tail to the concha cavum decreases the prominent lobule. Furnas advised plication of the fibrofatty tissue from the lobe to the insertion site of the sternocleidomastoid muscle. The posterior skin and subcutaneous tissue of the lobule may be excised in a "V," heart, or elliptical pattern and reapproximated for size reduction. The Spira technique combines an elliptical skin excision with dermal placation from the lobule to the conchal cartilage near the postauricular sulcus. A prominent, laterally projecting helical root can be pexied to the temporalis fascia for production of the temporal angle. Initially, a longitudinal incision is made medial to the helical root to expose both the root and temporalis fascia. At this site, a 4-0 clear nylon horizontal mattress suture can be placed to reduce the temporal helical angle. If excessive local tissue produces a buckled skin appearance, conservative excision of redundant tissue prior to Hatch suture placement should facilitate an aesthetic closure.

- Numerous postoperative regimens are available regarding otoplasty. One common recommendation is the use of a headband for six months during nonschool hours.

6. An overwhelming majority of postoperative patients report an improvement in self-confidence. However, despite the elective nature, sterile operative environment, and relatively uncomplicated nature of prominent ear correction, postoperative complications may be especially traumatizing to the patient. As with most surgical procedures, bleeding and infection comprise a majority of postoperative concerns.

  - **Malposition and recurrence** are the most notable complications. Often the result of excessive surgical zeal, prominence of the upper and lower poles despite an overly corrected middle-third frequently prompts further reconstructive efforts. A **telephone ear deformity** describes recurrence of the upper and lower pole prominence with a normal intervening middle-third.

  - Manifest as significant pain and swelling in the early postoperative period, local **hematoma** is treated with urgent suture removal and clot evacuation. The dressing may then be reapplied to minimize recurrence.

- Most frequently, the result of *Staphylococcus,* Streptococcal, or *Pseudomonas* spp., **cellulitis** is rare but requires aggressive therapy. The causative organisms are usually *Staphylococcus* and/or *Streptococcal* species and occasionally *Pseudomonas*. Treatment should include parenteral antibiotics and topical Sulfamylon to all exposed cartilaginous areas.

- With improper management, cellulitis may progress to involve underlying cartilage structure, or **chondritis**. Of special note, chronically draining sinus tracts may form as a result of permanent suture use. In addition to suture removal, the entire sinus structure requires excision as well. Treatment includes parenteral antibiotics and topical Sulfamylon, if areas of cartilage are exposed.

- **Sinus tracts** may form as a result of the use of permanent sutures. Treatment requires removal of the sutures as well as excision of the tract.

PRACTICAL PEARLS

1. Although "normal" values can be defined for almost any dimension of the external ear, the abnormal ear must always be viewed in context of an individual's facial structure.

2. From the scalp, projection of the helical rim of the ear may be remembered as roughly 10-15-20 at the superior, middle, and lower portions, respectively.

3. The timing and selection of surgical intervention should balance patient maturity level, appropriate ear development, psychosocial stress load resulting from deformity, and evolving auricular cartilage pliability.

4. Although hundreds of corrective maneuvers exist, the true art of structural ear correction is in the surgeon's ability to proceed with an algorithmic application of methods best suited to the specific auricular need. For effective conchal setback, cartilage-sparing techniques should precede any cartilage-cutting procedure.

References

1. Kelley P, Hollier L, Stal S. Otoplasty: Evaluation, technique, and review. *J Craniofac Surg*. 2003;14(5):643-653.

2. Mustarde JC. The treatment of prominent ears by buried mattress sutures: A ten-year survey. *Plast Reconstr Surg*. 1967;39(4):382-386.

3. Furnas DW. Correction of prominent ears by conchomastoid sutures. *Plast Reconstr Surg*. 1968;42(3):189-193.

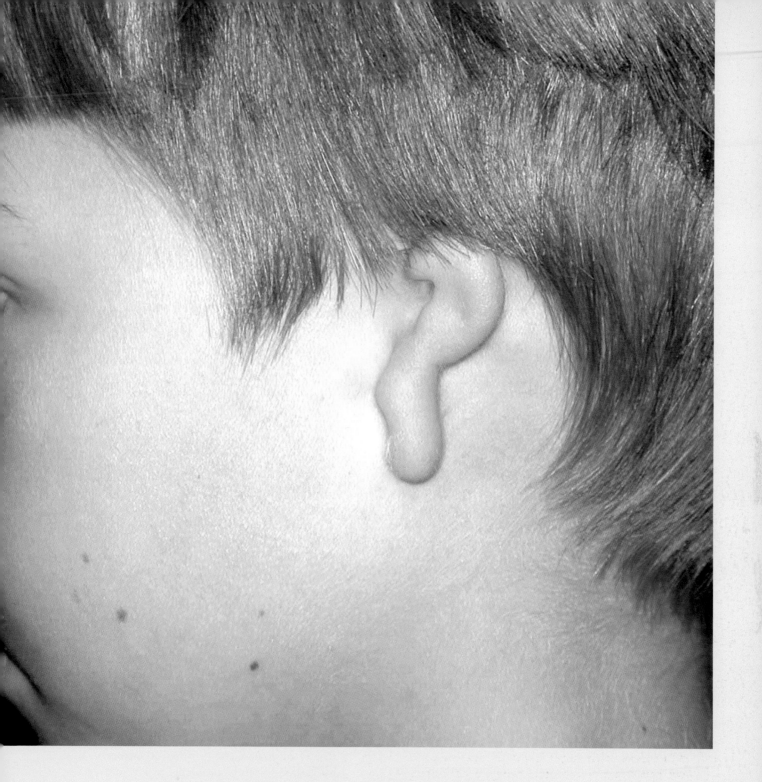

A 6-year-old boy presented to plastic surgery clinic with the ear deformity as shown above.

CHAPTER 19

Microtia

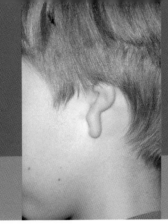

Mitchell A. Stotland

1. The patient shown has a partial absence of the external ear framework. When it is a congenital condition, it is termed microtia. The deformity is usually obvious and consultation may be arranged while the infant is still in the hospital. It may or may not present with middle ear involvement and may or may not be associated with related syndromes affecting the head and neck. Psychosocially, the deformity may have profound influence on a child's self-esteem and social integration. Several specific questions should be asked regarding the patient's history.

   • **What is the child's hearing status in each ear?** When meeting an infant with microtia for the first time, the greatest source of parental anxiety that needs to be addressed is the issue of hearing loss. It is important that the plastic surgeon recognizes this and takes the time to discuss the matter carefully before proceeding to a dialogue about reconstruction. It may be helpful to point out to the parents that the outer and middle ear derive embryologically from different tissue (first and second branchial arches) than does the inner ear (from ectodermal sensory placodes). The parents should understand that the visibly anomalous portion of the ear does not necessarily reflect aberrant inner ear structures (inner ear abnormalities occur in approximately 10% of microtic ears, and are usually minor). Patients with monaural hearing are at risk for delayed speech development and poor school performance but may be followed closely without a hearing aid.

   • **Has the patient had any ear infections?** Care should be taken to have an otolaryngologist routinely monitor the contralateral normal ear and promptly address any infections that occur.

   • **How is the patient doing in school?** While the vast majority of individuals with unilateral microtia will have highly functional hearing, affected children may benefit from strategic positioning in the school classroom. The development of true binaural hearing is only present if it is intact from birth. Bone-conductive hearing aids are indicated for severe bilateral hearing loss (typically for bilateral microtia) within weeks of birth. These devices are somewhat awkward and stigmatizing for an older child to wear, and so the implementation of a bone-anchored

hearing apparatus is an appealing option for many patients. It has been shown to be a reliable and successful intervention. Surgical exploration of the middle ear, involving drilling of the temporal bone to create a neocanal, and fabrication of a tympanic membrane using graft material, is an approach offered by some otologists with particular expertise in this area. Consideration of this challenging procedure is more common in cases of bilateral microtia, but not exclusively so. In cases of autogenous ear repair, the middle ear exploration should occur subsequent to the reconstruction in order to preserve the vascularity of the overlying skin pocket and allow for strategic placement of the otologist's incision.

   • **Is the patient being teased and does he/she try to hide the ear with hair or a hat?** As mentioned, the complete or partial absence of an ear may have profound influence on a child's self-esteem and social integration.

   • **Does the patient have any related congenital problems?** Several syndromes along the oculo-auriculo-vertebral (OAV) spectrum present with microtia in addition to anomalies of the spine, heart, and genitourinary system (ectopic or fused kidneys, reflux, obstruction, duplication). These include Goldenhar, hemifacial microsomia, Nager syndromes.

   • **What is the patient's general medical status?** Key clinical information should be obtained at the initial visit, including pregnancy and/or labor complications, maternal drug use or toxic exposure, and family history of craniofacial or other anomalies. A history of cardiorespiratory problems, prior surgery, use of medications, and presence of allergies will all determine whether the patient is an appropriate surgical candidate.

2. The physical examination of the child with microtia should certainly focus on the ear and which parts are deficient but must also search for concomitant malformations that would identify the presence of an associated malformation.

   • **What parts of the remaining ear are involved and which need to be reconstructed?** Various classification systems have been used to describe hypoplastic ear deformities. None of these necessarily need to be employed. However, it is useful when communicating findings, and in planning reconstruction, to outline the components of the auricle that are present or absent (e.g., lobule, tragus, constricted concha, severe helical constriction, etc.). In milder forms of auricular hypoplasia, the surgeon may recommend a subtotal reconstruction, salvaging the useful portions of the auricle and supplementing them with costochondral cartilage where needed.

- **Does the patient have associated auricular findings?** The presence of additional auricular anlagen such as preauricular tags, pits, sinus tracts, or other chondrocutaneous remnants may exist anywhere along the plane of the embryologic fault line from oral commissure to the temporal region.

- **Are there abnormalities of the hairline?** These may influence the placement of the ear framework, the need for management of hair-bearing skin overlying the reconstructed ear, or reveal the presence of anomalous sideburn placement that may be associated with Treacher Collins or Nager syndromes.

- **Are there defects of the eyelid margin?** Colobomas of the lid, iris, or retina may be present in these patients, as well as partial absence of the medial lower eyelid lashes, paucity of lower lid skin, or downsloping of the palpebral fissures. All may be associated with Treacher Collins or Nager syndromes. Epibulbar dermoid cysts may be present along the conjunctival surface of the lower lids that may be associated with Goldenhar syndrome.

- **Are there deformities of the orbitozygomatic contour or projection?** Hypoplasia in this region is characteristic of Treacher Collins and Nager syndromes.

- **Are there underlying temporal bone and/or soft-tissue hypoplasia on the microtic side?** Fabricating a good facsimile of the normal ear is only part of the reconstructive challenge when treating a patient with significant microsomia. The surgeon may find that the reconstructed ear sits hidden from frontal view within the concavity of a hypoplastic temporal region, or appears too caudad in relation to a hypoplastic mandible, or too anterior in relation to a midface constricted along the axial plane. Mandibular

distraction and/or soft-tissue augmentation need/needs to be considered in such patients.

- **Does the patient have full function of the facial nerve (CN VII)?** Asymmetry of the facial mimetic muscles is not uncommon in patients with microtia. Documenting this prior to embarking on the reconstructive process is important. Options for managing congenital facial palsy may be discussed depending on the severity of findings and motivation of the family.

- **Is there evidence of macrostomia?** This form of facial clefting (Tessier No. 7) reflects an error in fusion between the embryologic maxillary and mandibular processes. This presents along a spectrum of severity from a subtle transverse cheek crease, or mild lateral oral commissure displacement, to a complete cleft with commissure displacement extending far into the involved cheek. Infants with significant macrostomia may have some difficulty with feeding from non-cleft feeders because of problems with oral seal. Older children with macrostomia may suffer from oral salivary incontinence.

- **Is there an occlusal cant?** In the child with microtia, maturity may bring a progressive dental/skeletal occlusal canting, with asymmetric maxillary growth and dental eruption occurring in response to the mandibular hypoplasia on the side ipsilateral to the microtia. A simple clinical test used to demonstrate this is to have the patient bite down on a wooden tongue depressor that is placed horizontally into the mouth, as far posteriorly as is comfortable. Relative to the sagittal plane of the patient's face, the tongue blade will tend to cant upward toward the involved side. Following the occlusal relationship routinely through the early childhood years, both clinically and radiologically, will help to determine the possible need, and timing, for distraction osteogenesis.

- **Is the chin point in the midline?** Along with occlusal changes, the hypoplastic hemimandible is commonly reflected in a noticeable ipsilateral chin point in repose, with further lateral deviation of the jaw toward the microtic side evident when the patient opens mouth. Gentle palpation along the body, angle, and ramal regions, as the patient ranges the temporomandibular joint, may help reveal the extent of mandibular hypoplasia relative to the uninvolved side.

- **Is there any draining mass or sinus in the neck?** These may represent an associated branchial cleft cyst.

- **Is there evidence of torticollis?** Anomalies of the cervical spine should be recognized and addressed prior to operative intervention to prevent unwanted injury. Examine the patient carefully for the presence of congenital torticollis. This is a fairly common diagnosis in infancy, usually muscular in nature, and quite responsive to appropriate physical therapy. Significant congenital torticollis can cause marked facial asymmetry caused by external restriction in growth dynamics, and can exacerbate the underlying growth inhibition associated with microtia/craniofacial microsomia.

- **Is there evidence of cervical spine anomalies?** These may be seen in patients with syndromes along the OAV spectrum.

- **Does the patient have a murmur?** Ventricular or atrial septal defects and tetralogy of Fallot may be present in patients with syndromes along the OAV spectrum.

3. Several key diagnostic studies may be required for initial and preoperative evaluation of the patient with microtia. Some address the ear alone, while others search for associated anomalies.

- Congenital deformities of the cervical spine should be evaluated with preoperative **plain films** and/or a **CT scan of the neck**. Potential issues should be addressed prior to operative intervention to prevent serious injury.

- If an autogenous reconstruction is planned, **photographs** as well as a preoperative **X-ray film tracing** of the contralateral normal ear and its relation to the nose, oral commissure, and lateral canthus may be made. Intraoperatively, the inverted images are useful in determining the size, shape, and position of the reconstructed ear. Waterproof mirror-image digital photograph of the contralateral ear may also serve as a template. Correct placement of the pocket is critical to achieving an excellent surgical outcome. Measuring the cephalad and caudad extents of the normal ear, as well as its meatus and/or tragus, in relation to facial landmarks is valuable. However, some accommodation needs to be made in cases of significant facial asymmetry caused by hypoplasia. This necessary adjustment requires clinical experience as well as a careful attention to detail.

- **Ultrasonography** of the kidneys may be indicated in the presence of associated Goldenhar syndrome.

4. Like cleft patients, the long-term care of children with microtia requires a multidisciplinary effort.

- A developmental assessment should be made, specifically inquiring about the child's general behavior, school performance, social interaction with peers, and self-esteem. Evaluation by a **geneticist** may be indicated to identify any associated malformations (e.g., renal anomalies, any defects within the oculoauricular vertebral spectrum, mandibulofacial dysostosis syndromes, etc.).

- A **pediatric otolaryngologist** should assess children as early as possible to evaluate hearing and the potential need for hearing aids. Careful follow-up and possible, eventual middle ear reconstruction should also be considered in team approach.

- An **orthodontist** should participate in the routine evaluation of the patient with microtia, especially in the presence of a malocclusion or occlusal cant.

5. Reconstruction of the external framework may utilize either autogenous tissue or an alloplastic implant. Alloplastic reconstruction can generally be begun when the patient is as young as 4 to 5 years of age. Autogenous reconstruction is usually not performed prior to 6 years of age in order to allow for harvest of sufficient size donor rib cartilage. There are well-established advantages and disadvantages of each technique. The majority of reconstructive ear surgeons today still employ autogenous material, and this approach will be described in detail below. The modern technique of autogenous total ear reconstruction was developed by Tanzer, and popularized and modified by Brent, Nagata, and others. Reconstruction involves a variable staged approach. A common sequence is described below.

- **Stage one** involves the fabrication and insertion of a costochondral auricular framework.

    — The cartilaginous substrate for the framework is harvested through a slightly oblique incision measuring approximately 6 to 8 cm, located just above the contralateral costal margin. The synchondrosis of cartilages 6 and 7 is usually used for the auricular "base-block" of the reconstruction and the first free-floating rib is used in one or more sections for the helical rim. Prior to closing the donor site, the chest defect should be filled with saline while the lung is slowly expanded in a Valsalva-type maneuver in order to check for pneumothorax. The presence of air bubbles implies injury to the parietal pleura. This is not an uncommon occurrence during costal cartilage harvest and management is usually straightforward. A small red rubber catheter is placed into the parietal pleural defect. A figure-of-eight or purse-string suture is placed around the catheter. The wound is again filled with saline and the anesthesiologist is asked to provide another Valsalva expansion of the lung while the surgeon removes the catheter and draws the suture closed thereby stopping the air leak under direct vision. This is followed by a complete layered closure of rectus fascia, deep dermis, and skin. An upright radiograph is recommended to document any residual air in the pleural cavity.

— On a sterile back table, the framework is constructed. The base-block is trimmed and tailored using a template to guide shape and sizing. The free rib cartilage is carefully thinned and made delicate and flexible in order to wrap around the periphery of the base-block, fashioning a natural helical contour. The two components of the framework are spliced together using any of a variety of different suture materials. The author currently prefers to use a 4-0 braided polyester on double-armed straight needles. The base-block is placed onto a folded surgical towel and the double-armed needles are easily and precisely passed through the helical and base-block segments into the underlying towel upon exit. The knots are placed on the deep surface of the framework. It is important to exaggerate the contours of the framework since the overlying skin flap is thicker than that of a normal ear and will tend to obscure the sculpted detail. The back wall of the concha, antitragus, scapha, and triangular fossa may be carved with sharp gouges, fine curettes, and No. 15C and No. 11 scalpel blades.

— Finally, a pocket is created into which the framework will be placed. The incision for access may be placed anterior or superior to the microtic remnant. The skin flaps are kept as thin as possible to remove any hair follicles and to prevent concealment of the sculpted detail in the framework. Residual hair within the overlying flap may be treated subsequently with electrolysis. Any vestigial cartilage is removed at this time. The dissection is carried out beyond the immediate outline of the framework to facilitate draping of the skin over the cartilage and into its sculpted grooves and nooks. Suction drains should be placed beneath the framework, exiting peripherally within postauricular hair-bearing scalp, and should be left for 5 to 7 days. An adequate seal is imperative to maintain apposition of the skin to the framework. The ear is dressed with a soft Vaseline dressing to maintain contour.

- At **stage two**, at least 2 months later, the lobule is transposed with a Z-plasty. It is filleted open to receive the tip of the helix. This may be done concurrent with elevation of the framework for creation of a postauricular sulcus. An incision is placed several millimeters outside and all along the framework from the helical root to the lobular region. Care is taken to leave some soft tissue on the posterior surface of the cartilage to allow for skin graft take. The hairline is advanced into the postauricular sulcus and the remainder of the defect (the posterior surface of the framework) is closed using either a split- or full-thickness skin graft.

- At **stage three**, the conchal bowl is excavated and a tragus is created via an anterior "J-shaped" incision. Soft tissue is removed from the planned conchal bowl and lined with a full thickness skin graft harvested from the posterior lobule or posterior surface of the contralateral ear. The tragus is reconstructed by backing an anteriorly based skin flap with a composite chondrocutaneous graft harvested from the contralateral ear. Stages may be combined in the case of a bilateral microtia.

- The Nagata modification performs reconstruction in two stages. The created framework is inset through a Z-plasty incision designed to simultaneously rotate the lobule. Care must be taken to leave a small patch of undissected skin at the superior extent of the Z-plasty to preserve blood supply to the tips of the flaps. Necrosis in this area may lead to graft exposure and eventual loss. At the second stage, the conchal bowl and tragus are reconstructed.

- Alloplastic reconstruction utilizes an artificial material to reconstruct the ear. The components are assembled prior to insetting. The construct is wrapped under an inferiorly based flap of temporoparietal fascia and covered with a split thickness skin graft.

  — MedPor® (porous polyethylene) has been popular as an alternative to autogenous reconstruction. It is composed of porous polyethylene and is provided in two preformed pieces: a helical rim and combined antihelix, triangular fossa, tragus, and anti-tragus. The benefits of alloplastic reconstruction include reduced donor site morbidity, and the ability to perform reconstruction at a younger age. The disadvantages are increased framework exposure, concern over long-term permanence of the implant, and the necessary use of the temporoparietal fascial flap which sacrifices a valuable salvage procedure in the event of a complicated framework infection exposure.

  — Silicone is largely of historical note, but is still used by certain surgeons around the world.

6. Complications from ear reconstruction may be serious and may jeopardize the entire cartilage graft.

- **Pneumothorax** occurs with violation of the parietal pleura with harvesting autogenous rib cartilage, as discussed above. Because this almost surely only involves the parietal pleura, risk of tension pneumothorax is small. In the extremely unlikely event that a pneumothorax becomes symptomatic in the postoperative period, a repeat chest X-ray and/or immediate formal tube thoracostomy needs to be considered.

- **Infection**, when suspected, should be treated promptly with oral or intravenous antibiotics, depending on the extent and presence/absence of cellulitis. Incision and drainage of any purulence should be without delay.

- **Exposure of the cartilage framework** may be managed conservatively with meticulous cleansing and frequent application of 10% Sulfamylon cream, which effectively

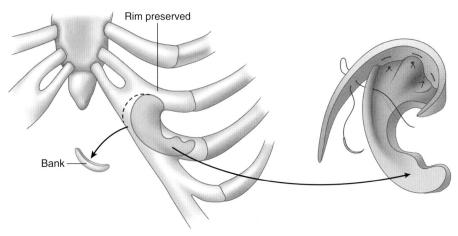

Rim preserved

Bank

Figure 19-1 Schematic drawing highlighting the donor site for reconstruction of the helical framework with costochondral cartilage.

penetrates cartilage. Areas of exposure larger than 2 to 3 cm, or showing no sign of granulation or wound contraction after several days may require either local flaps or ipsilateral temporoparietal fascia flap for larger defects. In the case of an alloplastic reconstruction, the TPF flap is no longer available, thus the implant either needs to be removed or a thin fascial flap needs to be transferred by microsurgical anastomosis from elsewhere.

- **Warping** only occurs with autogenous cartilage. It may be managed with a second cartilage graft, or with placement of an alloplastic framework.
- Long-term studies have noted **changes in the size of the implant** with time. Approximately half of the autogenous ear reconstructions grow at the same rate as the patient. Up to 40% may grow at a faster rate, while 10% grow slower.

PRACTICAL PEARLS

1. Most important of all for the treating physician is to convey a gentle compassion to the child and family in discussing the implications of both the deformity and the process that is involved in reconstruction. The physician should not lose sight of the psychological impact that a craniofacial anomaly may have on the patient and their family. Ascertain how much insight the child has into deformity and the influence it has had on self-esteem and social integration. It is rare for a child to demonstrate self-consciousness or anguish regarding their deformity prior to 5 years of age. Similarly, insults and ridicule from peers typically begins after 6 to 7 years of age.

2. The description of the surgical intervention may come across as mysterious, terrifying, or perilous. It is critical that realistic expectations regarding surgical outcome are established in advance for the patient and family. The use of drawings, pre- or postoperative photos of other patients, links to websites, and direct contacts with other patients may all be helpful in this regard. It is recommended that the patient and family understand that the product of any surgical reconstruction will never truly duplicate the delicately contoured, flexible, diaphanous structure of the elastic human ear.

3. It is helpful to converse directly with the child, describing in simple terms what the reconstructive process will entail including anesthesia, head bandages (with associated hearing limitation), drains, scars, activity restrictions, time out of school, and of course postoperative pain. Attempt to have the child articulate their motivations and/or concerns.

4. Be content in putting off surgery until the patient and family are comfortable with the issues presented and the treatment plan proposed. These efforts will help ensure that the patient and family will be more compliant and cooperative in the early postoperative convalescence period, and more satisfied in the long run.

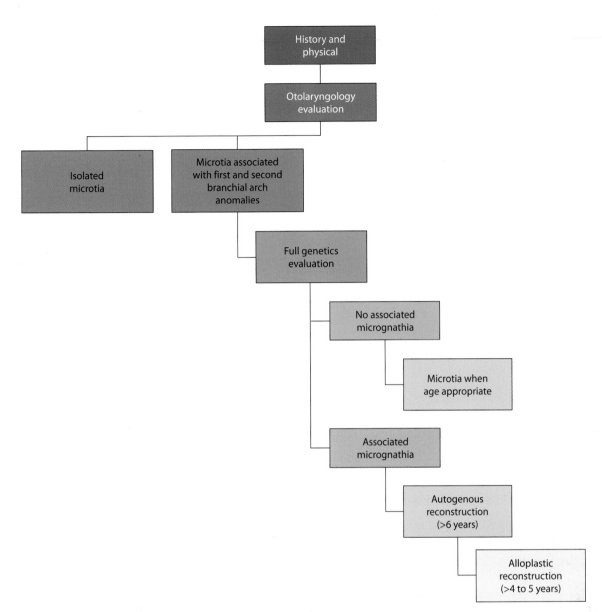

Algorithm 19-1 Algorithm for management of patients with microtia.

References

1. Moore KL, Persaud TVN. *The Developing Human, Clinically Oriented Embryology.* 7th ed. Philadelphia, PA: Elsevier Science; 2003.

2. Tietze L. Utilization of bone-anchored hearing aids in children. *Int J Pediatr Otorhinolaryngol.* 2001;58(1):75-80.

3. Jahrsdoerfer RA, Yeakly JW, Aguilar EA, et al. Grading system for the selection of patients with congenital aural atresia. *Am J Otol.* 1992;13(1):6-12.

4. Weerda H. Classification of congenital deformities of the auricle. *Facial Plast Surg.* 1988;5(5):385-388.

5. Aguilar EA III, Jahrsdoerfer RA. The surgical repair of congenital microtia and atresia. *Otolaryngol Head Neck Surg.* 1988;98(6):600-606.

6. Tanzer RC. *Reconstructive Plastic Surgery.* 2nd ed. Philadelphia, PA: WB Saunders;1977.

7. Stotland MA, Chang WT. A better template for microtia reconstruction: The waterproof, mirror-image digital photograph of the contralateral ear. *Plast Reconstr Surg.* 2007;119(7):2088-2091.

8. Wellisz T. Reconstruction of the burned external ear using a Medpor porous polyethylene pivoting helix framework. *Plast Reconstr Surg.* 1993;91(5):811-818.

9. Reinisch J. Ear reconstruction using a porous polyethylene implant, a twelve year experience. *ANZ J Surg.* 2003;73 Suppl 2:A185-A186.

10. Tanzer RC. Total reconstruction of the external ear. *Plast Reconstr Surg.* 1959;23:1-15.

11. Rueckert F, Brown FE, Tanzer RC. Overview of experience of Tanzer's group with microtia. *Clin Plast Surg.* 1990;17: 223-240.

12. Brent B. Microtia repair with rib cartilage grafts: A review of personal experience with 1000 Cases. *Clinics in Plastic Surgery* 2002;29:257-71.

13. Nagata S. Modification of the stages in total reconstruction of the auricle: Parts I-III. *Plast Reconstr Surg.* 1994;93: 221-253.

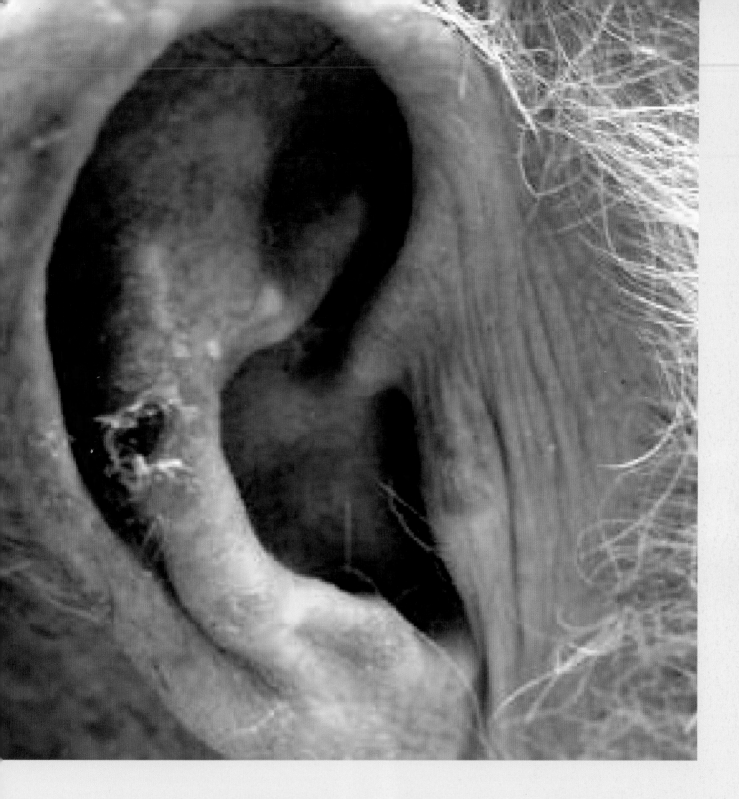

A patient is referred with a lesion

of the external ear.

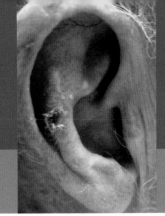

Ear Lesion

Larry H. Hollier, Jr.

1. Lesions of the auricular and periauricular regions may be benign or malignant. The latter are frequently associated with a history of excessive sun exposure and comprise approximately 5% of all skin neoplasms diagnosed annually in the United States. Primarily composed of basal cell cancer (BCC), squamous cell cancer (SCC), and rarely, melanoma, skin cancers originating on the ear continue to account for more than 25% of deaths caused by nonmelanoma skin cancers each year. Although treatment of these cancers has markedly improved in recent decades, closure of residual auricular defects continues to pose unique challenges to the reconstructive surgeon. As with all lesions, establishing an early diagnosis is essential to optimally managing tumors of the external ear framework. This is first performed with a directed patient history. Well-directed, initial questions should include:

- **How long has the lesion been present?** More chronic wounds are known to predispose to the development of squamous cell carcinoma.

- **Has there been any noticeable change in tumor appearance?** The patient's report of changes in the appearance of the lesion or the presence of any associated hearing problems should prompt increased concern.

- **Does the patient have a history of repeated sun exposure?** Sun exposure is the primary risk factor for the development of skin cancer. In addition, characterization of a potential chronic wound is essential. Marjolin's ulcer, or SCC arising from a chronically inflamed skin surface is well-documented occurrence.

- **Does the patient have any preexisting comorbid conditions?** In anticipation of probable resection and reconstruction, initial assessment should also note several important patient factors, such as medical history, skin type, history of prior tumors, environmental factors (e.g., where they work or whether they will continue to work outside), social factors, and patient expectations. Medical history alone may require extensive monitoring for a relatively slight procedure, and completely preclude more extensive surgical options. As always, the presence of hypertension, diabetes, or any potential vascular or immune compromise should be noted. Diabetic patients or those continuing to use tobacco must be advised to begin more appropriate blood-glucose management or quit smoking, as immediate improvements in either status facilitates likely surgical efforts.

- **Has the patient undergone prior surgical procedures in and around the head and neck?** Patients with previous local operations or tumors may have scars that obstruct the blood supply of potential flaps. In this event, a modified plan of reconstruction or delay procedure may be judicious.

- **Have other family members had similar lesions anywhere on their bodies?** A family history of malignancy, especially skin malignancy, is important to identify not only for the patient but also for other members of the family.

2. During the physical examination, the exact location of the lesion within the ear, as well as any appreciable adenopathy about the head and neck, must be accurately assessed.

- **Which part of the ear is involved?** The external framework of the ear is best divided into three areas: the superior third, middle third, and lower third. Because portions of the ear require differing reconstructive techniques based on tumor location, thorough clinical assessment of gross tumor extent often prevents surprises upon lesion resection. The site of the wound often dictates the choice of repair. While central defects with intact cartilage may do well with healing by secondary intention or skin grafting, advancement flaps are often utilized to return a normal curvature to the disfigured helix. More complex wounds, particularly those involving the middle and lower one-thirds may require slightly more extensive planning and closure techniques. Because each ear defect is unique, the surgeon must consider a wide range of reconstructive options to provide optimal aesthetic outcome.

- **Is the lesion mobile or fixed to underlying structures?** Fixation to underlying soft tissue or bone indicates malignant disease and generally presents a worse prognosis.

- **Are there concomitant lesions on the other ear or elsewhere on the head or neck?** Secondary lesions should be identified since they occur in areas of the head and neck that are exposed to similar amounts on sun exposure.

- **Are there enlarged lymph nodes?** Evaluation of palpable adenopathy within the head and neck is also imperative. As opposed to basal cell tumors, squamous cell tumors more frequently metastasize to lymph nodes of the face and neck area. The tragus, root of helix, and the superior helix arise from the first branchial arch and therefore drain to the parotid lymph nodes. Arising from the second branchial arch, antihelix, antitragus, and lobule drain to the cervical lymph nodes. Thorough evaluation of the regional lymph nodes cannot be overemphasized.

3. Suspicion of malignancy warrants a tissue diagnosis. Early determination of a lesion's identity and character is essential, and distinction between a benign process from one that is malignant is a priority.

    - Whether incisional or excisional, **biopsy** remains the gold standard for tissue diagnosis. Excisional biopsy is preferred when the resultant defect is amenable to primary closure with minimal tension. In cases of significantly large tumor or a very anatomically sensitive origin, an incisional biopsy may prove most useful.

    - In recent years, the course of external ear carcinoma has been appreciably improved by early diagnosis and treatment with **Mohs' microsurgery** (MMS). MMS is a technique that repeatedly provides a small amount of skin for diagnosis while excising the tumor cells to the margin of uninvolved tissue. If available, MMS provides both diagnostic as well as therapeutic management by excising tumor cells to the nearest tumor-free margin. While MMS may accomplish optimal margins in anatomically discrete areas that cannot afford extensive resection (i.e., lateral alar base or medial canthus), many discourage its use in the setting of melanoma since the true depth of the lesion holds important prognostic significance. Regardless of the technique, specimens sent for permanent sections more adequately show histopathologic detail, and should be more heavily relied upon than frozen section specimens.

    - In the event that MMS is unavailable, diagnostic confirmation and surgical management should be achieved with intraoperative frozen section despite the potential for added operating room time. This technique is a reasonable method in experienced hands. The obvious advantage of single-stage resection and reconstruction is the need for only one operative procedure.

    - In evaluation of regional involvement, thorough physical examination and appropriate imaging are critical. Further delineation of potential metastases may be made via **chest radiograph**, **CT scan**, or **MRI**.

4. Basal and squamous cell carcinomas of the ear are staged as follows

    T1: 2 cm or smaller.

    T2: 2 to 5 cm.

    T3: larger than 5 cm.

    T4: any size that demonstrates invasion.

    N0: no evidence of lymph node involvement.

    N1: spread to lymph nodes.

    M0: no distant metastases.

    M1: distant metastases.

    Stage I: T1 N0 M0

    Stage II: T2 or T3 N0 M0

    Stage III: T4 N0 M0 or any T N1 M0

    Stage IV: any T any N M1

    - Melanomas, on the other hand, are staged differently. Stage I lesions are up to 1.5 mm in depth with no lymphadenopathy. Stage II lesions are greater than 1.5 mm in depth with no lymphadenopathy. Stage III lesions have associated lymphadenopathy, while stage IV lesions present with metastatic disease.

    - Prior to attempting reconstruction, the potential need for adjuvant therapy should be discussed with an oncologist based on physical and diagnostic findings.

5. Following diagnosis, management involves surgical resection with reconstruction, adjuvant therapy if appropriate, and close follow-up.

    - While nonaggressive subtypes of BCC, such as nodular or superficial spreading, may be managed with 3 to 5 mm margins, the more aggressive morpheaform BCC variation requires 7 mm margins for sufficient extirpation. Adjunctive radiotherapy may be appropriate for more aggressive BCC tumors, and consultation of a radiation oncologist should never be delayed if concern is present.

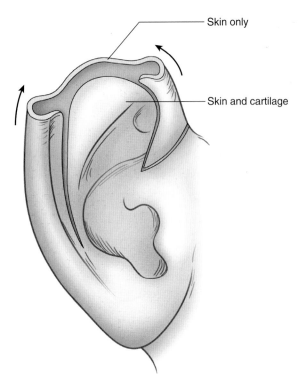

Skin only

Skin and cartilage

Figure 20-1 Schematic drawing highlighting Antia-Buch reconstruction of an upper one-third helical defect.

- Because of its more aggressive behavior, SCC requires a somewhat more extensive approach. In addition to a poorer prognosis, several studies have demonstrated a higher rate of recurrence and metastasis associated with invasive SCC of the external ear. These lesions should be resected with more liberal margins of at least 1 cm. Although radiotherapy is generally ineffective in SCC management, radiation is often advised for patients with significant risk factors, such as chemical exposure, viral infection, or immunocompromise.

- Although infrequent relative to BCC and SCC of the external ear, melanoma of this region warrants maximum concern. Subsequent to diagnosis, resection margins for melanoma are based on the depth of the lesion:

  — In situ lesions: 5 mm margins

  — Up to 1 mm in depth: 1 cm margins

  — 1 to 2 mm in depth: 1 or 2 cm margins

  — 2 to 4 mm in depth: 2 cm margins

  — >4 mm in depth: > 2 cm margins

- The need for further **lymphadenectomy** in cases of melanoma is also based on depth. Specimens greater than 1 mm in depth warrant a nodal staging procedure, such as a sentinel lymph node biopsy. As a result of a negligible risk of spread, lymphadenectomy is discouraged for lesions less than 1 mm in depth. Elective lymph node dissection is advocated for lesions 1 to 4 mm in depth; however, dissection is discouraged

for lesions greater than 4 mm in depth. Whereas the former case is associated with a 20% incidence of nodal metastasis, nodal bed involvement with lesions of the latter depth is a foregone conclusion. In these cases, with a 70% incidence of nodal metastasis, chemotherapy will always be given.

- Each ear defect is unique, and reconstruction must be based on defect size and location. It should be delayed until the resection margins are clear. Although several reconstructive options are available, planning should reflect principles of the reconstructive ladder, including primary closure, healing by secondary intention, and skin grafting. The major options may be broadly classified into two groups: wedge resection and direct advancement versus reconstruction with chondrocutaneous flaps. A variety of techniques have been used that are primarily dependent on whether the loss is partial thickness, full thickness, complete, or segmental. They are also dependent on the location of the defect. The ear may be divided into three topographic regions: antihelix/antitragus and helical rim (upper third), conchal bowl (middle third), and lobule (lower third).

- Lesions of the upper-third ear of the ear, such as those of the helical rim, are more amenable to either direct closure or a rotation flap

  — For many helical and antihelical defects less than 2 cm² in area, with or without perichondrial loss, direct closure with undermining of the surrounding edges following wedge resection is adequate. Although effective in maintaining relative proportions, wedge resection and extensive helical advancements will often shorten the vertical ear height.

  — For larger defects that are still less than 25% of total auricular area, a star-shaped excision, or anterior composite Burrow's triangle excision, can effectively redistribute tension throughout the ear to avoid "cupping" with primary closure. If these techniques fail to provide closure, use of a full-thickness skin graft may be preferred. Ideal skin graft donor sites include the periauricular, neck and supraclavicular areas.

  — Helical defects of between 25% and 50% may be managed with an Antia-Buch procedure. Lesions involving more than half of the framework often require borrowing postauricular skin over a cartilage graft. After freeing the entire helix from the scapha via an incision in the helical sulcus through underlying cartilage, the posteromedial auricular skin is undermined. Dissection just above the perichondrium further allows helical advancement from both directions to provide tension-free wound approximation. During this reconstruction, removal of a large portion of scaphoid may greatly augment closure of significant middle helical defects. Three stages are needed: (1) to tube

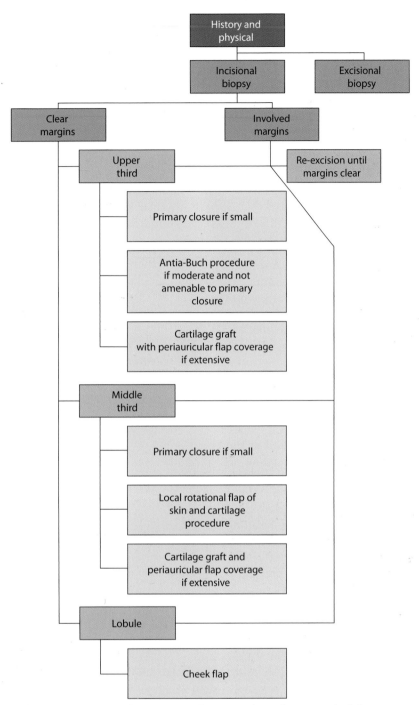

Algorithm 20-1 Algorithm for management of patients with external ear framework defects.

the postauricular skin vertically, (2) to release and inset 1 pedicle after 3 weeks, and (3) to release and inset the second pedicle 3 weeks later. The donor site may then be skin grafted.

— In reconstruction of larger full-thickness defects of the helix and antihelix, use of a composite-free graft up to 1.5 cm wide from the contralateral ear is an option. This technique involves harvest of a full-thickness wedge of skin and cartilage, approximately one-half the size of the defect, which is then replanted on the opposite ear. Theoretically, this should return symmetry to both ears.

- Middle and lower third defects often require direct closure, composite grafts or local flap reconstruction depending. Composite defects of the conchal bowl are often amenable to direct closure with or without helical advancement, secondary healing, full-thickness skin graft coverage, or retroauricular subcutaneous island flap replacement. Because exposed cartilage will eventually dessicate, three options are effective for cartilage coverage: local flap coverage, cartilage excision, or skin graft placement.

- Optimally, the defect is amenable to local rotational or advancement flap coverage. Local flap donor sites include the medial surface of the ear, preauricular, and postauricular tissue. Preauricular flaps for small antihelical defect coverage may be designed at the junction of the ear and face can receive inflow on either inferior or superior pedicles. This one-stage flap frequently leaves an inconspicuous temporomandibular surgery type scar. Flaps obtained from the medial surface of the ear are often simple, and the resulting scar very acceptable. Postauricular flaps are notably versatile and may be based superiorly, inferiorly, anteriorly, or posteriorly. In addition, cartilage previously placed inside the postauricular tissue may be raised along with skin and subcutaneous graft material. Coverage of a large lateral ear defect with a pedicled postauricular flap is a two-stage procedure. Following flap creation and placement over the auricular defect, pedicled flap division and closure is completed in conjunction with donor site coverage.

- Severe composite defects require much more extensive reconstruction, including new structural support in conjunction with vascularized skin coverage. Following creation of a structural framework using either auricular or costal cartilage, a temporoparietal fascial flap or skin grafting may provide adequate coverage.

- Over half of patients with skin cancer will develop a new cancer within 5 years. For this reason, close follow-up is strongly advised. Patients must also be informed that sun exposure is the probable cause of tumor growth, and a regimen including sun avoidance and sunscreens must be included in any postoperative plan.

6. As with all surgical procedures, **infection**, **bleeding**, and **scarring** may complicate an otherwise successful repair.

- Although local flaps utilized in larger defect closure may frequently show small areas of discoloration, significant **flap loss** is unusual when tissue tension, vascular flow, and sterile technique are managed appropriately.

- The tissue of the antihelix, helix, and crura is tightly bound by subcutaneous tissue to the perichondrium on the lateral surface. The tightly bound lateral tissues make these crura susceptible to irritations, such as **chondrodermatitis** following surgical manipulation.

PRACTICAL PEARLS

1. Never perform a shave biopsy to evaluate suspected melanoma.

2. A thorough evaluation of tumor extent, involvement of auricular structural units, and regional lymph nodes cannot be overemphasized.

3. Local undermining with direct closure, skin graft placement, and local flap creation permits coverage of a vast majority of auricular defects.

4. Auricular defects consisting of up to 50% of the upper structural third are frequently amenable to Antia-Buch reconstruction.

5. Over half of patients with skin cancer develop an additional tumor within 5 years. Close follow-up is strongly recommended, as is sunscreen use and sun avoidance if possible.

References

1. Reddy LV, Zide MF. Reconstruction of skin cancer defects of the auricle. *J Oral Maxillofac Surg.* 2004;62:1457-1471.

2. Silapunt S, Peterson SR, Goldberg LH. Squamous cell carcinoma of the auricle and Moh's micrographic surgery. *Dermato Surg.* 2005;31:1423-1427.

3. Manternach T, Housman TS, Williford PM, et al. Surgical treatment of nonmelanoma skin cancer in the Medicare population. *Dermato Surg.* 2003;29:1167.

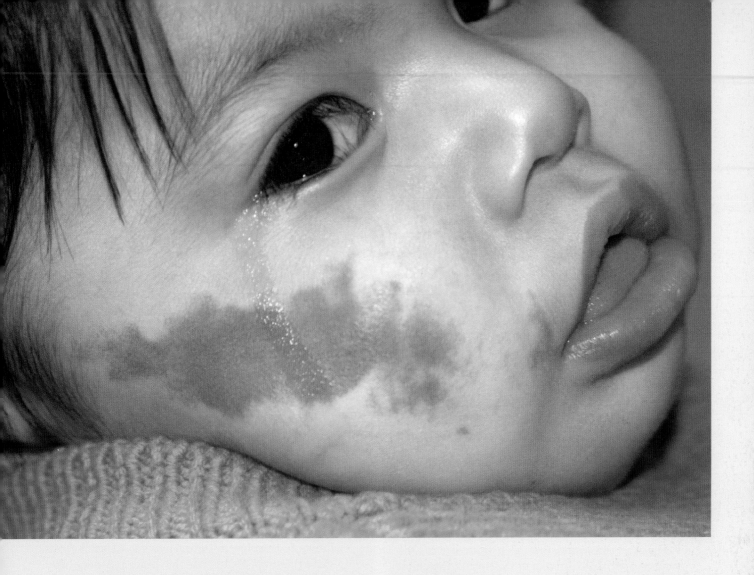

A 1-year-old boy is referred to your office

with a red lesion on the face.

CHAPTER 21

Venous Malformation

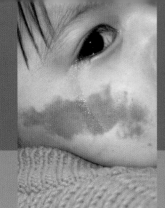

Robert Buka and Jessica Simon

1. The lesion in question appears vascular in nature. Congenital vascular lesions are a heterogeneous mixture of anomalies, which differ in both their clinical presentation and histopathological features. Historically, the nomenclature of these lesions has been inconsistent. In 1982, Mulliken and Glowaki addressed this by classifying vascular anomalies into two broad categories: **hemangiomas** are true tumors of endothelial cell origin, while **vascular malformations** are not tumors but rather normal cells arranged in an abnormal architectural pattern. The latter may be further characterized into capillary malformations, venous malformations, arteriovenous malformations, and lymphatic malformations, depending upon the predominant vessel type. The two major classes of vascular lesions continue to be confused, despite the clear difference in prognosis and treatment. Thus, a directed history is imperative to provide clues to the proper diagnosis.

- **When was the lesion first seen?** Vascular malformations are usually present at the time of the child's birth, but may or may not have been noted by the parents or clinicians. Hemangiomas usually appear sometime thereafter, often within the first couple of weeks.

- **Is the child male or female?** Hemangiomas are found more commonly in females while vascular malformations are equally distributed by gender.

- **How fast is the lesion growing? Is it growing commensurate with the patient?** Vascular malformations tend to grow commensurate with the child, showing a slow steady enlargement until puberty when pronounced expansion may occur with changes in sex hormone levels. Enlargement may also occur during physical activity or dependent positioning. By contrast, hemangiomas tend to grow rapidly during the early months of life, stabilize, and then regress slowly over the next several years. Once involuted, they often leave remnants, such as loose skin, telangiectases, and/or and fibrous fatty deposits.

- **Is there a history of recurrent infections?** Lymphatic malformations may be prone to recurrent bouts of local infection. This may be initially treated with antibiotics prior to any definitive intervention.

- **Is there a family history of similar lesions?** A family history of hemangiomas has been described in 10% of patients. Venous malformations and arteriovenous malformations have been found to be inherited in an autosomal dominant manner in a minority of cases. However, more often these lesions occur sporadically or appear as a clinical manifestation of congenital syndromes. Affected areas include the extremities as well as almost all other areas of the body. Both arteriovenous malformations and venular (port wine stain) malformations occur most frequently in the head and neck area.

- **Are there associated medical problems?** Associated complications are unique to each vascular lesion and depend on location and extent of the lesion.

- Vascular malformations within the V_1 and V_2 dermatomes may be associated with Sturge-Webber syndrome and involve the central nervous system. Venous malformations located in the head and neck may obstruct the airway, affect speech and/or dentition, or cause cosmetic defects. In such cases, ultrasound has been noted as the best method of determining the extent of the lesion. Complications of those in the limbs include pain, skeletal and skeletal muscle deformities, thrombosis and/or bleeding caused by localized intravascular coagulation, and phlebolith formation. Fast-flow arteriovenous malformations may produce high-output cardiac failure. Depending on the severity, treatment may consist of pharmacologic management, surgery, embolization or a combination of these.

- **Are there associated bleeding problems?** Bleeding is a complication of both vascular malformations and hemangiomas. In hemangiomas, this is usually a result of ulceration and can be controlled by compression of the affected area. More rarely, bleeding may be associated with Kasabach-Merrit syndrome, in which the vascular lesion—usually a kaposiform hemangioendothelioma or tufted angioma—triggers intravascular coagulation as a result of platelet trapping and release of cytokines (platelet-derived growth factor, for one), as well as a consumption coagulopathy. The thrombocytopenia is usually corrected when the tumor is controlled. The frequency of Kasabach Merritt syndrome in the United States is uncommon but it typically occurs in newborns or early infancy, rarely in adults. There is no racial or ethnic predilection and boys are affected slightly more often than girls. Prenatal cases may be diagnosed with the aid of ultrasonography.

2. The physical examination will help further clarify the diagnosis. Often, serial examinations are required to determine the growth characteristics of the lesion.

- **What color is the lesion?** With vascular malformations, and hemangiomas, the intensity of the color increases with proximity to the surface. Those in the superficial dermis may have a scarlet, red color while those in the deeper dermis have a darker, bluish hue. Midline, venular malformations (stork bites, nevus simplex) are usually lighter in color. Larger vessel lesions appear thick, purple, and cobblestoned.

- **Is the lesion flat or raised?** In the period of early proliferation, hemangiomas are often flat or macular. However, with proliferation, they may become raised off the surface of the surrounding skin. Venous malformations often present as flat patches. Arteriovenous malformations appear as firm masses which may be warmer or have a palpable thrill.

- **Does the lesion empty with compression?** Pressure on a hemangioma usually results in partial, but not complete, emptying when compressed. Venous malformations generally do not blanch when compressed.

- **Is there necrosis of the overlying skin?** Larger lesions may outstrip their blood supply and lead to ulceration in approximately 5% of lesions. This phenomenon is more commonly observed in hemangiomas.

- **Is there a particular distribution to the lesion?** Sturge-Weber syndrome consists of a triad of an upper facial venous malformation in the V_1 or V_2 distribution, vascular anomalies of the brain, and anomalies of the eyes (retinal detachment, glaucoma). The workup for a large hemangioma or venous malformation in the V_1 or V_2 distribution must include funduscopic examination and CT or MRI study of the brain.

- **Are there other physical symptoms?** A number of syndromes include vascular anomalies as part of the clinical presentation.

  — Blue rubber bleb syndrome includes skin and intestinal venous malformations so a thorough gastrointestinal examination, including digital rectal examination for blood in the stool, should be performed in suspected cases.

  — Klippel-Trenaunay syndrome involves venous malformations and limb hypertrophy.

  — Maffucci syndrome involves venous malformations and enchondromatoses.

  — Parkes-Weber syndrome involves arteriovenous malformations and soft tissue hypertrophy of an extremity.

  — Proteus syndrome involves vascular malformations and asymmetric gigantism, macrocephaly, epidermal nevi, and/or subcutaneous masses on the trunk (usually lipomas).

3. Appropriate tests/radiographic studies should be ordered to better delineate the nature of the lesion.

- Plain X-rays offer little information about the actual lesion, but should be obtained if there is any question of skeletal involvement.

- Ultrasound is a good initial study to document depth, extent, and flow within the lesion.

- MRI is perhaps the gold standard for evaluation and is usually preferred to CT in order to better evaluate the extent of soft tissue involvement.

- A biopsy of the lesion is rarely needed for diagnosis and may be problematic because of bleeding if performed in an office-based setting.

4. A management plan should be created that considers the input of clinicians from diverse specialties. Often, it is the best for patients with vascular anomalies to be seen in conjunction with a team well-versed in the diagnosis and management of these often challenging lesions, including:

- Plastic surgery.

- Pediatrics, hematology/oncology.

- Dermatology.

- Interventional radiology.

- Vascular surgery.

- Ophthalmology.

- Otolaryngology, for suspected lesions of the airway, some of which may cause sleep apnea.
- Gastroenterology, for suspected lesions of the GI tract.

5. The options for treatment differ by the diagnosis. Vascular malformations are often treated according to vessel type involved.

- **Venous malformations** respond either to sclerotherapy or laser treatment. Sclerotherapy involves intraluminal injury to the vessels with one of a number of agents including 5% sodium morrhuate, 95% alcohol, 1% to 3% sodium tetradecyl sulfate, or hypertonic saline. It is best used under general anesthesia and repeated every 4 to 6 weeks. Sclerotherapy alone is safest and most useful for lesions with no peripheral drainage or drainage into normal veins. It may be followed by surgical excision in extensive lesions. Sclerotherapy should not be used when there is a communication with the cavernous sinus (as seen in many upper and middle third of the face lesions via the superior and inferior ophthalmic veins, lower third lesions drain to the jugular system). Side effects include an allergic reaction, cerebral intoxication when alcohol is used, skin necrosis, and neuropraxia (from extravascular injection).*

  — Facial venular lesions ("port wine stain") never truly fade, but darken, thicken, and develop blebs. These lesions are often treated with the pulsed dye laser over several sessions, usually 4 to 5, separated by approximately 4-week intervals. Treatment success appears to vary with blood vessel diameter and density, where smaller vessel lesions (50 um to 150 um) respond better than do larger vessel lesions.

- **Capillary malformations** Nevus flammeus present very differently depending on their location. Most midline lesions disappear spontaneously by 1 year of age. However, those located on the nape of the neck may persist indefinitely. As transient lesions, treatment in most cases is not necessary. However, pulsed-dye laser may be used for cosmetic purposes if needed. The response to laser therapy is generally 15% for complete resolution, 65% for considerable resolution, and 20% for no improvement. Complications include hyperpigmentation, which usually resolves spontaneously or may be treated with 4% hydroquinone.

- Treatment of **arteriovenous malformations** involves super-selective embolization followed within 24 hours by an attempt at surgical resection the lesion. The inflow vessels should *not* be simply ligated since the lesions recruit new blood vessels. Surgical excision alone may be technically easier early, but is risky on

account of lower blood volume in the patient. For this reason, adjunctive preoperative embolization may be used prior to the anticipated procedure.

- **Lymphatic malformations** are primarily treated with surgery. Sclerotherapy reserved as an adjunctive option. The precise role for sclerotherapy has not been defined since alone it often leads to recanalization of the lesion. It may be useful for diffuse or persistent cases or macrocytic lesions. Good results have been seen with OKT3 and bleomycin, while inferior results have been noted with dextrose.

- Specific areas warrant special consideration.

  — Lesions involving the **lips** require an MRI to evaluate the extent of the lesion.

  — The **buccal fat** is a common site of involvement. Often, there is progressive enlargement of the lesion and surgical excision may require an extended parotidectomy incision and elevation of a flap superficial to parotid fascia but deep to SMAS. Here, it is important to identify the facial nerve (either antegrade or retrograde).

- Pulsed dye laser and surgical excision may be used in combination. Areas left with a paucity of tissue may require secondary soft tissue augmentation (autogenous fat, collagen, or hyaluronic acid).

6. Complications from the treatment of vascular malformations may be seen with surgery or less invasive modalities.

- With the use of the pulsed-dye laser, complications include **hyperpigmentation** seen in 10% to 20% of treated patients. This usually resolves spontaneously over time or may be treated with 4% hydroquinone.

- **Chronic hypopigmentation** is less common and may be managed with a topical concealer.

- The sclerosis seen with injection of lymphatic lesions may not be simply limited to the lesion but extend into the overlying skin and soft tissues. The resultant necrosis and **ulceration** may be initially treated with a topical dressing until it fully demarcates. Then, excision and further debridement will be required until the area is clean enough for eventual closure with either a skin graft or a soft tissue flap.

- Surgical excision may incompletely excise the entire lesion leading to **recurrence** or completely remove the tumor and leave a contour deformity. Both of these may be managed with follow-up procedures.

- Excision of any lesion in the face may cause injury to the facial nerve and temporary or permanent paralysis of the mimetic muscles of the face.

---

*Alternatively, the 595-nm pulse dye laser has assumed an equally prominent role in the noninvasive management for venous malformations. Directed laser energy serves to heat up vessels so rapidly as to induce their destruction and subsequent involution. These treatments may begin in infancy, are performed monthly, and may have a dramatic impact on eventual lesion size and cosmesis.

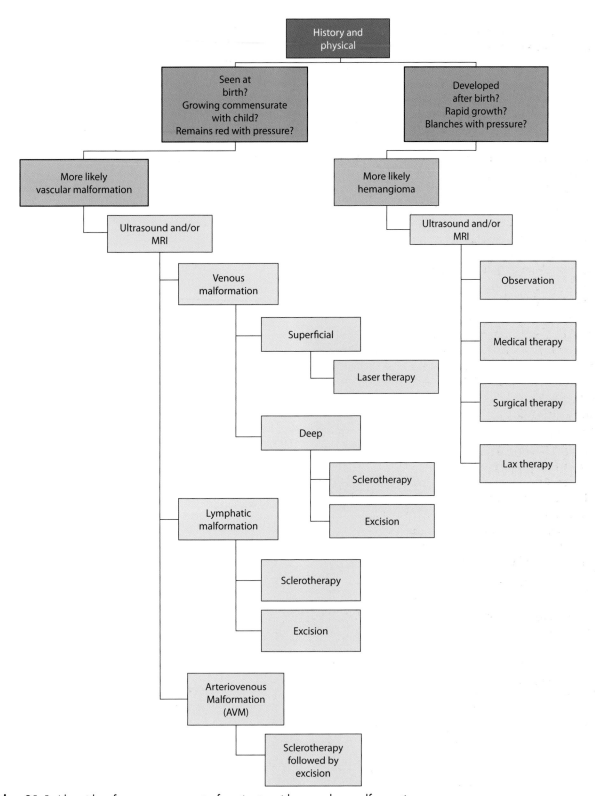

Algorithm 21-1 Algorithm for management of patients with vascular malformations.

PRACTICAL PEARLS

1. The proper diagnosis of a vascular lesion is of utmost importance, as there are distinct differences between the major classes of lesions in prognosis and treatment. Biologically, hemangiomas demonstrate hyperplasia of endothelial cells, up-regulation of growth factors (vascular endothelial growth factor [VEGF] and basic fibroblast growth factor [bFGF]) and activation of mast cells. Vascular malformations, on the other hand, demonstrate abnormal vessel architecture, with normal levels of growth factors and mast cells.

2. A thorough and directed history should be taken paying close attention to clinical behaviors of the lesion: hemangiomas tend to proliferate rapidly throughout the first 9 to 12 months of life, then slowly regress, while vascular malformations tend to grow as the child grows and may accelerate further in adolescence under hormonal influence.

3. For any lesion around the face, consultation by either an adult or pediatric ophthalmologist should be arranged to evaluate ocular involvement.

4. For the painful episodes seen with venous malformations, elastic compression (where possible) and low dose aspirin may be helpful.

5. Capillary malformations with smaller, more superficial vessels respond better to pulsed dye lasers, while venous malformations with larger, deeper vessel respond better to sclerotherapy and surgical excision.

References

1. Mulliken JB, Young AE, eds. *Vascular Birthmarks: Hemangiomas and Malformations*. Philadelphia, PA: Saunders; 1988.

2. Garzon MC, Huang JT, Enjolras O, Frieden IJ. Vascular malformations Part I. *J Am Acad Dermatol*. 2007;56:353-370.

3 Garzon MC, Huang JT, Enjolras O, Frieden IJ. Vascular Malformations. Part II: Associated Syndromes. *J Am Acad Dermatol*. 2007;56:541-564.

4. Astner S, Anderson RR. Treating vascular lesions. *Dermatol Ther*. 2005; 18(3):267-281.

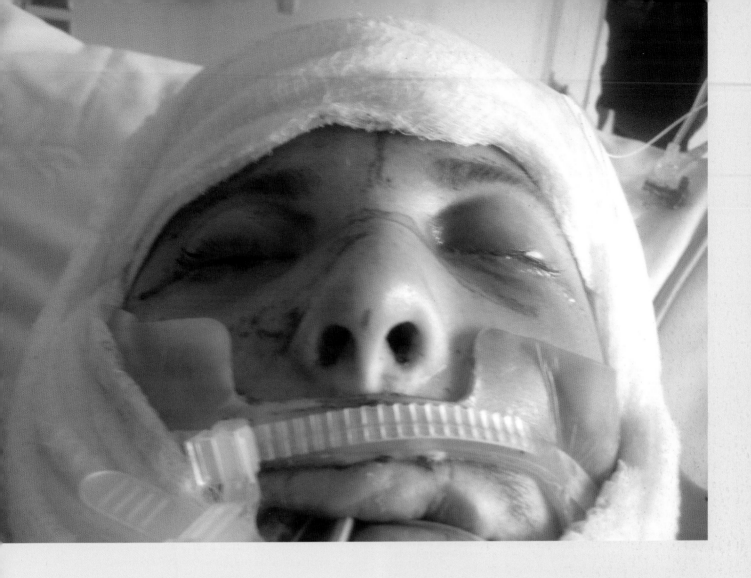

A 34-year-old man presents to the emergency department following a motor vehicle accident with suspicion of facial trauma.

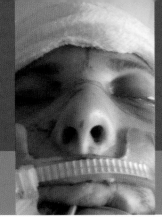

CHAPTER 22

Panfacial Fracture

Seth Thaller and David J. Pincus

1. The patient in question appears to have suffered unknown trauma to the head and neck. All trauma patients should be evaluated systematically, beginning with the **primary survey** to identify high priority problems. Recognition and acute treatment of concomitant life-threatening injuries is mandatory. Unseen blunt or penetrating trauma can be present in "facial trauma" patients, including intracranial injury, thoracic trauma, spinal injury, intra-abdominal trauma, pelvic, and long bone fractures, causing significant associated blood loss. Even prior to a detailed history the initial priority is the ABCs—airway, breathing, and circulation. Fractures of the facial skeleton are important in the primary survey as they may affect ventilation, either directly by fracture displacement or indirectly by causing bleeding.

- The first goal is to establish a patent **airway**. Signs of upper respiratory obstruction, such as crowing, stridor, or air hunger, usually signify significant injury to the hypopharynx and/or larynx and mandate immediate intubation, possibly via tracheotomy.

- With a patent airway, it is important to assess whether the patient is **breathing** effectively and provide ventilatory support in the way of CPR or mechanical ventilation if the patient is not. Adequate chest excursion should be noted with inspiration. No air should be heard over the stomach. And an end-tidal carbon dioxide monitoring device should be available to confirm tracheal placement of a ventilation tube.

- Adequate systemic **circulation** must be assured by palpating a pulse at either the carotid in the neck, the radial at the wrist, or the femoral in the groin. Administration of intravenous fluids will improve blood volume and perfusion pressure in the hypovolemic patient resulting from traumatic blood loss. Obvious areas of hemorrhage should be addressed in the primary survey with compression.

- A thorough history should be obtained from witnesses or rescue personnel. Information related to the specific traumatic event as well as the presence of any preexisting medical conditions or use of medications should be obtained.

- **Does the patient remember the entire event?** Failure to recall details of the trauma can be caused by loss

of consciousness which would indicate possible brain injury however minor. In such cases, diagnostic imaging and extended observation would be indicated.

- **Where was patient sitting?** Certain injuries are more likely depending on the patient's location in the vehicle. Steering wheel injuries occur almost exclusively in drivers. Back seat passengers are further from impact in the setting of a head-on collision.

- **Was the patient restrained or was the patient found outside the vehicle?** Airbags and shoulder/lap belts restrain passengers in their seats and prevent injury from movement within the vehicle and ejection from the vehicle.

- **Was the steering wheel or dashboard deformed? Was the windshield cracked?** Circumstances surrounding the injury can be quite valuable in directing the search for unrecognized trauma. Such information can identify the associated intra-abdominal, intrathoracic, neurosurgical, and/or orthopedic injuries.

- **Does the patient have any change from preinjury vision?** A basic ophthalmologic examination, including light perception, field of vision, and evaluation of extra ocular muscle movements, should be performed in addition to eventual consult by the ophthalmologist.

- **When was the patient last immunized for tetanus?** Current recommendations for tetanus immunization

- **Does the patient have a history of prior eye surgery?** Any previous eye surgery has the potential to increase the risk of globe rupture following a trauma.

- **Does the patient have any existing medical conditions, take any medications, or have any known drug allergies?** These are always important to note in the history as they may complicate resuscitative efforts.

- **Does the patient drink excessively, smoke, or abuse medications or drugs?** Significant information may be obtained from a review of the patient's social history. A history of smoking may compromise respiratory efforts while a history of alcohol abuse may have led to liver disease and problems with coagulation.

2. A thorough secondary survey should be performed to identify unrecognized injury and specific trauma to the facial skeleton.

- **Are there any areas of point tenderness or crepitus?** Point tenderness may indicate the site of a fracture.

- **Are there any palpable step-offs across the skull, around the orbits, within the midface, or along the mandible?** Step-offs indicate areas of displaced fracture fragments. Swelling may obscure any visible signs of fracture.

- **Is the maxilla mobile?** This can be ascertained by bimanually grasping the anterior maxilla and nasion and determining if the two move separately from one another.

- **Is there dental injury?** Loose teeth may be swallowed inadvertently. They may also need to be addressed by wiring or extraction depending on their nature of their injury. This may require chest X-ray.

- **What is the occlusal status?** Any change from the patient's preinjury occlusion may indicate either displacement of the maxilla, mandible, or both. Preinjury occlusion is judged by the normal wear patterns of the teeth that make "facets" in areas of longstanding contact.

- **Is the trachea midline?** Is there tenderness or crepitus of the cervical spine? Without removing the collar, palpation of the cervical vertebrae should be performed to identify any undiagnosed bony injury. Further radiographic images are imperative but an early examination is important.

- **Are there other associated injuries to the trunk and/or extremities?** Care of such injuries/extremities is exercised by taking precedence to any facial trauma.

3. Diagnostic tests should commence at the time of the primary survey and include cardiac monitoring and pulse oximetry.

   - A routine set of trauma laboratory values includes a complete blood count, serum chemistries (including liver function tests), coagulation parameters, and a type and crossmatch for blood products if necessary.

   - Imaging studies are invaluable in the diagnosis of facial trauma. Specific studies may be obtained at the time key trauma studies are ordered. Expeditious radiological examination of the cervical spine, chest, and pelvis are indicated in the presence of blunt trauma. Initial laboratory studies should be obtained for baseline and some repeated for comparison to identify ongoing hemorrhage.

     — Plain X-rays of the head and neck have largely been supplanted by **CT scanning** to evaluate head and neck fractures. In general, two-dimensional images in the axial and coronal planes with appropriate slices (1.5 to 2.0 mm slices) are sufficient to diagnose the vast majority of facial fractures. Additional three-dimensional reconstruction of the images provides a better understanding of the fracture patterns and communication with patients and families, as well as colleagues. In patients with frontal sinus fractures, it is important to perform a CT scan early because of the increased incidence of associated CNS injury which may be identified by the presence of pneumocephalus.

     — An **orthopantomogram** is helpful in the assessment of mandibular fractures. The entire bone is reproduced as a flat image as the device rotates around the head. The patient needs to be able to sit in an upright position to accomplish the study. While symphyseal area is often distorted, the more lateral areas of the mandible are well visualized.

4. Appropriate consultations should be considered based on each individual patient's clinical findings. All patients with severe trauma should be evaluated by the dedicated **trauma service** before all else.

   - Any evidence of head or spinal trauma warrants evaluation by the **neurosurgery** service.

   - Periocular trauma warrants evaluation by the **ophthalmology** service which should perform a posterior chamber examination despite its difficulty in an emergency department setting

5. Management of patients with facial trauma begins immediately with the arrival to the emergency department.

   - Nonoperative intervention includes initial **intravenous access** to handle fluid resuscitation requirements. Two large bore intravenous lines should be started and two liters of lactated Ringer's solution administered in an otherwise healthy patient. Excessive blood loss from soft tissue injuries of the head and neck may occur as a result of the significant vascularity in that region.

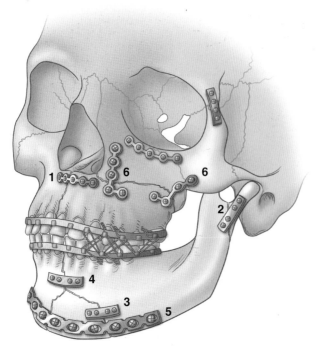

Figure 22-1 Schematic drawing highlighting placement of plates and screws for fixation of common fracture patterns.

— Oxygen is generally considered safe in any patient for a limited period of time and may be lifesaving.

— For patients with extensive injury, a **Foley catheter** should be inserted and urine output should be measured hourly.

— A **nasogastric tube** should be placed to suction to maintain gastric decompression.

— Analgesics and sedatives can be given as needed, but only after a thorough examination is completed to identify sites of pain or tenderness. They should be given intravenously only since intramuscular absorption is erratic. Small doses should be used, titrated to clinical response.

— Patients must be kept warm using warm intravenous fluids, warm gases if the patient is intubated, and adequate coverings. Hypothermia is a frequent and often serious problem in these patients. The patient's core temperature should be continually monitored.

• Operative management differs based on the site and complexity of the fracture:

— The management of **frontal bone and sinus fractures** depends on the status of the anterior and posterior tables of the sinus. These may present with obvious deformities or be obscured by other physical findings including contusions, lacerations, or hematomas. It is important to perform CT scan early because of the increased incidence of associated CNS injury with these fractures. A key finding is pneumocephalus or air within the cranial vault, often seen with disruption of the posterior table of the frontal sinus. Observation is generally satisfactory with nondisplaced anterior table fractures and posterior table fractures without CSF leak. Displaced anterior table fractures should be reduced and fixed. Displaced fractures of the posterior table with CSF leak require cranialization and an interdisciplinary approach with neurosurgery. For operative treatment, a coronal incision affords satisfactory exposure to inspect the anterior table and sinus. Often lacerations provide surgical exposure of the fracture pattern. The anterior table fragments are removed and kept in moistened gauze. If the nasofrontal duct is fractured, it is obliterated by removing the sinus mucosae, burring the bone, and filling the ducts with morcellized bone, fat, muscle, and/or artificial material such as tissue sealant.

— Indications for exploration in the presence of a pure **orbital floor fracture** include defects greater than 1 cm on the coronal CT scan, mechanical muscle entrapment, or acute enophthalmos. The floor is approached through any of a number of periorbital incisions. A transconjunctival incision is completely hidden since it is on the internal lamella of the eyelid. Dissection via this approach may be anterior or posterior to the septum and ends at the orbital rim. The floor is then exposed in a subperiosteal plane. Contents of the orbit that have herniated into the maxillary sinus are replaced into the orbit and the margins of the defect are identified circumferentially. Care is taken not to dissect into the orbit further than the extent of the posterior wall of the maxillary sinus to avoid injury to the optic nerve. A defect of the floor is bridged with either autogenous bone or alloplast. Bone from the fracture itself or from a remote site such as the outer table of calvarium, rib, or iliac crest may be used. Alloplastic materials include meshed titanium plates, sheets of silicone rubber, or discs of hydroxyapatite. These require no harvest procedure but remain foreign bodies that may or may not integrate with the host tissues.

— **Naso-orbital-ethmoid fractures** often require a coronal incision for exposure of the medial orbit and reconstruction of the medial canthus. Depending on the amount of bone that carries the medial canthus, the fracture fragments should be reduced and fixed. A medial canthal tendon that has detached from bone requires transnasal wiring to fix it to the contralateral side. Separate reattachment of the loose, if necessary, dorsal nasal support may be accomplished using a cantilever bone graft.

— **Nasal fractures** may be treated early with closed reduction using local anesthesia within the first 1 to 2 weeks. Associated hematomas of the septum should be immediately evacuated to prevent distortion and collapse. Internal packing and external

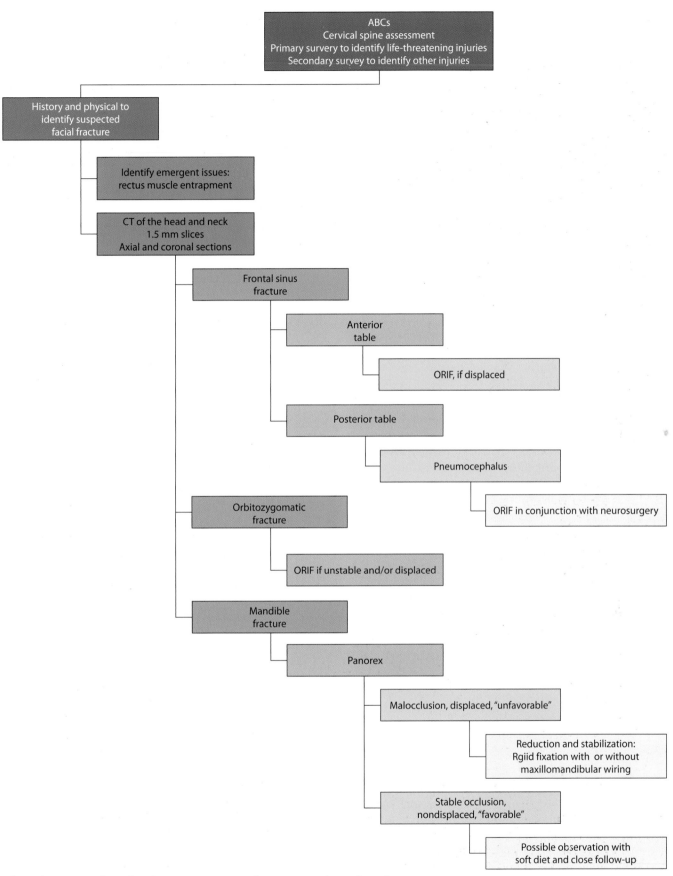

Algorithm 22-1 Algorithm for management of patients with panfacial trauma.

splints are applied following reduction and kept in place for 7 to 10 days. Repair of nasal fractures after bony union has occurred requires osteotomy and manipulation.

— The fixation of a **zygomatic fracture** following accurate reduction requires a minimum of three points of fixation for adequate stabilization. Exposure is achieved through a combination of upper and lower eyelid incisions and a gingivobuccal sulcus incision on the side of the fracture. Severely displaced fractures may require plating of the arch via a coronal incision. Visible deformities or trismus are indications for operative intervention in the presence of isolated arch fractures.

— **Maxillary fractures** are most often described with the Le Fort classification. If the occlusion is altered, intermaxillary fixation may be required to reestablish the preinjury dental occlusion. The medial and lateral buttresses are reduced and plated to restore the proper vertical and sagittal dimensions of the face. In the absence of suitable native bone, autogenous bone grafts may be required.

— **Mandible fractures** often result in malocclusion. A panoramic radiograph of the lower jaw is the most useful study because it allows evaluation of the entire mandible, including the condyles, in one image. The goal of operative repair is the accurate reestablishment of dental occlusion. Nondisplaced fractures may be treated with either maxillomandibular fixation (MMF) for 4 to 6 weeks or open reduction and internal fixation to allow early postoperative functioning. Displaced fractures generally require open reduction and internal fixation. Repair begins with placement of arch bars and IMF to align the fracture fragments and restore preinjury occlusion. After fixation, MMF is removed and alignment is checked. If the occlusion is adequate, the arch bars may be left and the patient left in simple vertical guiding elastics. After a stable period of 2 weeks, the arch bars may then be removed in the office. If there is any indication of misalignment, then reduction and fixation need to be repeated until satisfactory. Teeth that interfere with mandibular alignment or have associated periodontal involvement are extracted at the time of fracture repair.

— **Alveolar fractures** usually present with mucosal and palatal lacerations. These fractures demonstrate mobility of the maxillary dentition. Alveolar fractures require additional reduction and splinting along with the techniques used in fixation of Le Fort-type fractures.

6. Numerous complications are possibly following craniomaxillofacial trauma—some from the injuries themselves and some from the necessary interventions.

- Infectious complications specifically with frontal sinus fractures can include life-threatening complications such as **meningitis** and **osteomyelitis**. Mucopyocele can be a late complication.

- **Malunion** or nonunion of bone can occur with any fracture. Accurate reduction and rigid fixation can minimize the risk. Open internal fixation without proper reduction of the fracture fragments is often worse than no initial treatment at all.

- **Visual disturbance** should be identified and documented at the initial examination and then repeated frequently.

- **Lid retraction** may be a late complication from exposure of fractures around the orbit. Transconjunctival incisions are thought to produce less retraction than subciliary incisions but may not provide as much exposure.

- Malocclusion occurs with displacement of a segment of either the upper or lower jaw. Any discrepancy from the preinjury occlusion should be noted at the initial examination and investigated with the appropriate imaging tests. Following manipulation of the maxilla or mandible, confirmation that the adequate preinjury occlusion has been restored is imperative.

- The most common complication following repair of naso-orbital-ethmoid fractures is residual deformity, including **telecanthus**.

PRACTICAL PEARLS

1. Several key areas of bleeding should be noted as they relate to more important injury. Raccoon sign is periorbital hematoma, which results from a basilar skull fracture. Battle's sign is postauricular ecchymosis, which is an indication of fracture of the base of the posterior portion of the skull.

2. A key ophthalmologic finding is a Marcus-Gunn pupil, which is noted by absence of constriction of a unilateral pupil because of a lesion in the afferent visual pathway anterior to the chiasm.

3. Postinjury, enophthalmos may not be present despite significant displacement of the bony orbit on account of the edema. If the decision is made to observe the patient, then frequent follow-up is important to identify the development of orbital dystopia.

4. Fractures in the region of the symphysis and parasymphysis may be overlooked on a panoramic study of the mandible because of overlap causing blurring in this area.

5. Following naso-orbito-ethmoid fracture, accurate placement of transnasal wires requires positioning the wires as posterior as possible to restore accurate anatomic alignment.

References

1. Thaller,S, Blaisdell, FW. Trauma and Thermal Injury: Injuries to the Face and Jaw. In: *ACS Surgery: Principles and Practice*, 2008, on-line at http://www.acssurgery.com/acs/main.htm.

2. Edwards MC, Hollier LH. Facial fractures. In: Greer SE, Benhaim P, Longaker MT, Lorenz HP, eds. *Handbook of Plastic Surgery*. New York, NY: Marcel Dekker; 2004:223-235.

3. Manson P. Assessment and management of facial injuries. In: Weinzweig J, ed. *Plastic Surgery Secrets*. Philadelphia, PA: Hanley and Belfus; 1999:130-134.

4. Marsh JL. *Decision Making in Plastic Surgery (Clinical Decision Making Series)*. Mosby Year Book, 1993.

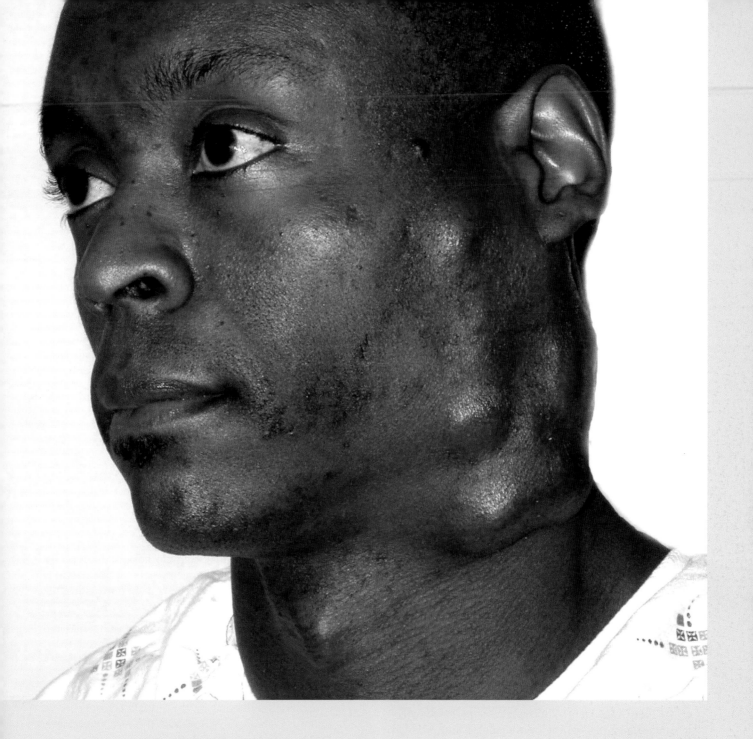

A 32-year-old patient presents with an enlarging mass as shown above.

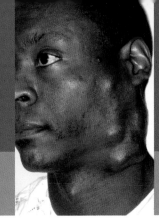

CHAPTER 23

Cheek Mass

Eric Genden

1. Because of its location, the mass in question likely of parotid origin. The gland itself lies anterior to the lobule of the ear and is most superficial over the ascending ramus of the mandible. Within its substance lie the branches of the main trunk of the facial nerve. In addition to location, a detailed history is important in the diagnosis of lesions in the cheek.

- **How long has the mass been present?** The majority of masses in the parotid gland are benign. Typically, they are slow growing tumors that are often incidentally discovered. Sudden enlargement is more common in cystic or malignant processes. A rapidly enlarging mass that is associated with pain and or facial weakness should raise concerns about the possibility of a malignancy. Tender masses are more likely inflammatory.

- **Does the mass interfere with swallowing or eating?** It is rare that a cheek or parotid mass will cause difficulty with mastication of eating; however, invasive lesions and malignancies involving the pterygoid musculature may result in trismus, pain, trigeminal deficit, or difficulty chewing.

- **Is the lesion painful?** Painful lesions often imply malignant invasion into the nearby peripheral nerves.

- **Is the lesion mobile?** Fixed lesions often imply malignant invasion of the tumor into surrounding structures.

- **Are there associated skin changes?** Superficial malignancies may invovle the overlying skin and produce an ulcer or a peau d'orange appearance.

- **Has the patient noticed recent weight loss?** As with other tumors, weight loss is more commonly associated with malignancy and portends a poor prognosis.

- **Is there facial weakness?** Facial weakness is commonly a result of malignant invasion of the facial nerve.

2. A physical examination of the head and neck is often sufficient to determine if a mass is present. It is also able to provide important clues as to the pathology of the lesion.

- **Where is the mass located?** Benign lesions of the parotid gland are most commonly located in the superficial aspect of the tail of the gland. Because the tail of the gland can descend below the angle of the mandible, it is not uncommon that tumors of the parotid are mistaken for a neck mass. Deep lobe parotid tumors are not usually palpable. Because they arise from the poststyloid fossa, as they enlarge, they impinge on the parapharyngeal space. This gives rise to fullness in the tonsil as seen on oral cavity examination.

- **Are there enlarged lymph nodes in the neck?** Once the primary lesion has been identified, the patient should be examined for secondary lesions and lymph node involvement. The lymph nodes of the neck (Figure 23-1) for the purpose of neck dissection are divided into six areas, or levels.

  — The submental triangle houses the **level IA** nodes and is bounded by the anterior belly of the digastric muscles (laterally) and the hyoid (inferiorly). The submandibular triangle houses the **level IB** nodes and is bounded by the body of the mandible (superiorly), the stylohyoid (posteriorly), and the anterior belly of the digastric (anteriorly).

  — **Level II** houses the upper jugular lymph nodes and is bounded by the inferior border of the hyoid (inferiorly), the base of skull (superiorly), the stylohyoid muscle (anteriorly), and the posterior border of the sternocleidomastoid muscle (posteriorly). Level II is divided by the spinal accessory nerve into A nodes (anterior) and B nodes (posterior). The upper jugular lymph node basin represents the first echelon of lymph nodes for the spread of malignant disease. Examination of the level II lymph node basin should be routinely performed to rule out metastasis. Additionally, the remainder of the gland should be carefully assessed as patients that have had prior surgery on the parotid gland are at risk for seed recurrence. This is most commonly a result of a seeding of the parotid bed during a prior parotidectomy for pleomorphic adenoma. Although not malignant, this tumor has a high risk of recurrence if there is tumor spill during the initial operation.

  — **Level III** houses the middle jugular lymph nodes and is bounded by the inferior border of the hyoid

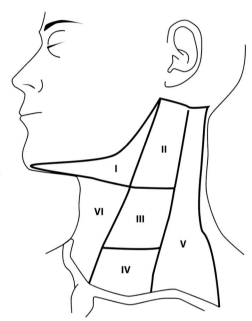

Figure 23-1 Schematic drawing highlighting the draining lymph node basins in the neck.

(superiorly), the inferior border of the cricoid (inferiorly), the posterior border of the sternohyoid (anteriorly), and the posterior border of the SCM (posteriorly).

— **Level IV** houses the lower jugular lymph nodes and is bounded by the inferior border of the cricoid (superiorly), the clavicle (inferiorly), the posterior border of the sternohyoid (anteriorly), and the posterior border of the SCM (posteriorly).

— **Level V** houses the posterior compartment lymph nodes and is bounded by the clavicle (inferiorly), the anterior border of the trapezius (posteriorly), and the posterior border of the SCM (anteriorly). Level VA lies above the level of the inferior border of the anterior cricoid arch, while level VB lies below.

— **Level VI** houses the anterior compartment lymph nodes and is bounded by the common carotid arteries (laterally), the hyoid (superiorly), and the suprasternal notch (inferiorly).

● **Is there facial asymmetry?** The presence of presurgical facial nerve palsy suggests malignancy. Each

branch of the facial nerve should be assessed for motion and strength:

— **Is the patient able to raise his brow?** Test frontal branch function and frontalis muscle innervation.

— **Is the patient able to close his eyes?** Test zygomatic branch function and orbicularis oculi innervation.

— **Does the patient have a symmetrical smile?** Test buccal branch function and buccinator muscle innervation.

— **Is the patient able to show his lower teeth?** Test marginal mandibular branch function and depressor anguli oris innervation (among others).

— **Is the patient able to tense the neck muscles?** Test cervical branch function and platysma innervation.

3. It is important to determine if the mass is benign or malignant. Clues to the pathology may be gained from imaging studies and/or tissue samples.

● Following a physical examination, **fine needle aspiration** (FNA) remains a useful diagnostic tool. A cellular aspirate can often confirm the diagnosis without the need for further intervention. Overall approximately 80% of parotid lesions are benign and 20% are malignant. The necessity of FNA is debated. While the information gained from an FNA is useful in counseling the patient, it seldom changes the approach to therapy. Most head and neck surgeons will consider an FNA if the mass is fixed, irregular on imaging, or painful. These findings suggest malignancy and a preoperative FNA will identify the diagnosis and the likely need for a neck dissection at the time of surgery.

— The most common tumor of the parotid is a benign pleomorphic adenoma (benign mixed tumor). These tumors presents as a mobile, painless, firm mass. Fixation to the underlying tissue may suggest malignancy.

— The second most common tumor is the Warthin's tumor (papillary cystadenoma lymphomatosum). It represents around 5% of all parotid tumors. The patients are usually male and the lesions may be multicentric or bilateral. Malignant degeneration in these lesions is rare.

— The most common malignant tumor of the parotid gland is the mucoepidermoid tumor.

— The second most common malignant tumor of the parotid is adenoid cystic carcinoma. Others include primary adenocarcinoma and metastatic lesions.

- **CT scan or MRI** of the head and neck should be able to clearly delineate the boundaries of the lesion and sites of potential invasion. Both imaging modalities are sensitive and specific. In rare cases where a malignancy is identified, a coregistered PET/CT is useful in identifying the extent of disease.

4. The diagnosis of malignancy should warrant consultation with an **oncologist** for evaluation of the need for adjuvant therapy.

- Adjuvant radiation is indicated in specific circumstances:

— Gross or microscopic residual disease.

— Disease close to the facial nerve.

— Documented lymphatic metastases.

— Extra-parotid extension of malignant tumors.

— It may also be applied to patients with multiple recurrent pleomorphic adenoma that has resulted in military seeding of the parotid bed.

5. The treatment of choice for most parotid tumors, either benign or malignant, is **parotidectomy**. Since most tumors lie in the inferior portion of the lateral lobe, they are amenable to removal of the superficial portion of the gland. Preoperatively, it is important to discuss potential injury to the facial nerve.

- During the procedure, paralytic agents should be avoided and a nerve stimulator should be available to identify branches of the facial nerve.

- Parotidectomy is performed through an extended face-lift incision with the submuscular aponeurotic system (SMAS) layer included in the flap.

- The proximal facial nerve is carefully identified cognizant of its course through the face. The nerve exits from stylomastoid foramen. It can be identified by dissecting out the pointer of the tragal cartilage, the tympanomastoid suture line, the anterior border of the sternocleidomastoid muscle, and the posterior belly of the digastric muscle. Using these landmarks, the nerve can be identified adjacent to the tympanomastoid suture line. Once the main trunk of the facial nerve has been identified, the peripheral branches can be dissected free from the gland as the tumor is resected.

6. The more common complications following parotidectomy include bleeding and wound infection; the more serious ones are related to injury to branches of the facial nerves.

- **Bleeding** is rare; however, meticulous hemostasis prior to wound closure is essential since elevations in blood pressure with emergence from anesthesia can incite new bleeding.

- The incidence of **wound infection** is similarly low but usually involves common organisms from the skin. A dose of preoperative antibiotics is prudent.

- **Facial nerve injury** is the most worrisome complication. Postoperative paresis occurs in less than 5% of patients. The nerve should be sacrificed if invaded by malignant disease and microneural reconstruction should be performed at the time of the initial surgery. A nerve graft can be harvested from the greater auricular if a single cable of nerve is required, or from the lateral sural nerve if the multiple cables are necessary. **Facial paralysis** is a devastating complication that requires careful postoperative management. Most importantly, incomplete eye closure requires careful attention to detail. A moisture chamber, eye lubrication, and daily assessment for dry eye and scleral injection should be performed. Thereafter, gold weight implant and canthopexy may be necessary for incomplete eye closure and lagophthalmos. Failure to manage the incomplete eye closure can result in exposure keratitis, infection, and blindness.

- The parotid normally receives parasympathetic fibers from the auriculotemporal nerve which triggers the release of saliva with chewing. Division of the small nerve fibers with parotidectomy followed by aberrant reinnervation of the overlying sweat glands of the skin leads postoperative sweating of the cheek during swallowing or eating ("Frey syndrome"). It is seen in approximately 5% to 10% of postoperative patients. The diagnosis may be made by painting the skin with starch iodide and observing the cheek for bluish discoloration with eating. Treatment options include topical anticholinergics, such as atropine, fascial grafts interspersed beneath the skin flap, and injection of dilute botulinum toxin which may be 80% to 100% effective.

- **Injury to the greater auricular nerve** is an inevitable side effect of parotidectomy since the greater auricular nerve traverses the gland and must be sacrificed during the operation. Patients should be made aware that they will experience numbness of the inferior ear lobe for 2 to 3 months.

- **Salivary fistula** and/or **sialocele** are rare complications that results from a communication between the remaining parotid tissue and the skin. Salivary fluid, high in amylase, may collect under the skin flaps. A conservative regimen of observation usually results in spontaneous closure; however, in some case surgical intervention is necessary.

- **Deformity of the cheek** following surgery may result after the excision of a large parotid tumor. Fat grafting or augmentation with acellular dermis provides appropriate techniques for management.

- With complete excision and meticulous surgical technique, **tumor recurrence** is rare.

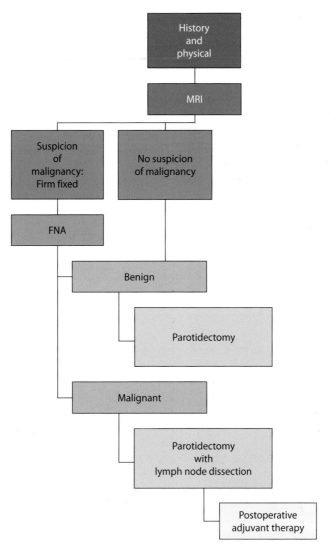

Algorithm 23-1 Algorithm for management of patients with parotid lesions.

PRACTICAL PEARLS

1. While the vast majority of parotid masses are benign, pain, facial weakness, and fixation suggest malignancy.

2. Diagnostic imaging with MRI provides essential information regarding the extent and character of a parotid mass.

3. Facial nerve paralysis is rare; however, when it occurs, management of the incomplete eye closure is a priority.

4. When nerve grafting is required, the best results occur with immediate reconstruction.

References

1. Howlett DC. Diagnosing a parotid lump: Fine needle aspiration cytology or core biopsy. *Br J Radiol.* 2006;79(940): 295-297.

2. Carlson GW. The salivary glands. Embryology, anatomy, and surgical applications. *Surg Clin North Am.* 2000;80(1): 261-273.

3. Carlson GW. Surgical anatomy of the neck. *Surg Clin North Am.* 1993;73(4):837-852.

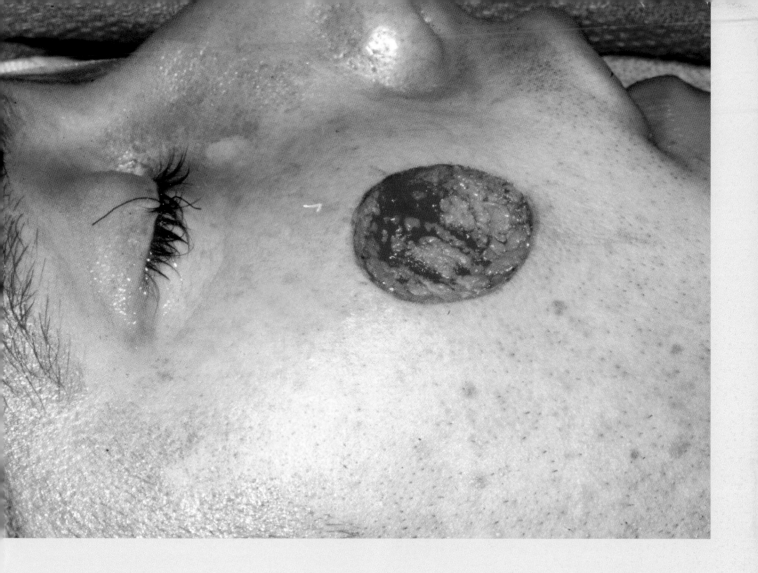

A Mohs' surgeon refers a 35-year-old man in whom he just removed a lesion of the cheek and left the defect as shown.

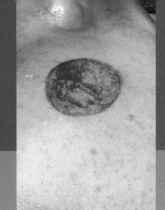

Lesion of the Cheek

Gregory R.D. Evans

1. The cheek is both a cosmetic and functional structure whose loss can lead to significant alterations in the quality of life. Mastication, deglutition, and communication are just a few of the critical elements that the cheek provides. Defects resulting from surgical resection must be restored with rapid, functional and aesthetic tissues. In patients who present with changing or nonhealing lesions of the skin of the cheek, cancer must be the primary concern. Cancer of the skin is the most frequently diagnosed cancer in the United States and is even more common in countries with high exposure to ultraviolet rays such as Australia. Of these, approximately 80% are basal cell carcinoma (BCC) and 20% are squamous cell carcinoma (SCC). The primary goal of treatment is the eradication of benign or malignant lesions and wound closure by return of form and function, while minimizing structural deformity, xerostomia, anesthesia, and facial paralysis. Defects in this area may affect patient's quality of life and alter their ability to interact socially.

   - **How old is the patient and how much sun exposure has the patient had over lifetime (outdoor occupation or avocation)?** Older patients with more chronic exposure to ultraviolet radiation logically have a greater chance of developing skin cancer.

   - **Has the patient been exposed to risk factors for the development of carcinoma?** Exposure to chemical carcinogens, such as arsenic or polyaromatic hydrocarbons, should be questioned with the patient.

   - **How long has the lesion been present?** Lesions present for years with little change are less suspicious for malignant degeneration. Concerning characteristics include changes in appearance, large size, variable color, and irregular boundaries.

   - **Does the patient have paresthesias?** Paresthesias are indicative of nerve involvement and may portend a worse prognosis.

   - **Does the patient have risk factors in the past medical history that suggest a higher risk of development of skin carcinoma?** Immunosuppression from infection (human immunodeficiency virus) or medication (posttransplant), ionizing radiation, infection (human papilloma virus), genetic susceptibility (xeroderma pigmentosum), or a history of chronic inflammation (Marjolin ulcer).

2. The boundaries of the cheek are the buccal mucosa medially, the lips anteriorly, the pterygomandibular raphe posteriorly, the upper alveolar ridge superiorly, and the lower alveolar ride inferiorly. Every patient with a suspicious lesion of the cheek should undergo a comprehensive head and neck examination. The overall appearance of any skin lesion must be detailed.

   - **What is the patient's skin type and hair color?** Fair skin, blonde or red hair, and light-colored eyes are characteristics that predispose to the development of carcinoma.

   - **Where is the lesion located?** The cheek itself may be divided into three distinct zones or aesthetic units. The suborbital region is from the anterior sideburn to the nasolabial line and from the lower eyelid to the gingival sulcus. The preauricular region is from the superolateral junction of the helix and the cheek to the mandible and the buccomandibular region is the remaining lower anterior cheek.

   - **What is the size of the lesion?** Tumor size and location affect the cosmetic and functional outcome of surgical excision.

   - **Is the lesion flat or raised?** The classic presentation of a SCC is that of a shallow ulcer with heaped-up edges, often covered by a plaque. Of course, the presenting appearance of each SCC varies according to the site and extent of disease.

   - **What is the status of the branches of the facial nerve?** The presence of presurgical facial nerve palsy suggests malignancy. Evidence of cranial nerve dysfunction should raise concern of significant perineural invasion, most frequently involving the facial and trigeminal nerves. Each branch of the facial nerve should be assessed for motion and strength:

     — **Is the patient able to raise his brow?** Test frontal branch function and frontalis muscle innervation.

     — **Is the patient able to close his eyes?** Test zygomatic branch function and orbicularis oculi innervation.

     — **Does the patient have a symmetrical smile?** Test buccal branch function and buccinator muscle innervation.

— **Is the patient able to show his lower teeth?** Test marginal mandibular branch function and depressor anguli oris innervation (among others).

— **Is the patient able to tense the neck muscles?** Test cervical branch function and platysma innervation.

- **Are there any palpable lymph nodes?** Regional lymphatic drainage should be assessed for metastatic spread. The most frequently involved lymphatics include those located within the parotid gland and upper cervical lymph node levels. Rarely, SCC presents as a parotid or neck mass because of lymphatic spread. The risk of metastasis correlates roughly with tumor size and differentiation.

3. The preoperative workup must obtain tissue for histologic examination in order to determine whether the lesion is benign or malignant.

- The type of **biopsy** performed depends on the size of the lesion. Small skin lesions in noncritical areas may be amenable to excisional biopsy, where the entire area of concern is removed. This method has the benefit of being diagnostic as well as potentially therapeutic without the need for a second procedure. For larger lesions or those located in cosmetic or functionally critical areas, confirming the diagnosis before embarking on surgical excision that may be extensive and require reconstruction is often preferable. In these cases, an incisional or punch biopsy should be performed initially with further treatment based on the pathology results. Whatever biopsy method chosen, several principles should be followed. The biopsy should contain the full thickness of the skin in order to evaluate the depth of the lesion. Therefore, a shave biopsy is generally not recommended when malignancy is suspected. The biopsy should be centered over the transition point between normal and involved skin, thereby providing a reference for comparison by the pathologist.

— **BCC** originates in the basal cell of the epidermis. Risk primarily associated with sun exposure. It grows slowly in a radial fashion with little chance for vertical growth or lymphatic or hematogenous spread.

— **SCC** originates in the spindle cell layer of the epidermis. Risk of development associated with sun exposure, chronic wounds, and chemical exposure (cytotoxic drugs). It is seen in older male patients most commonly and presents with induration, inflammation, or ulceration. It may be slow or fast growing.

— The rising incidence of **melanoma** is related to sun exposure, especially if chronic and intermittent. The incidence is ten times higher in whites. The earlier the detection the better the prognosis. The diagnosis is suggested by pigmentary changes, an indistinct border, a variegated color, and growing size. The current 5-year survival is 80%. Depth of invasion is the most important factor, therefore, biopsies that yield shaved specimens, such as Mohs' technique, are *not* indicated. Four growth patterns exist. Superficial spreading melanoma is the most common (70%) and portends the best prognosis. Nodular melanoma is the second most common type (20%) and portends the worst prognosis because it lacks a radial growth phase. Five percent of these may lack pigmentation. Acral lentiginous melanoma is characteristically seen on the palms and soles, while lentigo maligna melanoma develops slowly and appears later in life usually appearing as a large, flat lesion on the face in elderly patients.

- Certain basic tests may also be indicated in the face of malignancy.

— With BCC, there is a low risk of metastases making chest X-ray and liver function tests (LFTs) unnecessary.

— With SCC, chest X-ray and LFTs are indicated. In advanced-stage SCC, imaging with CT or MRI can be helpful in defining the extent of disease. CT is better able to identify the presence of bone or soft tissue invasion and for evaluating cervical lymph nodes at risk for metastasis. MRI is preferred to evaluate perineural invasion or extension into surrounding structures.

— With melanoma, chest X-ray, LFTs, and possibly endoscopy and funduscopy for stage III and IV disease are indicated.

- The TNM staging system for nonmelanotic skin cancer is as follows:
  — Primary tumor (T)
    a. T0: No evidence of primary tumor.
    b. T1: Tumor 2 cm or less.
    c. T2: Tumor larger than 2 cm but smaller than 5 cm.
    d. T3: Tumor larger than 5 cm.
    e. T4: Tumor invades deep extradermal structures (bone, muscle, cartilage).
  — Regional lymph nodes (N)
    a. N0: No regional lymph node metastasis.
    b. N1: Regional lymph node metastases.
  — Distant metastasis (M)
    a. M0: No distant metastasis.
    b. M1: Distant metastasis.
- From the TMN classification, a stage can be determined:
  — Stage I: T1, N0, M0
  — Stage II: T2 or T3, N0, M0
  — Stage III: T4, N0, M0, or any T, N1, M0
  — Stage IV: Any T, any N, M1

4. Consultation with an oncologist may be required to determine the need for adjuvant therapy.

- BCC—treated primarily by surgery. Diffuse cases may be managed with topical antineoplastic agents, such as Effudex (5-FU).
- SCC—treated primarily by surgery. Chemotherapy reserved for metastatic cases.
- Melanoma—stage III patients appear to benefit from Interferon alpha-2b, while the use of radiotherapy in this setting is *not* well defined.

5. Reconstruction is based on the location of the defect, the extent of tissue loss, functional loss, and comorbid medical conditions. One must consider not only the external requirements but also the need for lining. There are a variety of techniques and donor materials available to reconstruct the complex three-dimensional defects of the cheek that may involve one or more tissue types. Small mucosal resections not requiring extensive fat or muscle removal should be closed primarily. Defects that are larger may require mucosal flaps or skin grafts for reconstruction. Occasionally defects involving the entire buccal mucosa, especially after radiation therapy, may necessitate skin and/or muscle to reduce the incidence of trismus or xerostomia. Full-thickness defects present a significant challenge for the reconstructive surgeon. The creation of a functional oral cavity with internal and external epithelial coverage of the underlying bone must be achieved to reach the primary goal of an aesthetically acceptable closure with resumption of an oral diet and normal verbalization. Reconstruction of full-thickness cheek defects is not considered completely successful unless oral sphincter and vermilion sensory functions are reestablished, improving food handling, verbalization and preventing drooling. It is vital to reestablish orbicularis oris muscle ring continuity to maintain sphincter function by suturing vermilion advancement flaps to the folded aspect of the free flaps forming a neocommissure. Further, with the loss of facial motor function, the use of fascial slings can also assist with a decrease in drooling and reestablishment of the oral commissure by fixation of the commissure to temporalis fascia. Frontal branch resection may also necessitate addressing brow position or lagophthalmus.

- For any malignancies, one must take an adequate margin, which might include underlying cartilage and bone. The final reconstruction should be delayed until *after* the final pathology and margins are known. In the cheek, the superficial parotid may need to be excised to adequately remove the draining lymph nodes while preserving the branches of the facial nerve below. Nerves that are involved should be sacrificed and the surgical plan should include a sural (or other) nerve graft, if necessary.
- Adequate margins for **BCC** are 2 mm, while those for **SCC** are at least 1 cm. Adequate margins for **melanoma**, on the other hand, depend on the depth of the lesion. For in situ lesions, 5 mm is adequate. For lesions up to 1 cm, 1-cm margins are used. For lesions between one and 2 cm, one or 2 cm are used. For lesions two to 4 cm, 2 cm are used and for larger lesions, margins greater than 2 cm are preferred.
- With melanoma, the need for **lymphadenectomy** is also based on depth. All patients with a depth >1 mm should have a nodal staging procedure. Sentinel lymph node dissection (LND) is performed 2 to 4 hours after radionuclide injection and immediately after local dermal injection of lymphazurin dye. If the sentinel node is positive, completion of regional LND would be performed. Some areas, such as the head and neck, may still be better treated with traditional elective lymph node dissection (ELND).
  — For lesions less than 1 mm, the risk of spread is too low.
  — For lesions 1 to 4 mm, there is a 20% risk of spread and ELND recommended.
  — For lesions greater than 4 mm, there is a 70% risk of spread and ELND is *not* felt to be of benefit since patients do poorly and will receive treatment anyway.
- **Primary closure** is the preferred method of repair of small, superficial oral cavity wounds. Depending on the extent of the resection, defects larger than 3 cm should be closed with a random local tissue transfers or mucosal flap, skin graft or a pedicle musculocutaneous

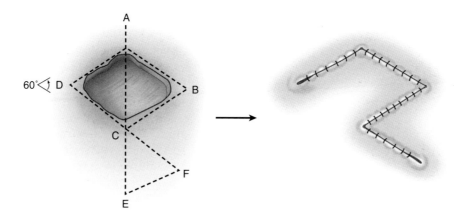

Figure 24-1 Schematic drawing highlighting the planning of a rhomboid flap for reconstruction of a skin defect on the cheek.

flap to minimize the incidence of wound contraction leading to trismus. Defects involving the entire buccal mucosa that are reconstructed with insensate grafts may develop xerostomia and numbness that may impair food handling, swallowing, and quality of speech. Rehabilitation for swallowing and speech is necessary in these patients. These large defects may occasionally require the transfer of sensate or lubricating free grafts to improve function, particularly when significant amounts of underlying soft issues are resected or metastatic lesions to regional lymph nodes prevent the use of local flaps.

- The advantage of locally advancing neighboring tissue is that it provides good color match, similar tissue and, although additional scars are placed, skin laxity usually yields a good result. Local tissue advancement is ideal in the cheek area for reconstruction. It is less conspicuous than skin grafting, which may lend itself to color mismatch. In elderly patients, skin laxity allows closure with minimal donor site complications. Patients with a history of smoking or preexisting medical conditions may have compromised vasculature to the skin

and soft tissues warranting an initial delay procedure. The ultimate design of these flaps can be slightly smaller than the defect itself to allow for the incorporation of surrounding tissue in the flap closure. Common designs include one or more rhomboid shapes, whose sides mirror those of the defect. Redundant tissue at the margins (dog ears) may require further resection to allow a more tailored closure. Alternatively, if resection may hamper vascular compromise, resection can be performed at a later time.

- Full-thickness cheek defects present unique challenges for the reconstructive surgeon. These defects are frequently associated with loss of oral sensation, lubrication, facial motor function or other reconstructive concerns such as loss of mandibular continuity. Traditional reconstructive techniques using **pedicle flaps** of muscle and skin, such as the pectoralis major, trapezius and latissimus dorsi effectively provide wound coverage. However, contraction of the base of the pedicle of these flaps and their bulk may not be the ideal form of reconstruction. Even though free flaps clearly have superior aesthetic and functional

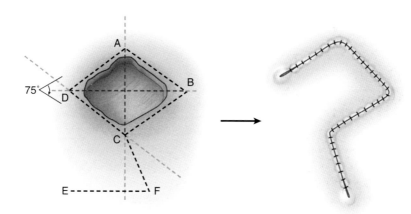

Figure 24-2 Schematic drawing highlighting an alternate rhomboid flap using different angles to reconstruct a skin defect on the cheek.

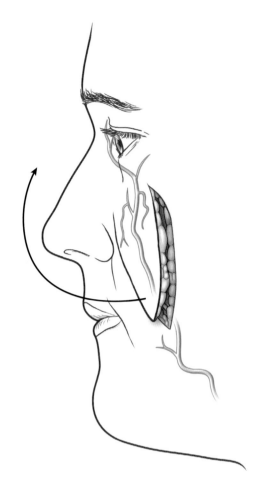

Figure 24-3 Schematic drawing highlighting the elevation of a nasolabial flap for reconstruction of a local skin defect cheek.

It is simple to harvest and has minimal aesthetic impact on the neck. Care must be taken to avoid kinking of the pedicle that results from rotating the flap through the 180-degree arc of rotation necessary for inset.

— The **sternocleidomastoid myocutaneous flap** may also be used for cheek reconstruction, especially in the reconstruction over the mandible. Because of its tenuous and segmental blood supply, care must be utilized in its rotation.

— Full-thickness defects may require alternative flaps. The temporalis, upper trapezius, pectoralis major, and latissimus dorsi can provide full-thickness coverage.

• Large cheek defects can be reconstructed with **free flaps** that provide epithelium-lined soft tissue with the potential for sensation or lubrication. Unfortunately, no flap currently offers both the structural and functional equivalents to the native tissue. Prospective randomized trials have not yet demonstrated improved functional outcomes when sensation is restored earlier with primary neurorrhaphy. However, conceptually, the concept of early sensation does appear appropriate. The characteristics of the defect and the desires of the patient are taken into account when determining which flap should be utilized for the reconstruction as well as whether sensation should be utilized.

— The most reliable flap for intraoral and cheek reconstruction is the **radial forearm flap**. It is a pliable, thin, and durable with a long vascular pedicle and consistent anatomy. The radial forearm tissue may be transferred as a sensate flap by anatomizing the sensory nerves in the forearm to the lingual or inferior alveolar nerves. Other flaps that can be utilized in this area include the lateral arm, and the anterolateral thigh.

— Mucosal free flaps have been demonstrated to prevent xerostomia in patients with decreased salivary secretion after radiation therapy. The preferred mucosal free flap for intraoral reconstruction is the **transverse colon** because it provides an adequate pedicle, is durable, and has pliable tissue plus it secretes mucin, even after radiation therapy.

— Other flaps that can be utilized include the **lateral thigh** based on the third perforating branch of the profunda femoris and may regain sensory function by performing a neurorrhaphy with the lateral cutaneous nerve.

— The **rectus abdominis flap** is perhaps the most versatile and sturdy flap available as a result of its rich vascularity but is generally limited to the reconstruction of large maxillary defects. The skin and fat may be removed if the cutaneous flap is too bulky. Skin grafting on the muscle can be performed for intraoral closure or alternatively reepithelialization can occur.

outcomes, pedicle flaps should be considered in selected patients when comorbid medical conditions preclude the use of free flaps or when surgeons lack the technical skill and equipment to perform free tissue transfers. Some of these patients may however require free tissue transfer to avoid increased complications frequently seen in with rotational flaps. Cervical pedicle myocutaneous flaps, such as the platysma and sternocleidomastoid, provide small to medium-sized skin paddles that can cover most buccal defects. These flaps readily reach many areas within the oral cavity and aesthetically acceptable closure of the donor site can usually be achieved. The cervical pedicle flaps, however, are not acceptable for larger tissue defects or when metastatic tumors, radiation therapy or previous surgery involve the proposed donor site. The vascular supply of these flaps is often segmental and unreliable. Surgeons should be familiar with reconstruction using platysma and sternocleidomastoid flaps, although other reconstructive options that have fewer limitations are usually available.

— The **platysma myocutaneous flap** has a wide arc of rotation and provides thin, pliable tissue that can replace buccal mucosal defects up to 5 cm × 7 cm.

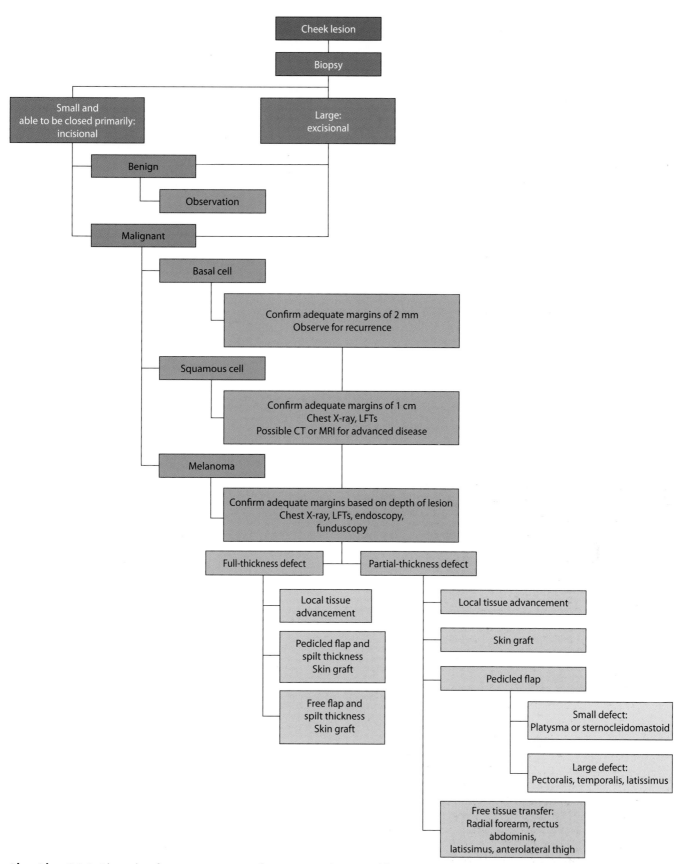

Algorithm 24-1 Algorithm for management of patients with parotid lesions.

— The **latissimus dorsi flap** is a thin, flat, and broad muscle that will occasionally provide coverage for large cheek defects but more commonly is used during orbitomaxillary reconstruction for replacement of tissue bulk. Again, because of the size of the muscle it may be split to allow a more aesthetic closure.

6. The complications of excision and reconstruction should not be common.

- **Bleeding** and **infection** are uncommon but must be considered with any surgical procedure.

- Tight closure or excessive scar formation with healing may lead to the development of an **ectropion**. Mild cases may respond to massage, more severe cases require release and reconstruction.

- Because of the proximity of the branches of the facial nerve, **nerve injury** should be identified preoperatively and prevented during reconstruction.

- **Incomplete resection and recurrence** should not be sacrificed at the expense of primary closure. The primary goal is excision of the tumor with adequate margins followed by functional and aesthetic reconstruction.

References

1. Harii K, Asato H, Takushima. Midface reconstruction. In: Mathes S, ed. *Plastic Surgery*. Philadelphia, PA: Saunders Elsevier; 2006.

2. Bunkis J, Mulliken JB, Upton J, Murray JE. The evolution of techniques for reconstruction of full-thickness cheek defects. *Plast Reconstr Surg.* 1982;70:319-327.

3. Juri J, Juri C. Cheek reconstruction with advancement-rotation flaps. *Clin Plast Surg.*1981;8:223-226.

4. Crow ML and Crow FJ. Resurfacing large cheek defects with rotation flaps from the neck. *Plast Reconstr Surg.* 1976;58:196-200.

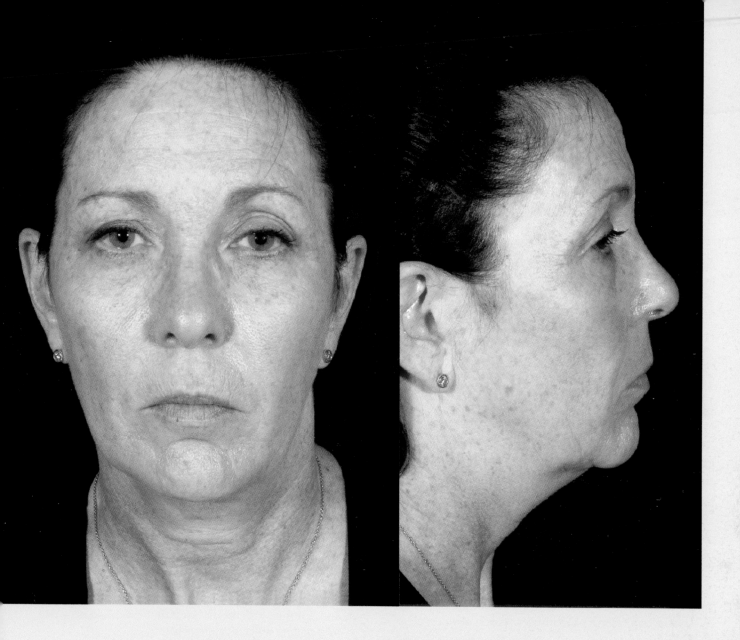

A 55-year-old woman pictured above is concerned about the aging appearance of her face. She recently underwent a facial rejuvenation procedure.

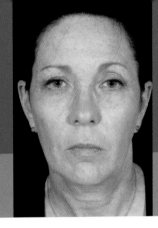

CHAPTER 25

Subjective Facial Aging

Richard Skolnik

1. Perhaps, the most difficult preoperative interview involves the patient desiring facial rejuvenation. Noticeable aging in the face and neck can be seen in the forehead, eyebrow, periorbital skin and soft tissue, nasolabial creases, jowls, and neck among other areas. In addition to determining the required procedures, preferred techniques, and medical suitability for surgery, the physician must also determine the patient's motives and emotional stability. Unlike with reconstructive procedures, a feeling of easiness about performing surgery on a given patient should not be taken lightly and often should lead to recommending another surgeon.

   - **How long has the patient being considering facial rejuvenation?** The patient's personal motivation is important to address before proceeding. Spur of the moment decisions or those related to a displeasing event in one's life may often present dissatisfaction postoperatively.

   - **What specific problems does the patient find troubling?** Specific concerns about the jowls, neck, brow, etc. should be noted. Wrinkling around the eyes is not well addressed with a standard facelift. Do not fall into the trap when a patient states "Isn't it obvious?"

   - **Why is the patient considering surgery at this time?** Surgery should not be a reaction to an adverse event in one's life, such as death or divorce. Better candidates are those that have been considering one or more procedures for some time and perhaps have even had a friend who had undergone a similar procedure.

   - **Has the patient had a previous facelift?** The presence of existing facial scars may influence subsequent surgical options.

   - **Does the patient have any associated medical conditions?** Certain special conditions predispose to unacceptable wound healing problems; others do not.

     — **Cutis laxa** produces a degeneration of the dermal elastic fibers. It may be autosomal dominant (type I) in which the symptoms are confined to the skin or recessive (type II) in which patients may develop abdominal wall hernias, pulmonary emphysema, intestinal diverticula, and/or vascular aneurysms. Rhytidectomy in these patients may be used to improve appearance.

     — **Ehlers Danlos** is an X-linked or autosomal recessive disorder marked by joint hypermobility and thin, fragile, hyperextensible skin. Patients have many wound healing problems after surgery, such that rhytidectomy is contraindicated.

     — In patients with a history of previous **keloids**, rhytidectomy may also be contraindicated.

   - **Does the patient smoke?** Tobacco use impairs wound healing and presents a higher risk of skin flap slough with certain procedures. The ability to discontinue tobacco use preoperatively is frequently difficult for the patient. The surgeon must consider this in deciding whether to proceed and what type of procedure (limited vs. extended facelift) is indicated.

   - **Is the patient currently using a nicotine patch or nicotine gum?** These have the same effect as smoking and may not be volunteered by the patient.

2. As in all aspects of medicine, making the proper diagnosis is key to choosing the correct procedure for the patient. The physical examination should start with the appropriateness of a facelift for the patient in question and continue with specific areas of the face and neck that may require different approaches.

   - **What is the patient's overall skin quality?** Preexisting sun damage might warrant a preoperative skin regimen to improve the overall result. Are there perioral rhytids that would benefit from a simultaneous skin resurfacing?

   - **Are there any associated lesions on or around the face that appear suspicious for malignancy?** The presence of associated lesions around the face should be addressed beforehand. Suspicious lesions, that may turn out to be a malignancy, may be biopsied in the office. It is never prudent to improve a patient's appearance by resection of lax skin only to be faced with a midcheek squamous cell carcinoma 6 months postoperatively.

   - **Are there any preexisting scars around the face?** Facial scars may interfere with symmetrical repositioning of the elevated skin flaps. Preexisting scars may also compromise the vascularity of the skin flaps and must be taken into consideration in your preoperative planning. Also, planning one's incisions must take into consideration the position of the hairline and sideburn. Modification of the incisions will prevent abnormal elevation of the temporal hairline and place the incisions in the most inconspicuous spots.

- **What is the patient's facial shape and how will that affect the result?** Round full faces have less dramatic results than angled faces and this must be pointed out to the patient preoperatively.

- **Are there coexisting problems in the forehead and periorbital region that need to be addressed?** Aging in the upper face may require repositioning of the brow and/or procedures on the eyelids. The latter may include resurfacing only or involve skin resection or fat removal. Rhytids around the glabellar region may be addressed with neuromuscular blockade with botulinum toxin A. Deeper furrows may be addressed with soft tissue fillers such as fat, collagen, or other dermal and subdermal products.

- **Has the cheek fat descended with age?** Descent of the malar cheek pad leads to the aging appearance of the face and would require repositioning.

- **Are the nasolabial folds problematic?** With descent of the cheek complex, deep furrows in this area become noticeable and worrisome to many patients. Upward pull on the superficial muscular aponeurotic system (SMAS) alone will often tend to worsen the fold. These may be better addressed with soft tissue fillers or even direct excision.

- **Is the chin hypoplastic?** Chin augmentation or sliding genioplasty can be combined with a facelift to improve the facial balance and therefore improve the final result. If the patient has lip incompetence, chin augmentation might be contraindicated.

- **Is there excess submental fat?** Direct excision and/or liposuction to improve an obtuse mandibular-cervical angle must be considered in the preoperative planning. Subplatysmal fat must also be identified and possibly resected if excessive.

- **What is the status of the platysmal bands?** Prominent, divergent bands along the leading edges of the platysma muscle may need direct approximation through a submental incision.

- **Are there prominent submental salivary glands?** These must be pointed out to the patient

preoperatively because they may become more prominent postoperatively.

- **What is the condition of the pretragal skin?** Planning a pretragal or a posttragal incision will depend upon the texture, quality, and the presence of vellus hair in this region.

- **Is the ear lobule attached or hanging?** The position of the earlobe should be noted since its position should be recreated when closing the incisions.

3. In the healthy patient, few preoperative studies are required. Specific laboratory values will be determined by the patient's medical history. A chest X-ray and electrocardiogram will be required in older patients in certain facilities.

- Well-lit preoperative **photographs** should be taken in several views: AP, lateral, and oblique. Additional photographs may be warranted if additional procedures are being performed.

- There are no specific studies to obtain for a facelift procedure. A **lateral cephalogram** should be obtained if an adjunctive chin augmentation is planned.

4. Consultations for the patient contemplating a facelift procedure should relate to the patient's suitability for surgery. The primary care physician should review the patient's medical history, current medications, and exercise tolerance. Often, a cardiac workup is indicated.

5. With every patient, the nature, benefits, risks, alternatives, and expectations of surgery should be discussed at one or more sessions beforehand.

- A **preoperative skin care** regimen is advised to maximize the surgical result. Beginning the patient on a preoperative regimen of retinoids and/or bleaching creams, such as hydroquinone, will improve the appearance of the skin. A youthful appearing complexion will add to the overall result of facial rejuvenation surgery.

- Perioperatively, certain medications may be ordered to ameliorate the patient's anxiety or minimize the potential for postoperative complications.

  — Sedatives may be ordered that the patient can take with a sip of water the night before and the morning of surgery to minimize anxiety.

- The patient's own antihypertensive medication should be taken the morning of surgery again with a sip of water to lessen the incidence of perioperative blood pressure elevation that could lead to bleeding and hematoma formation.
- Steroids may be used around induction to minimize swelling and augment the effects of any other medications being administered.

- In modern facelifting, a natural youthful appearing result depends on facial shape modification rather than stretching and pulling the skin. Repositioning the facial fat is the key to achieving an excellent result. Youthful faces are round and full with soft curves and a full midface and malar region. To obtain these results several surgical options are available:
  - The **skin only** facelift is the oldest technique and perhaps the simplest.
  - Descent of the deeper structures of the face may be addressed by redraping the skin and repositioning a composite flap of the cheek fat and SMAS layer. Simple **SMAS plication** involves placing sutures anterior to the retaining ligaments of the cheek/malar complex.
  - More extensive **SMAS elevation** and rotation involves developing the SMAS and platysma layers to various degrees and directions to reshape the face. Various authors have described different procedures (extended SMAS, high SMAS, auto cheek augmentation with the SMAS, etc.) to accomplish these changes.
  - Excision of a strip of SMAS anterior to the retaining ligaments followed by plication ("**SMASectomy**") may also be employed.
  - The **deep plane facelift** elevates the forehead, eyelids, and SMAS layer in continuity.
  - The **subperiosteal facelift** elevates the soft tissues of the face at the subperiosteal plane. It may be combined with another type of facelift.

- Adjuvant procedures and modalities are often considered to augment the effect of surgery. The surgeon should always weigh the appropriateness of performing additional facial (browlift, blepharoplasty, rhinoplasty, chin augmentation) or body procedures (mastopexy, abdominoplasty) as a single stage or as the first of additional stages.
  - Laser resurfacing.
  - Chemical peel.
  - Fat injections.
  - Botox injection.

6. The best tact for managing a **complication** following a facelift is to acknowledge what has occurred. Hopefully, the risk of complications was reviewed in preoperative visits. The surgeon must recognize and deal with these problems early. The surgeon must also make himself available for daily visits, if necessary.

- The etiology of a **hematoma** is multifactorial but correlates most closely with perioperative hypertension. Pain is unusual following an uncomplicated facelift so its occurrence must be regarded as a sign of fluid under tension until proven otherwise. Early recognition is the key to preventing disaster (flap necrosis). Drains cannot prevent the development of an expanding hematoma.
  - Small hematomas (2 to 20 mL) are not apparent until edema begins to subside and occur in 10% to 15% of patients. Initially, a small area of firmness is palpable followed by ecchymosis in the overlying skin, and depending on the amount of hematoma present, the skin surface may become irregular. Between the 7th and 10th days small hematomas liquefy, making it possible to express most of the blood by fingertip manipulation through a small stab incision. Sometimes small hematomas can be aspirated using a 5-mL syringe and an 18-gauge needle. Either technique may require repetition on 2 to 4 successive days to remove as much blood as possible. Hematomas not detected and evacuated during the period of liquefaction result in skin firmness, irregularity, and discoloration that may persist for several weeks to months. Occasionally, hemosiderin deposits in the skin result in permanent discoloration. Patients who must return to the office frequently for aspiration of small hematomas require especially supportive care from the surgeon and the staff. Warm compresses and gentle daily massage may be helpful by making the patient an active participant in the healing process. Early intervention with injection of dilute steroids after aspiration can also be considered.
  - An **expanding hematoma** occurs in 1% to 8% of patients, twice as common in males. Hematomas occur most frequently in the first 6 to 8 hours postoperatively. Patients should be observed and monitored closely following the procedure. This is a surgical emergency. Causes include inadequate preoperative evaluation of the patient, inadequate intraoperative hemostasis/management of blood pressure, and/or inadequate postoperative management of pain, blood pressure, and nausea. As such, many instances may be prevented with thorough preoperative screening for patients at risk, especially adequate perioperative blood pressure control. Clonidine may be used at a dose of 0.1 to 0.3 mg 1 hour before surgery and lasts 10 hours. Intraoperatively, parenteral labetalol and/or Vasotec may be used. Of course, adequate hemostasis intraoperatively is important. Postoperatively, the patient should be kept pain free (the flaps may be irrigated with bupivacaine) and nausea free (continue NPO and administer Zofran 4 mg IV or Compazine 10 mg). Management involves removing the dressings and evaluating the wounds for

bluish discoloration and hardness. Prior to returning to the operating room, the sutures should be released at the bedside as a means of decompression. All clots should be removed and all bleeding points cauterized. The wound may be closed as before without any difference in the rate of healing.

- **Postoperative edema** may be managed with elevating the head of the bed (pressure dressings are of doubtful significance and may compromise the flaps). Postoperative steroids can also be considered.

- **Ecchymosis** may persist for many weeks.

- Nerve injury is the most dreaded complication.

  — The **greater auricular nerve** is the most common avoidable sensory nerve injury during rhytidectomy. With the head turned 45 degrees to the opposite side, the greater auricular nerve crosses the superficial surface of the sternocleidomastoid muscle; below it's fascia 6.5 cm below the caudal edge of the bony external auditory canal. It is found just posterior to the external jugular vein. The vein and nerve lie deep to the SMAS/platysma layer. Injury to the main trunk of the nerve as it passes over the sternocleidomastoid muscle may produce dysesthesia or neuroma symptoms of the lower two-thirds of the ear, the preauricular area, and the cheeks. For the first 2 to 6 weeks postoperatively, some numbness is unavoidable. When recognized during surgery, injury to the main trunk should be immediately repaired.

  — The frontal branches of the **facial nerve** emerge from beneath the parotid gland on a line extending from 0.5 cm below the tragus of the ear to a point 1.5 cm above the lateral brow, passing deep to the SMAS over the zygomatic arch. They enter the frontalis muscle on its deep surface. The most common branch of the facial nerve, which is injured, is the buccal branch, with expected return of function in 3 to 4 months. Injury to the frontal branch tends to produce longer lasting facial weakness. Fortunately, permanent injury to the facial nerve branches is rare. Most patients regain full motor function after injury to a branch of the facial nerve within a few weeks to a year, although an occasional patient may take longer. The reported incidence of facial nerve injury of 0.9% (from before the era of extended SMAS dissections and composite rhytidectomies and the incidence of nerve injuries is almost certainly higher now). If transection of the facial nerve branch is detected during the procedure, immediate microsurgical repair must be performed. It is more likely, however, that nerve injury is not recognized during surgery, and the surgeon and patient are placed in the difficult position of waiting for return of function.

- **Hypertrophic scarring** is rare but does occur. The postauricular incision is the most frequent site of hypertrophic scars. It is most commonly caused by vascular compromise of the skin flaps (i.e., hematoma) and excess tension on the closure. The two points of maximum skin tension are in the temporal scalp just above the ear and at the apex of the postauricular incision. The remaining skin flaps are trimmed conservatively so there is minimal tension on the closure. This point is especially true in the preauricular area and around the earlobe, where the slightest tension widens the scar and distorts the earlobe. Management includes small-volume injections of dilute insoluble steroids which helps flatten these scars. Care is taken when placing the submental incision to minimize its length, so that when the skin flaps are advanced laterally the incision remains hidden underneath the jawline. The submental incision should not be placed in a deep submental crease but should be placed distally. If placed within the crease, normal scar contracture will exaggerate the crease causing a "witch's chin" deformity. Elliptical skin excision in the submental area tends to produce "dog ears" and is avoided if possible.

- Superficial **skin slough** of the epidermis usually heal with little or no residual scarring; however, hyper -or hypopigmentation may occur. Full-thickness skin slough always result in some degree of permanent scarring. The postauricular and mastoid areas are the most frequently involved, presumably because the skin is thinnest in this area and is furthest from adequate circulation. Fortunately, small sloughs in this area are concealed by the ear and hair. Full-thickness slough in a visible area of the face and neck is a devastating complication. In most series, the incidence of skin slough after rhytidectomy is 1% to 3%. It is not known why some patients develop skin sloughs, whereas most have no such problems. Most likely causes of skin slough are undiagnosed hematomas, skin flap that is too thin or that is damaged during flap dissection, excessive tension on wound closure, and cigarette smoking (Rees and colleagues demonstrated a risk of skin slough 12 times greater in smokers than nonsmokers. For this reason patients are required to abstain from smoking for at least 2 weeks, preoperatively).

  — All facial skin sloughs, even when in a highly visible area, are treated by careful observation—not surgical intervention. Areas of skin slough epithelialize and contract dramatically. The resulting scar is almost always better than would be anticipated from the initial wound appearance. Depending on the size of the sloughed area, it may be possible to excise the scar and readvance the facial skin, but it is generally years before sufficient skin laxity allows a secondary lift.

- **Seroma** results from fluid collection in small pockets beneath the flaps, most commonly in the neck.

These should be aspirated in the same fashion as small hematomas.

- **Contour irregularities** are seen more with extensive defatting during platysma surgery. They are caused by improper defatting of the flaps. Approximately 5 to 7 mm of fat should be left on the undersurface of the cervical skin flaps. A masculinized neck can also occur with a completely transected platysma.

- **Wound infection** is rare, with an incidence less than 1%. Most commonly, the organism is *Staphylococcus aureus*, which is managed with antibiotics.

- Some degree of **alopecia** can occur after rhytidectomy. Excessive tension and thin flaps are the most common reasons. Management involves either revision of the scar or hair transplantation

- **Hyperpigmentation** is caused by hemosiderin deposits in the dermis and occasionally epidermal sis. Small, unseen hematomas that become apparent after edema subsides are frequent sites of hyperpigmentation. The discoloration is slow to resolve, occasionally taking 6 to 8 months. Rarely, the color change is permanent. If the cause is postinflammatory pigmentation then retinoids and fading creams are useful in eliminating the problem.

- **Apposition** of the ear and/or hairline is caused by an error in surgical technique, excess tension, and/or excision of too much skin.

- **Patient dissatisfaction** may be the hardest to avoid. The physician should have a good sense of the patient's maturity and understanding of reasonable results. Operating upon a patient with whom the surgeon has trepidation is never wise.

PRACTICAL PEARLS

1. Facial shape is the key to modern facelifting.

2. A drain should always be left postoperatively in male facelifts.

3. Do not undertake any procedure without a complete understanding of the anatomy. Most complications occur immediately after a conference or course.

4. Do not distort the hairline—rather vary your skin incisions.

5. Perioperative blood pressure control will prevent you from having to do a secondary facelift the same day as the primary.

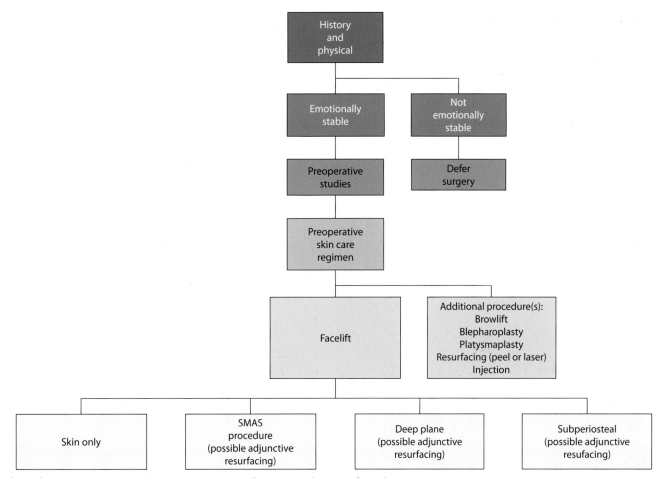

Algorithm 25-1 Algorithm for management of patients desiring facial rejuvenation.

References

1. Stuzin JM. Restoring facial shape in face lifting: The role of skeletal support in facial analysis and midface soft-tissue repositioning. *Plast Reconstr Surg.* 2007;119(1):362-376.

2. Ramirez OM. Classification of facial rejuvenation techniques based on the subperiosteal approach and ancillary procedures. *Plast Reconstr Surg.* 1996;97(1):45-55.

3. Gosain AK, Yousif NJ, Madiedo G, Larson DL, Matloub HS, Sanger JR. Surgical anatomy of the SMAS: A reinvestigation. *Plast Reconstr Surg.* 1993;92(7):1254-1263.

4. Baker TJ, Gordon HL, and Stuzin JM, eds. *Surgical Rejuvenation of the Face.* 2nd ed. Philadelphia, PA: C.V. Mosby; 1996.

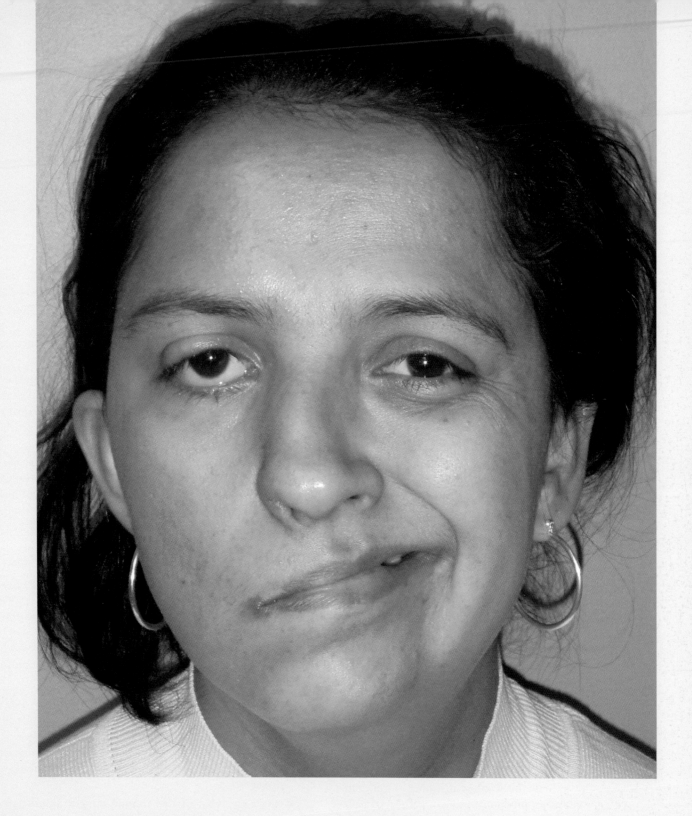

A 17-year-old student is referred to you

with facial asymmetry.

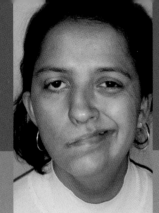

CHAPTER 26

Facial Paralysis

Jin K. Chun

1. The cause may be congenital (Moebius syndrome), traumatic (either at birth from molding or forceps delivery or later from basal skull or facial fractures or penetrating lacerations), infectious (chickenpox, coxsackie, influenza, herpes zoster, Lyme disease, malaria, mumps, syphilis, tuberculosis), metabolic (diabetes, hyperthyroidism, vitamin A deficiency), neoplastic (facial nerve tumors, parotid gland tumors, or carotid aneurysms), toxic (thalidomide, alcohol, arsenic, tetanus, diphtheria, or carbon monoxide), or idiopathic. Of course, iatrogenic injury is also a cause, such as during excision of either a primary or secondary acoustic neuroma or parotid gland tumor. The most obvious deformity in the photograph shown and the one that causes the most concern is the profound asymmetry made worse with animation. A thorough history should begin with the origin of the deformity.

- **When and how did the deficit appear?** In patients with ipsilateral paralysis of the mimetic muscles, the etiology may be congenital or from subsequent injury to the nerve. Injury may be the result of trauma—either at birth or secondary to laceration—or of prior infection, such as an unresolved Bell's palsy.

- **How old is the patient?** Younger patients tend to respond to procedures that improve facial animation better than older patients.

- **How long has the deficit been present?** The timing of muscular inactivity has important treatment implications. Muscles that have been denervated from birth or have been nonfunctional for more than a year are generally not able to be reinnervated with nerve graft alone. In such cases, free muscle transfer is required.

- **Does the patient drool when drinking?** Oral competence is a major functional concern with facial palsy and an indication for intervention.

- **Does the patient complain of facial distortion with smiling?** While less problematic from a functional standpoint, an asymmetric smile is of significant concern to most patients.

- **Does the patient experience dryness of the eyes at night?** This is particularly concerning because drying of the cornea and sclera can lead to irreversible globe injury. In many patients, a Bell's phenomenon is present in which the globe rotates upward to project the visual axis. If absent, steps must be taken to lubricate and protect the eye at night.

- **What prior steps have been taken to correct any or all associated problems?** Attempts at prior slings, nerve transfer, and/or muscle transfer—either pedicled or free—should be ascertained.

- **What is the patient's level of motivation?** Since surgery to improve facial animation is often complex and recovery requires therapy and cooperation, effort on the part of the patient is critical to achieving satisfactory results.

2. The physical examination of patients with facial nerve injury should focus on separate areas of the face as well as on each of the major branches of the nerve to determine which are functioning and which are not, noting whether or not there is some overlap.

- **Is the patient able to raise his/her brow?** This tests frontal branch function and frontalis muscle innervation.

- **Is the patient able to close his/her eyes?** This tests zygomatic branch function and orbicularis oculi innervation.

- **Does the patient have a symmetrical smile?** This tests buccal branch function and buccinator muscle innervation.

- **Is the patient able to show his/her lower teeth?** This tests marginal mandibular branch function and depressor anguli oris innervation (among others).

- **Is the patient able to tense his/her neck muscles?** This tests cervical branch function and platysma innervation.

- **Does the size of the tongue appear symmetrical and does it move adequately?** Prior transfer of the hypoglossal nerve as a source of innervation will negatively affect the appearance and motion of the tongue.

- **Are there any preexisting scars?** The presence of scars in the preauricular region or in areas commonly used as donor sites, such as the lower leg for sural nerve grafts or the upper leg for fascial grafts, is important to note since a history of prior surgery may be omitted in the patient's history.

3. Certain key studies are of value in the preoperative evaluation of patients with nerve palsy.

- **Electromyogram** (EMG) and **nerve conduction velocity** (NCV) studies, performed initially and at subsequent intervals, help determine the extent of paralysis and the prospect for recovery so that surgical planning can be initiated before muscle atrophy becomes permanent. The spontaneous release of acetylcholine provides resting tone to the muscles. Following denervation by 2 to 3 weeks, extrajunctional sensitivity to acetylcholine develops as indicated by the onset of fibrillations on EMG, which may persist for years. Fibrillations are pathognomonic for denervation, but their absence does not rule out viability. The small facial muscles do not completely degenerate for several years and may be capable of being reinnervated for many months after the event.

- In patients with a history of malignancy, further imaging of the head and neck may be important to rule out residual or recurrent tumor.

4. Preoperatively, it is important to consult with those clinicians who will follow the patients postoperatively and partially determine the final outcome.

- Most notable of these is the **therapist** who will work with the patient and use techniques in biofeedback to retrain the nerves to function in concert with the contralateral side at the appropriate time.

- The patient's **otolaryngologist** should be involved to determine the appropriate timing of intervention. Reconstruction should be entertained when the patient is felt to demonstrate no further improvement in function and, in the case of malignancy, be free of disease.

- An **ophthalmology** consult is warranted to examine the globe and provide adjunctive treatment for any sequelae of corneal exposure.

5. The primary objectives of surgical reconstruction are: first, protection of the cornea from exposure and second, restoration of oral competence of the paralyzed side to prevent drooling. The secondary objective is the restoration of normal resting balance to the face, and creation of a dynamic symmetrical smile. The latter is often difficult to achieve. There are several treatment options for

management of the paralyzed face. The surgical strategy for each patient should be tailored to individual need of the patient based on their age, overall medical condition as well as the patient's desired treatment objective. The surgical planning should factor in the experience and technical expertise of the operating surgeon to select reliable operation and to set a reasonable expectation of the patient.

- **Immediate nerve repair** with or without a nerve graft is the treatment of choice when injury to the nerve is discovered at the time of surgery. Direct repair is usually possible for immediate repair when the cut ends reapproximate without tension. Repair is best performed using a grouped fascicular technique where groups of fascicles are repaired. In a delayed repair, interpositional nerve grafts are often needed to avoid tension in the repair. The sural and greater auricular nerves most commonly serve as donor nerves. In proximal facial nerve transaction, the nerve is subdivided into upper and lower axonal groups repaired with two cable grafts. The rate of regrowth is approximately 1 mm/day and the progress can be followed clinically by eliciting a Tinel sign along the nerve (tapping on the skin over the nerve should elicit a tingling sensation in the region of the advancing reinnervation). Postoperative occupational therapy and the use of biofeedback are essential in optimizing reanimation of paralyzed face. They may provide less involuntary motion on speaking and swallowing than with hypoglossal transfer.

- A small **gold weight**, approximately 1 to 1.2 g, is used to assist in closure of the affected upper eyelid. It is placed in a pretarsal position via a lid crease incision under local anesthesia. The proper weight should be chosen preoperatively to weigh down the lid by gravity but not significantly reducing eye opening. When supine, it does not protect the cornea and patients often have to tape the eye when sleeping.

- **Cross-face nerve grafting** is indicated when a proximal ipsilateral facial nerve stump is unavailable, as is the case following excision of an acoustic neuroma, a distal nerve stump is present, and the facial muscles are felt to be capable of reinnervation. The donor facial nerve branch on the unparalyzed side is identified by careful intraoperative electrical stimulation. Facial nerve branches are mapped by stimulation and duplicate branches supplying zygomaticus major are taken for cross-face nerve grafting. The chosen nerve branch is transected and repaired to proximal end of the nerve graft which is tunneled across to the paralyzed side. At a second procedure, the distal end of the nerve graft is repaired to the nerve stumps of the paralyzed muscles in 6 to 9 months when axonal growth has traversed the nerve graft. Up to three cross-face nerve grafts are placed to reanimate the paralyzed zygomaticus major, orbicularis occuli, and depressor anguli oris in that order. Denervation and atrophy of the end muscles determines the limitation of this technique. Therefore, the period of denervation and the age of the patient are important determinants for a successful outcome. Direct muscle stimulation has been attempted to slow the muscle atrophy but the results have been mixed.

- **Hypoglossal-facial nerve transfer** is used if the proximal central stump is unavailable for transfer. This is indicated if there is complete interruption of the proximal facial nerve stump and lack of availability of the central stump for repair yet extracranial facial nerve is intact and mimetic muscles are available. Repair is possible within 1 year of injury. It is contraindicated in the presence of a contralateral deficit of the vagus nerve or hypoglossal nerve caused by paralysis and atrophy of the ipsilateral tongue. Postoperatively, the patient may experience, involuntary grimacing with normal tongue movement (synkinesis), articulation errors of speech, ophthalmologic problems (dryness, irritation), and absence of spontaneous facial movement. Improvement in resting tone begins around 4 to 6 months after surgery and progresses. Variations in the technique by using partial hypoglossal transfer and end-to-side anastomoses have lessened morbidity to the tongue. Hypoglossal transfer is sometimes combined with cross-face nerve graft as a "baby-sitter" to maintain innervation while the conduction signal advances across the nerve graft.

- In addition to placement of a gold weight, static procedures, such as a **browlift and blepharoplasty** are beneficial for older individuals where facial paralysis amplified the existing soft tissue ptosis of the aging face. They are often performed bilaterally where more skin and soft tissue are excised from paralyzed face than normal side. Slings to support and reposition the midface and lower lip using fascia lata or Gore-Tex are reliable in controlling the facial distortion at rest that results from an acute onset from traumatic and postsurgical nerve injury especially in elderly patients. Static slings do not provide a smile but help to control drooling from the corner of the mouth. Overcorrection in anticipation of postoperative relaxation is recommended.

- Dynamic muscle transfers using the temporalis or masseter muscles are able to provide improved symmetry and some function.
  - The central one-third of **temporalis** muscle may be reflected inferiorly either with or without a fascial graft or pericranial strip to provide length. The distal end is insetting at the modiolus as well as the corner of upper and lower lips. Postoperatively, hollowing in the temporal region is the result of muscle harvest and abnormal muscle bulk over the zygomatic arch. Alloplastic implant correction is often needed. Overcorrection of the paralyzed face is needed to account for postoperative relaxation of the muscle. Although the muscle provides pull in the smile vector, activation while eating (dyskinesia) makes it a secondary choice for smile reconstruction, especially in younger patients.
  - Transfer of the **masseter** muscle provides pull in a more lateral vector. Transfer of the digastric muscle, on the other hand, produces pull on the modiolus in a more inferior vector, reproducing the action of the depressor anguli muscle. These ancillary muscle transfers are beneficial in fine-tuning the vector of smile pull and should be employed in addition to Botox injection to contralateral normal side to modulate symmetric smile.

- When the mimetic muscles are atrophied from a long period of denervation, **free muscle transfer** can be neurotized by the proximal stump of the facial nerve or be combined with first-stage cross-face nerve graft when proximal facial nerve stump is not available. The gracilis muscle was the first muscle transferred for smile reconstruction. The ease of harvest and relatively hidden donor site makes it a popular choice. A portion of the muscle containing the neuromuscular unit is selected by stimulation of obturator nerve and is harvested for use.

- **Cross-face nerve graft and secondary free muscle transfer** can be performed with the gracilis, latissimus dorsi, serratus anterior, or pectoralis minor muscles.
  - The gracilis muscle is most popular choice because of its ease of harvest and its acceptable donor site scar. A small segment containing obturator nerve and medial circumflex vessels is transferred to paralyzed side and repaired to the distal end of cross-face nerve graft.
  - The latissimus dorsi muscle is an alternative choice because it is also relatively easy to harvest through posterior axillary incision. The thoracodorsal nerve and the vascular pedicle large enough to make the repair technically easy. The muscle tends to be large and may require revisional debulking.
  - The pectoralis minor muscle may be approached via a small anterior axillary incision which leaves

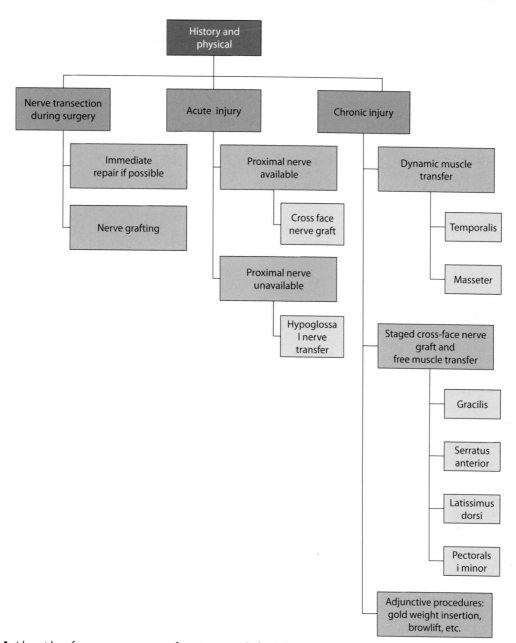

Algorithm 26-1 Algorithm for management of patients with facial palsy desiring reanimation.

an excellent donor site incision but is technically more difficult to harvest. The medial pectoralis nerve innervates the muscle and the vascular pedicle, especially the vein, maybe variable making the dissection challenging.

— Two to three slips of the serratus anterior muscle may be harvested with the long thoracic nerve and vascular pedicle to provide a thin, flat muscle for transfer to the face. This technique may be more difficult but provides multiple vectors of pull.

6. The greatest concern following facial reanimation is perhaps a less than ideal result. Patients have to be cautioned that improvement is more common and a symmetrical, spontaneous smile is unlikely. In addition to generic complications, such as hematoma or seroma formation or infection, several specific complications should be recognized.

- The most frequent complication involves inadequate axonal regeneration across the nerve repair and distal **muscle atrophy** following functional muscle transfer resulting in inadequate muscle pull. External muscle stimulation may prevent muscle atrophy but can also cause muscle fibrosis and contracture.

- **Poor axonal regeneration** and failure of reinnervation is a result of technically poor repair. Additionally, tension across the nerve repair, postoperative sheer forces, and movement can disrupt and impair axonal regrowth.

- **Synkinesis**, or mass movement of the muscles, is a frequent finding that results from cross innervation of regenerating axons. The more proximal the injury, the greater the degree of synkinesis is to be expected.

- Overly active pull of the transferred muscle combined with fibrosis of the muscle may result in **facial contraction** on the reconstructed side which is difficult to correct. Secondary debulking and denervation maybe needed.

PRACTICAL PEARLS

1. A thorough history and physical examination is essential in establishing the etiology and timing of the deficit and formulating a surgical plan for the paralyzed face.

2. Functional protection of cornea and control of drooling should be the priority of reconstructive plan.

3. Static procedures are generally practical and reliable for older patients with facial paralysis especially when there is significant deformity at rest.

4. Dynamic smile reconstruction is highly technique-dependent and should be performed by experienced microsurgeons familiar with facial reanimation.

5. Tension, along with poor technical apposition, is the most common cause of incomplete axonal regeneration.

References

1. Chun JK. Facial paralysis. In: Rose EH, ed. *Aesthetic Facial Restoration*. Philadelphia, PA; Lippincott Williams & Wilkins; 1998.

2. May M. *Facial Paralysis: Rehabilitation Techniques*. New York, NY: Thieme Medical Publishers; 2002.

3. Jackson CG, von Doersten PG. The facial nerve. Current trends in diagnosis, treatment, and rehabilitation. *Med Clin North Am*. 1999;83(1):179-195.

4. Mersa B, Tiangco DA, Terzis JK. Efficacy of the "baby-sitter" procedure after prolonged denervation. *J Reconstr Microsurg*. 2000;16(1):27-35.

5. Terzis JK, Noah ME. Analysis of 100 cases of free-muscle transplantation for facial paralysis. *Plast Reconstr Surg*. 1997;99(7):1905-1921.

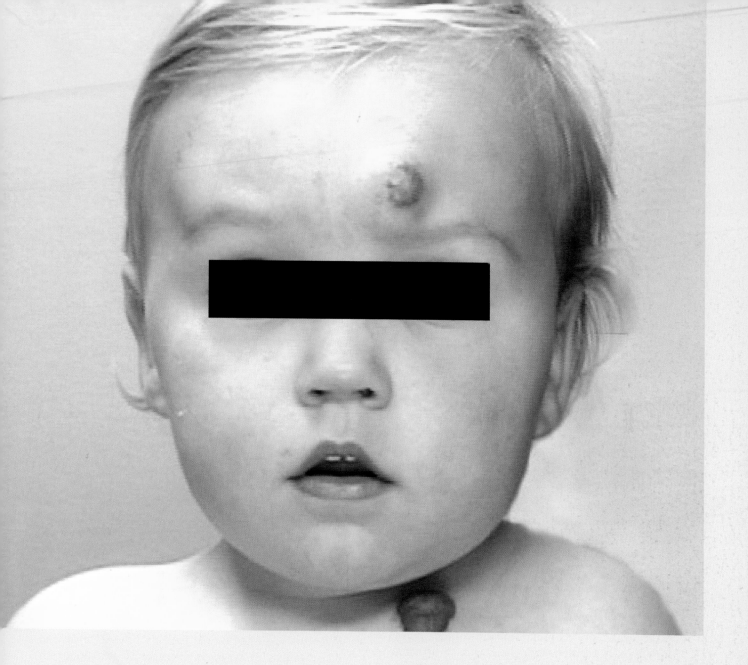

A 14-month-old boy is referred to you with three lesions on the forehead and torso.

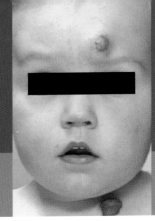
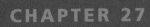

CHAPTER 27

Hemangioma

Corey S. Goldberg, Mark M. Urata, and John F. Reinisch

1. The lesions in question appear to be vascular in origin. Vascular anomalies are a heterogeneous mix of lesions that differ greatly in their presentation and treatment options. It is important to make a correct diagnosis, before proceeding with treatment. Most of the lesions fall into one of two broad categories, as described by Mulliken and Glowacki. **Hemangiomas** represent true neoplasms of endothelial cells. In the past, colloquial terms were used by clinicians to describe these lesions which today should be avoided (e.g., "strawberry nevus" and "cavernous hemangioma"). **Vascular malformations**, by contrast, are not tumors but rather remnants of embryonic tissue. They may be categorized by their components parts: arteries, veins, capillaries, lymphatic vessels, or a mixture of vessel types (combined). These can be further categorized as high flow or low flow.

- **When was the lesion first seen?** Hemangiomas are rarely present at birth (congenital hemangioma), but typically appear within the first 2 months of life. They often first appear as a "scratch" or a "pimple" on the surface of the skin, but then continue to grow over the first months of life ("early proliferative phase"). Vascular malformations are usually present at birth.

- **Is the lesion growing proportionally with the child's growth or at a faster rate?** The growth of hemangiomas usually plateaus by 6 months of age, and then continues unchanged until 12 to 18 months of age ("late proliferative phase"). A period of progressive atrophy then begins that takes years to complete ("involutional phase") and finally remain dormant. Vascular malformations tend to grow proportionally with growth of the child.

- **Does the lesion ulcerate or bleed?** Local complications are indications for treatment. Local complications include ulceration with or without infection of the overlying skin, bleeding, anatomic destruction and deformation, hypopigmentation or hyperpigmentation, and obstruction of nearby structures (airway, vision, auditory).

- **Is there respiratory compromise, failure to thrive, fatigue, or other symptoms of congestive heart failure?** Systemic complications may include congestive heart failure, failure to thrive, and/or a coagulopathy.

Kaposiform-hemangioendotheliomas can clinically appear similar to hemangiomas, but can cause consumptive coagulopathy known as Kasabach-Merritt phenomenon, which has a high mortality rate. The workup includes CBC, PT/PTT, and fibrin-split products. Clinicians should limit platelet and blood product transfusions to that which is absolutely necessary, as excess transfusions can exacerbate platelet consumption. Antifibrinolytic agents such as epsilon–aminocaproic acid may limit bleeding. A steroid regimen of prednisolone (5 to 10 mg/kg over 4 weeks, then taper) may be effective. An alternative is interferon (3 mU/m2 subcutaneously daily for 6 to 8 months). Medical failure warrants surgical debulking, if technically possible.

- **Are there psychosocial sequelae of the lesion?** Facial hemangiomas reduce self-esteem in children at an early age, cause a sense of loss and grief in parents, and can impair parent-child interaction.

- **Is there a family history of similar lesions?** Certain congenital syndromes have vascular lesions as part of their clinical spectrum.

2. A thorough physical examination serves to validate the diagnosis suggested by the patient's history. Superficial hemangiomas involve the papillary dermis, and can stretch overlying epidermis. This is worsened by abundant mast cell degranulation, producing elastolysis. Ectatic vessels within the lesion are lined with plump endothelial cells and a multilaminated basement membrane. These endothelial cells later flatten out as the lesion atrophies, leaving behind loose fibro-fatty tissue. Rapidity and completeness of involution is not altered by lesion size, location, ulceration, depth, gender, or age at presentation. Early onset of involution is the only factor that predicts an improved outcome. Historically, 50% complete involution by age 5% and 70% by age 7 years. Improvement may continue until 12 years of age. However, even when a hemangioma involutes "completely," there is often a remnant area of hypopigmented atrophic skin, or a subcutaneous mass of fibro-fatty tissue. These are often large and disfiguring and benefit from surgical treatment.

- **What are the vital signs?** Rarely, vascular anomalies can cause ventilatory compromise as a result of airway obstruction or congestive heart failure.

- **How many lesions are there?** Three or more lesions may indicate diffuse neonatal hemangiomatosis, and suggests the risk of visceral hemangiomas. Look for signs of congestive heart failure and examine the liver for enlargement. If symptomatic, consider an abdominal ultrasound.

- **Is there a particular distribution of the lesion?** Sturge-Weber syndrome consists of a triad of an upper facial capillary malformation in the V_1 and/or V_2 distribution, ipsilateral brain vascular anomalies, and eye anomalies (retinal detachment, glaucoma).

- **What color is the lesion?** Color is largely determined by depth and blood flow. More superficial lesions and those with high flow appear redder, while deeper lesions and those with low flow appear bluer. Larger vessel lesions appear thick and purple.

- **Is the lesion flat or elevated?** In the early proliferative phase, hemangiomas are often flat (macular). With time, they may become raised (nodular). Cobblestone skin is more common with late venous malformations.

- **Is there necrosis of the overlying skin?** Lesions may ulcerate, causing pain and potentially getting infected.

- **Is there obstruction of the visual axis?** This requires urgent treatment to prevent amblyopia, a developmental problem in the occipital cortex caused by either absent or poor transmission of visual images to the brain for a sustained period of time.

- **Are there other physical symptoms?** Hemangiomas may be part of one or more larger syndromes. PHACE syndrome includes posterior cranial fossa malformations (such as Dandy-Walker), large facial hemangiomas, arterial abnormalities, coarctation of the aorta, and eye abnormalities. Other findings in the extremities should be sought since they might point toward the presence of vascular malformations rather than hemangiomas.

3. Clinically significant hemangiomas and vascular anomalies are best managed with a team of experienced clinicians on an individualized basis.

— Plastic surgery.

— Pediatrics, hematology, and medical oncology.

— Dermatology.

— Interventional radiology.

— Vascular surgery.

— Ophthalmology.

— Orthopedic surgery (in cases of limb hypertrophy).

— Otolaryngology (in cases of airway compromise).

— Psychology and support groups.

4. The workup must include a CT or MRI of the brain and annual funduscopic examinations.

- **Plain X-rays** are indicated if the clinician suspects that the lesion is causing a deformation of the surrounding osseous structures. Otherwise, little information is gleaned.

- An **ultrasound** is the initial study to differentiate high flow from low flow lesions. A specific abdominal ultrasound should be obtained if there is a suspicion of visceral hemangiomas or diffuse hemangiomatosis. It may be obtained with the child awake and produces no pain.

- **MRI** is the gold standard for cases of uncertain diagnosis or for complex anatomic regions. Their appearance is mediated by their growth phase. During the **proliferative phase**, they have a mixed signal intensity with filling defects. In the **involuting phase**, the fibro-fatty tissue is most apparent. Unfortunately, patients must be still for a period of time to obtain the study so monitored sedation or general anesthesia is required.

5. Patients with a hemangioma should be regularly examined in the first 3 months to identify any complications in a timely fashion. In the absence of complications or significant cosmetic deformity, lesions may be observed until involution. Once the involuted phase is reached, any residual stigmata can be addressed surgically.

- Medical therapy is mostly in the form of steroids.

— Intralesional steroids can shrink hemangiomas, but are most effective during the proliferative phase. One possible regimen is triamcinolone 3 to 5 mg/kg (maximum dose), for up to 5 treatments at 6- to 8-week intervals. Complications include hypopigmentation, ulceration, and systemic effects such as adrenal suppression and growth restriction.

Intralesional chemotherapeutic agents, such as bleomycin, are alternatives.

— Systemic steroids are the first line of treatment for large destructive or life-threatening lesions. They are also useful for cosmetically deforming lesions that are too large for injection or excision. One possible regimen is prednisolone 5 mg/kg per day for 2 weeks, then tapered every 2 to 4 weeks by 1 mg/kg per day. Some lesions may have rebound growth after discontinuation of steroids, or may be completely resistant. In cases of rebound, failure to respond, or other steroid complications, Interferon may be used as second line treatment. One possible regimen is 2 to 3 mU/m^2 subcutaneously daily for 6 to 12 months. Response to treatment is noted after 1 to 2 months. Complications include flu-like illness, hypotension, and late spastic diplegia (5%). The first 24 hours should be monitored because of the risk of hypotension. Vincristine and other chemotherapeutic agents are alternatives, and may be useful for kaposiform-hemangioendotheliomas.

- Laser therapy makes use of blood within the lesion carries oxyhemoglobin, which absorbs light in three peak frequencies: 415 nm, 540 nm, and 580 nm. This can be exploited for selective photoablation. In the **proliferative phase**, the superficial, telangiectatic macules may be treated with a yellow light laser (5 mm spot size, 6.5 to 7.5 J), which is repeated every 4 to 6 weeks for up to 6 treatments. Papular lesions 1 mm above the surface can be treated with a flashed lamp pulsed dye laser (FLPD) (590 to 600 nm, 1.5 ms pulse width, 5 mm spot size, 6.5 to 7.5 J). In early involution, superficial, small vessel lesions may be treated with the FLPD laser and larger vessel lesions with the frequency-doubled Nd:YAG laser (1 to 50 ms pulse width, 12 J). During late involution, residual epidermal atrophy may be tightened with a CO_2 laser. Elevated, thick, and deeper lesions are out of the range of effective laser penetrance.

- Surgical excision is the standard of care for cosmetically deforming lesions that can be removed and closed primarily without deforming or damaging local anatomy. Although the natural history of these lesions is involution, even complete "resolution" often yields a cosmetically unacceptable result and the early psychosocial impact on the patient and parents is neglected. In the involuted phase residual skin atrophy from superficial lesions and remnant fibro-fatty tissue from deeper lesions merit excision and revision if cosmetically or functionally problematic.

6. Not infrequently, complications from either the lesion or the treatment may be encountered.

- Lesions within the aerodigestive tract may produce problems with **airway obstruction** that require urgent intubation or tracheostomy. Great care must be exercised to avoid bleeding. MRI is useful. Often requires urgent debulking surgically or with the CO_2 laser. Unresectable lesions require systemic treatment.

- **Obstruction of the visual axis** also requires urgent ophthalmology consultation and treatment to prevent amblyopia. Deep lesions benefit from intralesional steroids, with a small risk of blindness caused by retinal artery thrombosis. More superficial lesions may be excised. Large lesions not amenable to injection or excision require systemic treatment.

- **Ulceration**, especially in sensitive areas such as the perineum, can be painful. Local wound care, Sitz baths, and topical anesthetics are useful. Failure to heal or repeated ulceration indicate surgical excision or debulking. Large ulcerated areas that are beyond excision can be closed with skin grafting, although it is best to test the suitability of the underlying bed with allograft first. Ulcerated lesions should not be injected with steroids, as this most often exacerbates the problem.

PRACTICAL PEARLS

1. Not all strawberries are hemangiomas. Not all hemangiomas are strawberries.

2. If it is bleeding, put pressure on it.

3. Facial hemangiomas make babies and parents unhappy, and should be considered for excision.

4. Visual axis obstruction demands rapid treatment and ophthalmology consultation.

5. Life-threatening lesions refractory to systemic steroids should receive interferon.

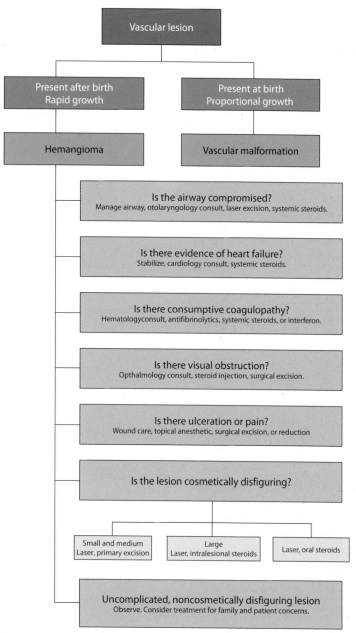

Algorithm 27-1 Algorithm for management of patients with a hemangioma.

References

1. Mulliken JB, Glowacki J. Hemangiomas and vascular malformations in infants and children: A classification based on endothelial characteristics. *Plast Reconstr Surg.* 1982;69(3):412-422.

2. Maguiness S, Guenther L. Kasabach-Merritt syndrome. *J Cutan Med Surg.* 2002;6(4):335-339.

3. Calonje E, Wilson-Jones E. Vascular tumors: Tumors and tumor-like conditions of blood vessels and lymphatics. In: Elder E, ed. *Lever's Histopathology of the Skin.* Philadelphia, PA: Lippincott Williams & Wilkins; 2005:1015-1059.

4. Gampper TJ, Morgan RF. Vascular anomalies: Hemangiomas. *Plast Reconstr Surg.* 2002;110(2):572-585.

5. Tanner JL, Dechert MP, Frieden IJ. Growing up with a facial hemangioma: Parent and child coping and adaptation. *Pediatrics.* 1998;101(3 Pt 1)446-452.

6. Ranchod TM, Frieden IJ, and Fredrick DR. Corticosteroid treatment of periorbital haemangioma of infancy: A review of the evidence. *Br J Ophthalmol.* 2005;89(9):1134-1138.

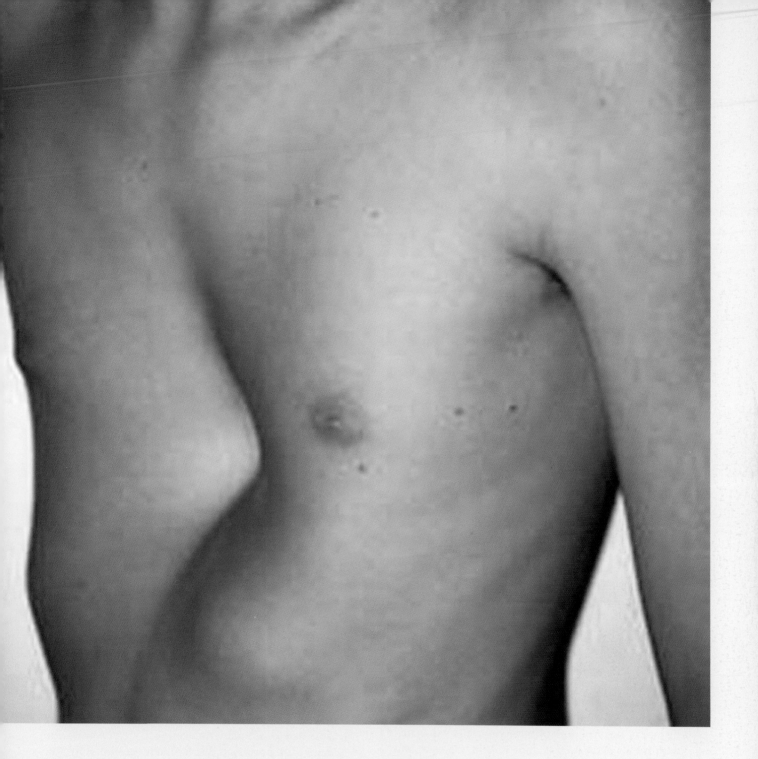

Your local pediatrician refers you a 14-year-old patient with the chest deformity pictured above.

CHAPTER 28

Congenital Chest Deformity

Michael L. Bentz

1. The patient shown in the photograph has a deformity of the chest referred to as **pectus excavatum**. This is the most common congenital chest wall deformity, appearing in 1 in 300 live births and representing 90% of congenital chest wall deformities. There is male predominance by 3:1. By contrast, **Pectus carinatum**, characterized by a prominence of the lower sternum, is less common. Both deformities result from abnormal costochondral overgrowth of unknown cause.

   - **Does the patient experience localized pain?** Some patients experience chest and/or back pain. This is usually musculoskeletal in origin, with the exact cause poorly understood.

   - **Does the patient suffer from any cardiac or respiratory symptoms?** Controversy exists regarding the degree of cardiopulmonary impairment caused by either lung compression and/or cardiac displacement. Exercise tolerance is frequently reported as normal, and the majority of patients are asymptomatic. However, severe cases may be associated with respiratory and cardiac dysfunction. It is possible that some patients become symptomatic during their teenage or early adult years.

   - **Does the patient have any other congenital anomalies?** Pectus excavatum is associated with Marfan syndrome in 25% of cases. The disorder is autosomal dominant with wide variability. The genetic defects may be because of mutations in the fibrillin (FBN1) gene located on chromosome 15. Often, there is a family history of the syndrome. Other syndromes associated with pectus excavatum include Poland, Noonan, and Leopard syndromes.

2. Physical examination should focus on the chest, but should also evaluate other structures commonly affected in patients with associated syndromes.

   - **What is the patient's visual status?** Visual disturbance resulting from lens dislocation is common in patients with Marfan syndrome.

   - **Where is the defect located?** The depression in the chest usually begins below the sternal angle and is most obvious toward the xyphoid.

   - **Are the heart sounds located in their normal location?** Auscultation of the chest should evaluate the location of the heart and lung sounds. Heart sounds are often displaced to the patient's left side (as a result of abnormal rotation of the heart). There may also be evidence of a cardiac murmur consistent with either aortic or mitral valve insufficiency in patients with Marfan syndrome. The lung sounds are usually clear, but may be diminished because of lower tidal volumes.

   - **Are the structures of the chest wall and upper extremities normally developed?** Patients with Marfan syndrome usually have an unusually large and thin stature with joint laxity and scoliosis. Absence of the sternal head of the pectoralis major muscle and associated distal anomalies, such as brachysyndactyly are seen in patients with Poland syndrome.

   - **What is the patient's posture?** In many patients, there is an anterior curvature of the thoracic spine causing the shoulders to rotate forward, a position that can also be voluntary to try to hide the deformity. While postural adjustments tend to conceal the deformity, they can also generate secondary problems of the spine. Correction of this posture is difficult, even following successful repair of the pectus excavatum.

3. Imaging and function studies can be important in the initial assessment of any patient with a chest wall deformity.

   - Baseline AP and lateral **chest radiographs** should be obtained in all patients. This will demonstrate the degree of posterior displacement of the sternum, particularly in relation to the spine, but will not visualize the appearance of the affected cartilaginous ribs. In severe (and rare) cases, the posterior sternum may contact the vertebral bodies. Plain films will also document the amount of associated scoliosis.

   - A **CT scan** of the chest is useful in determining the anterior and posterior diameters of the chest so that a CT index may be obtained. A greater index has been correlated with a more severe deformity requiring surgery. It may also provide valuable information for planning operative intervention. A three-dimensional CT scans may be used for surgical planning, but are not necessary.

- **Echocardiography** and/or **pulmonary function tests** are not mandatory, and are obtained only if indicated based on the medical history and physical examination findings. The presence of mitral valve prolapse is not unusual in patients with pectus excavatum and can be evaluated with an echocardiogram. Several physiologic/functional studies have demonstrated reduced stroke volume in the sitting or upright position that normalizes when the patient is supine.

- Pulmonary function tests may be useful in determining either preoperative or postoperative pulmonary volumes, ventilation, and exercise tolerance. They may demonstrate variable, if any, decrease in pulmonary volume and reserve.

4. A specific history of visual disturbance may be because of the lens dislocation and should be evaluated by an **ophthalmologist**.

5. There are no reasonable nonoperative strategies for the correction of severe pectus excavatum. Historically, the surgical options have been either invasive or non-invasive, and may involve camouflage by an implant placement, resection of the abnormal chest wall structures, or simply displacement of the cartilage by bending it into a more desirable contour. Specifically, the surgical approaches have included subperiosteal exposure, V-shaped osteotomy high on the chest within the intercostal space (where the curvature begins), and resection of cartilages below. The pectoralis muscles are then brought together over the repair (Ravitch procedure). Currently, many pectus excavatum deformities are commonly treated by the less invasive Nuss procedure.

- Operative correction should be considered in patients presenting with a pectus deformity and cardiopulmonary impairment. Appearance of the chest wall can be particularly important in younger patients who may have significant problems related to self-esteem. Other indications include limited exercise tolerance, cardiac and/or pulmonary dysfunction, chest pain, and psychological distress. (Adult patients with pectus excavatum can have significant displacement and rotation of the heart into the left chest. This can make operative approach to the heart quite difficult and challenging. As a result, elective repair prior to open heart surgery may occasionally be advisable.)

- Camouflage with a custom submuscular silicone implant (sometimes fixated by Dacron mesh backing) is possible, but not the mainstay of definitive therapy. The implant may be custom fabricated from the data sets and images acquired during a CT scan of the chest.

- The open repair of pectus excavatum has been used in adults and children over decades with excellent results. The **Ravitch procedure** is the most common procedure employed, which involves removal of all abnormal costal cartilages (usually 3 to 5 on each side) with preservation of the costochondral junction and repositioning of the sternum by a transverse osteotomy. Internal support can be provided across the lower ribs with a temporary bar, plate, or pins. Additional fixation modifications include the use of a vascularized 7th rib as a strut based on the anterior intercostal artery (Hayashi), bioresorbable struts (Matsui), or plate fixation. Fonkalsrud advocates resection of the lower 4 to 5 cartilages, creation of a transverse wedge osteotomy through the anterior table of the sternum so that it may be greensticked, and support with either periosteum from each side sutured together, or a thin steel strut for 6 months.

- The minimally invasive approach is recommended for a wide variety of patients with an ideal age between 8 to 12 years capitalizing on the malleability of the chest wall. (Experience in adult patients has been more limited.) The **Nuss procedure** leaves all the existing costal cartilage intact. Through bilateral transverse incisions, the dissection is carried subcutaneously and substernally with a clamp. The clamp is then replaced with a pre-bent metal fixation bar that is advanced across the chest and rotated 180 degrees to displace the pliable rib cartilage into the opposite configuration. The use of thoracoscopy has decreased the incidence of mediastinal trauma from blind dissection. The principal advantages of the minimally invasive approach are the absence of the more significant anterior chest wall incision, rib cartilage resection, and sternal osteotomy. The result is a shorter operating time, less blood loss, and an earlier return to full activity.

179

6. Objective, comprehensive corroboration of long-term outcome after surgical repair is lacking. Several large series have been reported that examine complications and outcomes of the minimally invasive approach. In those reports, patient and family satisfaction were found to be very good, with excellent and good results reported as 72% and 20%, respectively. However, the only multi-institutional study, which reviewed 251 cases, demonstrated a significant rate of complications (overall incidence of complications was almost 20%).

The most common complication requiring reoperation was **displacement of the retrosternal support bar**, initially reported to occur in 9.5% of all patients. Current stabilization methods have resulted in a current incidence of less than 2.5%.

- Injury to surrounding mediastinal and intrathoracic structures is possible and should be discussed with the patient and/or family preoperatively.
- Of course, bleeding and infection have also been reported following the operative intervention.

PRACTICAL PEARLS

1. Pectus excavatum is a depression of the sternum caused by costochondral overgrowth; the etiology is unknown.

2. Indications for operative repair of pectus deformities include cardiac and/or pulmonary impairment, and cosmetic concerns.

3. Chest X-rays should be obtained in all patients; CT scans may aid in operative planning; cardiac and pulmonary function tests are only indicated based on history or physical examination findings.

4. Surgical options include the open Ravitch technique, the minimally invasive Nuss procedure, and silicone implants that camouflage the deformity.

5. The most common complication of the Nuss procedure is bar displacement.

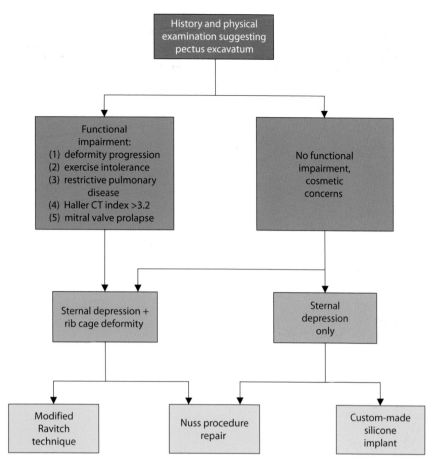

Algorithm 28-1 Algorithm for management of patients with pectus excavatum.

References

1. Ravitch MM. *Congenital Deformities of the Chest Wall and Their Operative Correction.* Philadelphia, PA: W. B. Saunders; 1977.

2. Croitoru DP, Kelly RE, Goretsky MJ, et al. Experience and modification update for the minimally invasive Nuss technique for pectus excavatum repair in 303 Patients. *J Pediatric Surg.* 2002;37(3):437-445.

3. Nuss D, Croitoru DP, Kelly RE. Review and discussion of the complications of minimally invasive pectus excavatum repair. *Eur J Pediatr Surg.* 2002;12:230-234.

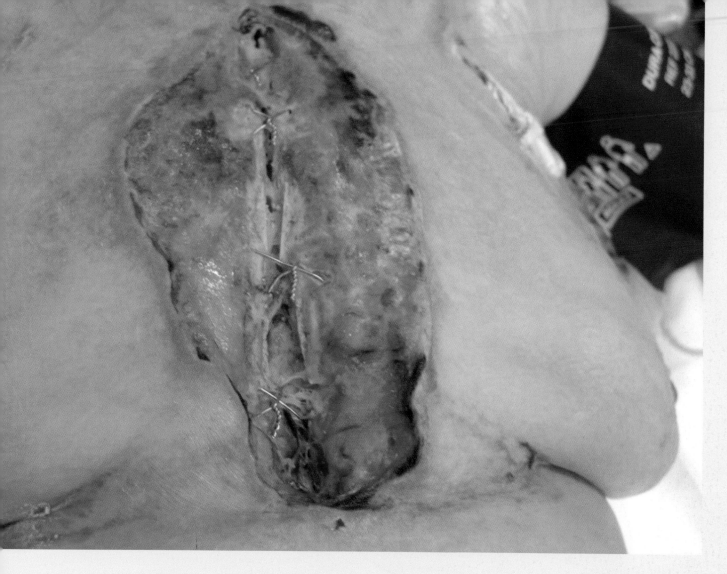

The cardiothoracic intensive care unit requests your consult regarding a patient with a chest wound 1 week following open heart surgery.

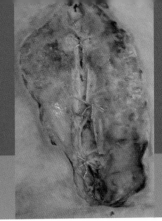

CHAPTER 29

Sternal Wound Infection

Norman H. Shulman

1. Sternal wounds result from either infection or dehiscence following a median sternotomy approach for cardiac surgery—the vast number from infection. Dehiscence, when it occurs, is usually in the early postoperative phase resulting from mechanical problems in closure or in the patient with severe chronic obstructive pulmonary disease (COPD) who may literally "tear himself apart." The cause of most infections, as in other surgical procedures, is commonly unclear but is more likely to occur in diabetics, overweight, or poorly nourished patients, or those with a history of immunocompromise or ischemia either preexisting or related to the specific cardiac procedure. Introduction of the organism is hardly ever clear and although infection prevention is important by the time the plastic surgical wound consultant is called, infection is already established.

- Sternal wounds result from either infection or dehiscence following a median sternotomy approach for cardiac surgery. The vast number results from infection. Dehiscence, when it occurs is usually in the early postoperative phase resulting from mechanical problems with the closure or in the patient with severe COPD who may literally "tear himself apart." The cause of most infections, as in other surgical procedures, is commonly unclear but is more likely to occur in diabetics, overweight, or poorly nourished patients, those with a history of immunocompromise or ischemia either preexisting or related to the specific cardiac procedure. Introduction of the organism is hardly ever clear and although infection prevention is important by the time the plastic surgical wound consultant is called, infection is already established.

- **How long ago was the procedure?** To guide therapy, sternal wounds may be divided into one of the three categories: Acute—occurring in the first two postoperative weeks, subacute—between the second and fourth week, and chronic—any time after that. Acute wounds require early, if not emergent, intervention especially if fresh coronary bypass grafts are exposed. Subacute and chronic wounds may tolerate an interval of wound preparation prior to the reconstruction.

- **Was internal mammary artery used for bypass grafting?** The internal mammary artery courses along the internal aspect of the sternum and supplies perforators to the overlying pectoralis muscle. The muscle cannot be used as a turnover flap based on these vessels if the artery has been sacrificed for cardiac revascularization.

- **Does the patient have other comorbidities?** Many patients with cardiovascular disease have other comorbid conditions that preclude major reoperative surgery. In such cases, drainage/debridement and extended wound care may be a more prudent strategy.

- **Has the patient undergone other surgical procedures?** Use or compromise of local muscles must be considered when outlining a treatment plan. For instance, prior to the thoracic surgery via a posterolateral thoracotomy may have sacrificed the latissimus dorsi muscle as a source of donor muscle.

- **Is the patient on anticoagulant medication?** It is always beneficial to discontinue anticoagulants at least 1–2 weeks prior to the surgery. In many instances, this is not possible or desirable. Coordination with the patient's cardiologist, intensivist, and cardiac surgeon can develop a plan to either discontinue nonessential anticoagulants or convert the patient to a more rapid-acting medication (heparin) that may be reversed in a more rapid time frame.

- **Does the patient smoke?** This is important to note since smoking affects the vascular anatomy and can impair circulation to pedicled flaps.

2. To institute proper treatment, a correct diagnosis must be established concerning the wound. The diagnosis is established by the presentation of the wound, the time interval from sternotomy and the nature of the cardiac surgery. Treatment protocols are dependent on these same factors plus the medical status of the patient, exposure of underlying structures or devices, and the extent of the infective process. For the sake of therapy the wounds are divided into one of the three categories—acute, occurring in the first 2 weeks postoperative, subacute, between the second and fourth week and chronic, and any time after that. The acute category requires early if not emergent intervention, especially if fresh coronary bypass grafts may be exposed, the subacute an interval of adequate wound preparation for repair, and the chronic semielective. A thorough physical examination of the patient and specifically

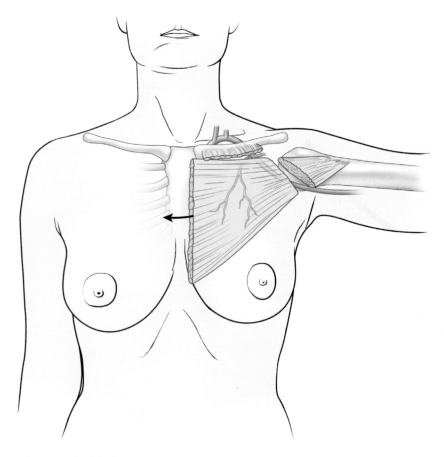

Figure 29-1 Schematic drawing highlighting pectus major muscle flap for sternal wound reconstruction.

the wound with any dressings removed should be performed.

- **Does the patient seem septic or febrile?** Evacuation of infectious material may be life-saving in the presence of sepsis. Emergent drainage of fluid may be done at the bedside but is often most thoroughly done in the operating room.

- **Is there gross purulence or necrotic material?** The presence of grossly purulent fluid requires urgent drainage to prevent sepsis and minimize further contamination.

- **Is there exposed hardware or bone?** This needs to be removed in the operating room during debridement to eliminate the presence of bacterial contaminants.

- **Are there preexisting scars?** As mentioned previously, prior surgery may have compromised sources of donor tissue. A midline abdominal incision may indicate that the omentum is no longer a viable option for reconstruction if it is scarred or has been removed.

- **What is the patient's body habitus?** Thin patients usually have thin, unsupportive fat stores, such as omentum, and therefore may not be the good candidates for omental reconstruction.

3. Necessary studies must include a current ECG and chest X-ray.

- The ECG should be compared with any preoperative tracing and great care placed on determining any irregularity especially indicating arrhythmia and possible status of the coronary circulation following bypass grafting.

- The chest film will reveal any plural fluid or pulmonary condition such as pneumonia. The X-ray will also be helpful in reconstruction as to the location and condition of sternal closure wires. Other parameters such as cardiac output or ejection fractions can be ascertained with appropriate measurements and if the patient has had valve surgery then transesophageal sonography is helpful in determining the condition and function of the cardiac valves.

- CT scans were routine for sternal wounds at one time but are not usually productive unless a particular circumstance exists such as a suspected substernal collection—manifest if a patient is sicker than the wound suggests. In the chronic wound, a SPECT CT, a new study combining standard CT technique utilizing a radioisotope labeled substance which collects only in an inflamed area, may pinpoint an infective foci which may then be surgically approached. SPECT CT is currently available only in a handful of institutions but can be extremely helpful.

- Culture and sensitivity of the wound is the simplest, along with the standard chest X-ray, and most important of necessary studies.

4. Prior to definitive therapy, it is important that the cardiac and general medical status of the patient be clearly and completely understood. The cardiologist or internist must evaluate and treat any underlying contributing conditions such as diabetes, respiratory insufficiency, and renal disease. Consultants must include these specialists plus an infectious disease expert to administer proper antibiotics, and not infrequently a neurologist as many patients who have been on cardiac bypass have neurologic sequela which must be recognized and treated.

5. The periopeative treatment plan should include decontamination with serial debridements until it is felt that the defect is suitable for closure. Removal of the wires used to close the sternum is best left for the operating room.

- At the time of debridement, all nonviable tissue should be removed, as well as any foreign material such as surgical wires, and the wound irrigated with pulsed antibiotic solution. Exposed bone and myocardium should be covered with healthy vascularized tissue, while attempting to minimize any dead space. The surgical procedure should include:
  - Cover exposed bone and myocardium with healthy vascularized tissue; also to minimize dead space.
  - Prolonged aggressive postoperative wound suction (wall suction set to 100 mm Hg negative pressure) to facilitate flap adhesion and obliterate dead space.

- Airtight and watertight wound closure.

- The interim dressing may be initially with wet-to-dry gauze in the presence of gross purulence and then changed to negative pressure therapy when cleaner. Chest wall stability can be supported by Velcro binders and "coughing pillows."

- Once clean, the exposed sternum and myocardium should be covered with vascularized muscle, which should also minimize any dead space. Coverage options include the following:
  - The **pectoralis muscle** comprises the most commonly used muscle flaps. Numerous iterations have been described, including a unilateral muscle pedicled on the dominant acromioclavicular pedicle, which is visible along the medial border of the underlying pectoralis minor muscle. In this instance, the muscle is freed from its bony origin along the sternum and planes are developed above and below the muscle. The insertion along the humerus may also be taken down to facilitate mobility and coverage of the sternum. Bilateral pectoralis muscles may also be used and sutured to one another in the midline. If mobility is not a problem, the plane above the muscle may be left intact to improve viability of the overlying skin. The "turnover" pectoralis flap has generally been discarded because the blood supply to the muscle in this instance comes from the sternal pedicles which arise from the internal mammary artery, which is frequently used for the primary coronary artery bypass procedure. The contralateral muscle may still be usable but often has inadequate reach and therefore limited application.
  - One or both **rectus abdominis muscles**, based on the superior epigastric pedicle, may be used either as a primary option or a secondary option. This is not an option if the ipsilateral internal mammary artery has been used for the bypass.
  - The **latissimus dorsi muscle** is usually a secondary or teriary option for sternal reconstruction. While the muscle based on the thoracodorsal pedicle is reliable and large enough to cover large defects, harvesting the muscle requires a lateral decubitus or prone position, as well as extensive mobilization in order to allow the muscle to be transposed anteriorly.
  - A flap of **omentum** may be used in the absence of existing muscle to cover fresh grafts and as a "rescue" flap in cases of severe infection and necrosis where earlier muscle flaps were not successful.
  - Any combination of the above options may be used as well as nonoperative treatment with extended VAC (KCI Corporation) therapy. Microvascular

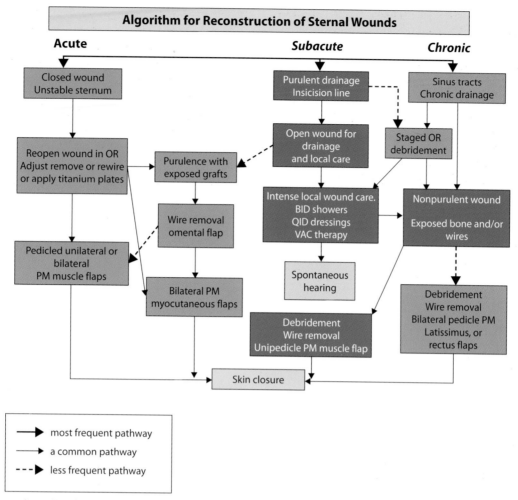

Algorithm 29-1 Algorithm for management of sternal wound infections.

free tissue transfer may also be used when the above flaps are contraindicated.

6. Postoperative complications:

- **Hematoma** formation is infrequent, most commonly seen with early resumption of anticoagulation. Most clinical situations can bear up for at least 72 hours before anticoagulation becomes critical. Consultation with the cardiologist and cardiac surgeon often permits early, safe anticoagulation intervention with either low dose aspirin or Heparin (no more than 300 mL/h) in the most critical cases. Warfarin may be started as early as 48 hours, without a loading dose, and clopidogrel not before 72 or 96 hours.

- **Seroma** formation usually results from the presence of large raw surfaces beneath the muscle flap mobilization. Wall suction for up to 5 days with size 19 French drains minimizes residual dead space and promotes early flap adherence.

- Best strategy to prevent recurrent infection prevention is the use of intense preoperative wound care consisting of incision and drainage and evacuation of gross pus, frequent dressing changes and/or VAC (KCI Corporation) therapy, and appropriate antibiotics after culture and sensitivities. Information gathered from culture of the wound in the OR before surgical prepping is particularly important when treating postoperative recurrent infection. With the exception of the omentum, flaps should not be placed in areas of frank pus any earlier than 48 hours after cleansing. Intraoperative pulsatile antibiotic irrigation, for example, orthopedic joint solution should be used in a volume of at least 2 liters after debridement and preceding the flap placement. Wounds reinfected after reconstruction must be opened for drainage and will usually heal by secondary intention, often aided by VAC therapy. Secondary flap reconstruction is rarely called for.

PRACTICAL PEARLS

1. Initial intervention should categorize each wound as acute, subacute, or chronic.

2. Purulent fluid should be drained and nonviable material debrided as soon and as thoroughly as possible before definitive operative reconstruction.

3. A final, thorough debridement, including wound edges and walls, should be done in the OR at time of reconstruction.

4. Intraoperative pulsatile antibiotic irrigation should be used in a volume of at least 2 L after debridement and preceding the flap placement.

5. With the exception of the omentum, flaps should not be placed in areas of frank pus any earlier than 48 hours after cleansing.

6. Any dead space should be minimized at the time of final closure to reduce the chance of fluid accumulation and subsequent infection.

References

1. Arnold PG, Pazolero PC. Use of pectoralis major muscle flaps to repair deficits anterior chest wall. *Plast Reconstr Surg.* 1979;63:205.

2. Nahai F, Rond RP, Hester JR, Bostwick J III, Junkiewicz MT. Primary treatment of the infected sternotomy wound with muscle flaps. A review of 211 consecutive cases. *Plast Reconstr Surg.* 1989;84:434.

3. Hugo HE, Sutton MR, Ascherman TK, Patsis MD, Smith CR, Rose EA. Single stage management of 74 consecutive sternal wound complications with pectoralis major myocutaneous advancement flaps. *Plast Reconstr Surg.* 1994;93:1433.

4. Schulman NH, Subramanian V. Sternal wound reconstruction—252 consecutive cases. The Lenox Hill experience. *P last Reconstr Surg.* 2004;114:44.

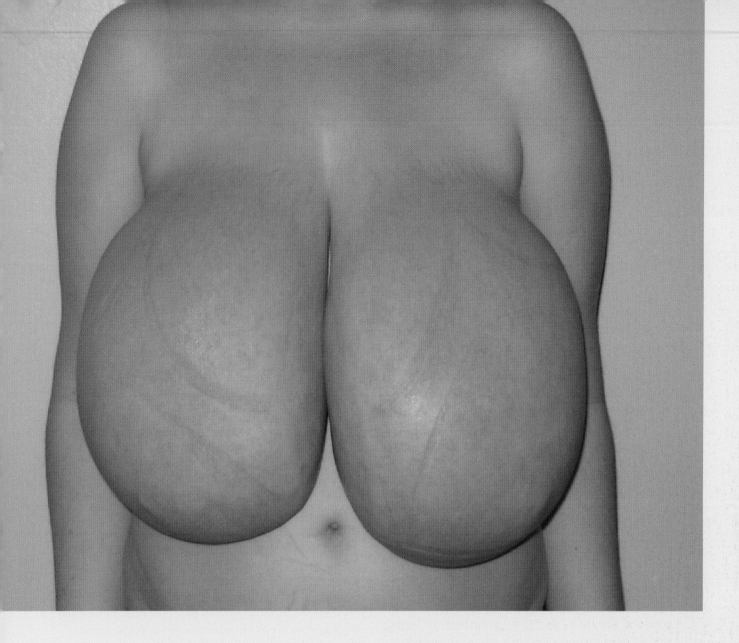

A 14-year-old girl presents with discomfort related to her significant breast development over a relatively short period of time.

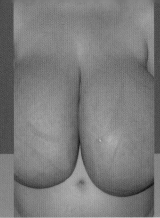

CHAPTER 30

Juvenile Virginal Hypertrophy of the Breast (Gigantomastia)

Joseph M. Serletti

1. The patient described likely has juvenile virginal breast hypertrophy. The change in breast size is rapid and bilateral and usually interferes with normal activities of daily living. The etiology appears to be multifactorial. Body weight does not appear to play a significant role. Pathologic examination of the involved breast tissue usually reveals either no proliferative changes or mild hyperplasia. As with any breast concerns, any and all related symptoms should be sought. Many of the following symptoms are more important in standard breast hypertrophy but they take a back seat in someone this young who has had such a massive rapid breast development.

- **At what age did the rapid change in breast size begin?** The rapid enlargement of the breasts usually appears during adolescence in the face of otherwise normal puberty.

- **Does the patient suffer from back pain or shoulder pain?** The weight of the breast tissue over time produces understandable pain in the upper torso, specifically the cervical and thoracic spine and shoulders. Bra straps place constant pressure across the lower neck and shoulders. The rapid growth of the breast volume in virginal hypertrophy can result in numerous musculoskeletal symptoms in growing young adolescent.

- **Does the patient experience rashes in the skin beneath the breasts?** A warm, moist area creates an environment for the development of dermatitis caused by contact of two adjacent epithelial surfaces and possibly secondary fungal infection. Patients may need to use dry gauze pads beneath the breast or antifungal creams.

- **Does the patient smoke?** With any patient, and especially those contemplating breast surgery, a history of smoking should be sought. Smoking has a negative effect on tissue flap survival, ultimate wound healing, and most importantly nipple–areola survival.

- **Does the patient desire to breast-feed in the future?** The surgical options for macromastia may interfere with the patient's ability to breast-feed, but in patients with this amount of excess development, the choice for breast-feeding will not take precedence.

- **Is there a prior family of breast disease?** With any issue regarding the breast, a family history of either benign or malignant disease is important to ascertain.

- **Does the size of the patient's breasts interfere with her activities of daily living?** The patient and her parents should be queried with respect to psychological issues related to the rapid breast enlargement since this plays a role in management. Patients often try to cover up their breasts, have poor posture, and do not participate in sports. They are upset with derogatory comments and people staring at their chests. This can lead to a poor self-image as well as other psychological manifestations.

2. Breast tissue enlarges under the influence of the hormonal challenges associated with puberty and pregnancy. No one knows why these young patients develop so rapidly. Juvenile breast hypertrophy is different from the usual breast development. Breast tissue contains adipose, glandular, neurovascular, and connective tissue components. The amount of fatty tissue is variable by weight, genetics, age, and hormonal status but there is very little fat in these young patients with juvenile breast hypertrophy. A thorough breast examination should be performed.

- **What is the patient's height and weight?** Although the breasts are large, patients are usually of normal height and weight.

- **What size are the breasts?** The breasts are heavy, solid, and difficult to examine. Not only are they massively large, but the skin is clearly under tension and may appear edematous. The patient's current bra size should be noted. Irrespective of the torso dimension, patients with symptomatic macromastia usually have a cup size in excess of a D cup. The change is breast size over time should be documented and photographs taken. Any asymmetries should be noted.

- **Are there any marks on the shoulders from the patient's bra straps?** Deep indentations in the skin are more likely in patients with normal macromastia who have tolerated the excess weight for a long period of time.

- **Are there any rashes beneath the breasts?** A warm, moist area creates an environment for the development of dermatitis caused by contact of two adjacent epithelial surfaces and possibly secondary fungal infection. Patients may need to use dry gauze pads beneath the breast or antifungal creams. A history of treatment and/or medications should be sought.

- **Are there any masses palpable?** This should be a systematic examination of each breast, looking for any discrete masses or areas of tenderness. It should be noted that the upper outer quadrant may extend into the axilla as the tail of Spence and examination of this area should not be omitted. Patients with juvenile breast hypertrophy appear to have breasts that feel as if they are composed of one solid mass.

- **Are there changes in sensation to the breast, including the nipple-areola complex?** Sensation to the superior portion of the breast is supplied by the supraclavicular nerves (C3, C4), which are branches of the cervical plexus. The medial breast skin is supplied by the anterior cutaneous divisions of the second through seventh intercostal nerves. The dominant innervation to the nipple appears to derive from the lateral cutaneous branch of the fourth intercostal nerve. It pierces the serratus anterior and travels medially and makes a right angle turn. Other sources of innervation include the intercostobrachial nerve, the inferolateral intercostal nerves, and the anteromedial intercostal nerves. Each of the nerve territories has an overlapping area of supply. While uncommon, the rapid development seen in these breasts can result in neuropraxia such that some of these patients will present preoperatively with decreased or absent nipple–areola sensation. Patients with juvenile breast hypertrophy need to be informed about the potential for postoperative changes in nipple sensation as well as sensation to the surrounding breast skin. They should also be counseled on the potential for an inability to breast-feed.

- **Are there any skin changes noted in the breasts?** Although certain parenchymal cancers of the breast will present with changes in the superficial skin ("peau d'orange texture), any skin changes in these patients is more likely due to the edema that is associated with the rapid development of the breasts in juvenile hypertrophy. A consequence of the rapid breast development in these patients is a commensurate rapid expansion of the overlying skin envelop. This can result in striae, which may be permanent despite some skin resection with reduction mammoplasty.

- **Is there any discharge from the nipple?** Tumors of the ductal system may produce bleeding from the nipple as a presenting symptom. This is not likely to be an issue in these juvenile hypertrophy patients.

- **Is there any adenopathy palpable in either the axillary or supraclavicular lymph nodes?** The axilla and the supraclavicular area are the common pathways for lymphatic egress from the breast. Nodes in the axilla may be quite high and should be sought.

3. The diagnosis of juvenile macromastia is mainly clinical since patients have normal levels of circulating hormones. The problem is due to a possibly familial, abnormal end-organ response to a normal level of circulating estrogen.

- Suspicious lesions should be biopsied for examination. On histological examination, there is increased connective tissue with little fat and possibly ductal hyperplasia.

- Mammography is difficult because of the dense glandular tissue and therefore not indicated in younger patients.

4. If the patient is obese, there is no question that a **weight loss program** is an important first step but surgical treatment may also be indicated. Many patients experience loss of significant breast volume when they are successful with weight loss but this is not likely to occur in these patients. On the other hand, a patient who is not overweight but has breast hypertrophy will not respond to weight loss. These young breasts are very fibroglandular with only a minimal amount of fat present. The recommendation for breast reduction surgery will depend on how much of a problem it is for the patient, how rapid the breast growth has been, and the patient's maturity. Breast reduction in a teenager will depend on the patient's understanding of the nature of the problem, the expected results (such as scarring, potential loss of sensation, and potential inability to breast-feed), and the potential complications (infection, wound healing, necrosis, etc). In these patients, surgical intervention may be needed on an urgent basis and is less elective in nature.

5. The major issue with treatment is timing. The surgeon needs to ascertain whether the symptoms are disabling enough to warrant surgery at a young age. Symptoms that would force patients to consider breast reduction surgery are both psychological and physical. If the patient is avoiding normal social activities (which can lead to weight gain), breast reduction may well be a good option. Physical symptoms include back and neck pain, shoulder grooving, rashes in the skin under the breasts, and even headaches. Some patients will also get numbness and tingling in their hands. Reduction mammoplasty can contribute significantly to a woman's quality-of-life. In younger individuals operated before the completion of growth, the prospect of reoperation may outweigh the benefits of more normal psychosocial development. If the patient's symptoms are not severe, then it is worth postponing the surgery to see if there is further development. A single operation would be preferable once the patient has finished puberty, but sometimes it is better to proceed knowing that a second reduction may be indicated. A thorough discussion with the patient and her parents is always necessary. The patient needs to be informed that the potential for breast-feeding may be compromised with surgery.

- Initial hormonal manipulation is usually of little benefit. Recurrence following surgery would more clearly warrant hormonal therapy in the form of a potent progesterone. Dydrogesterone 10 mg orally for 12 days of each menstrual cycle is suggested. It does *not* interfere with lactation or ovulation and has rare side effects. It has not been shown to be carcinogenic. Clearly, this type of treatment needs to be directed by an endocrinologist.

- A thorough discussion regarding the surgical options should be entertained. There are several common surgical approaches for breast reduction. Each must address several specific elements: parenchymal reduction, skin reduction, preservation of the nipple–areolar complex viability, and creation of a natural shape. The best procedure is one that is reliable and consistent in that surgeon's hands. All surgeons should, however, have a range of possibilities to consider so that they can offer the patient a procedure that is most suitable to her.

    — **Liposuction-only**: This technique addresses only the parenchymal portion of the breast, relying on the skin to contract secondarily. It may produce an acceptable result with a lower risk for circulatory or healing problems, but it is not an option in patients with juvenile hypertrophy. Breasts of these younger patients are solid and consist of dense, glandular tissue. Resection of sufficient parenchyma is difficult. Liposuction alone may have a role in older patients where the breasts consist of more adipose tissue and where only a small elevation in nipple position is required.

    — **Circumareolar technique**: The circumareolar technique addresses largely the skin envelope. A doughnut of skin is removed from around the areola, breast tissue freed circumferentially, and the concentric incisions gathered together with a nonabsorbable purse-string suture. Reduction by a circumareolar technique is generally reserved for smaller reductions and may result in flattening of the breast shape.

    — **Vertical skin incision with various pedicles**: A mosque-shaped incision is made in the skin, which ultimately produces a scar around the areola and straight down the breast toward the inframammary fold. The nipple–areola complex is preserved on an underlying pedicle that maintains a viable blood supply to the remaining tissue. The three chief sources of vascularity to the breast include the internal mammary artery to the medial portion through perforators near the sternal border, the lateral thoracic artery to the lateral portion, and the anterior and lateral branches of the intercostal vessels to the remainder. Common pedicle choices are superior, inferior, and medial. A lateral pedicle is less common since this is where tissue usually needs to be removed. In a young patient, a full thickness pedicle would be preferable to preserve the best potential for sensation and breast-feeding.

    — **Inverted-T skin incision (Wise pattern) with various pedicles**: This approach best addresses both excess skin and parenchyma. It is most appropriate for the patient who is too large for a circumareolar reduction but not large enough to require an amputative technique with free nipple grafting. The inverted-T, or Wise pattern, skin incision should be marked preoperatively with the patient standing and not drastically changed in when the patient lies down (Fig. 30-1). The initial marking is a vertical line down the central breast meridian from clavicle to inframammary fold. This line follows the aesthetic axis of the breast and specifically ignores the occasional nipple–areola complex that may fall medially or laterally off this line. The most critical determination remains is that of the desired level for the nipple–areola. It is imperative not to mark the new nipple–areola position too high. Superior malposition of the complex is easily the most common significant error during reduction mammoplasty by any technique and remains the most difficult to correct secondarily. The one acceptable landmark for use in the determination of nipple–areola position remains the inframammary fold. The fold should be marked beneath the breast and the new nipple position transposed to the intersection of the breast meridian and the level of the inframammary fold transposed on the surface of the breast. In the case of modest level disparity between the inframammary folds of asymmetric breasts, the higher position is selected; for greater disparity, a compromise setting is recommended. With the position of the new nipple chosen, the two infra-areolar limbs of the "T" are drawn at an angle determined by the amount of desired skin excision. The greater the desired skin excision, the wider the angle and vice versa. The ends of the limbs are then connected to the medial and lateral ends of the inframammary line. Any underlying pedicle may be chosen. The medial pedicle technique retains tissue near the cleavage and may minimize bottoming out seen when an inferior pedicle is chosen (Fig. 30-2). The pedicle may be drawn on the skin to remind the surgeon which areas will be de-epithelialized rather than resected. Tissue surrounding the de-epithelialized pedicle is resected until the desired volume is achieved. The scars will ultimately lie around the areola, down the inferior meridian of the breast, and within the inframammary fold.

— **Inverted-T techniques with free nipple grafting**: In patients with larger breasts or poor skin quality, an inverted-T approach will be needed to manage the excess skin. However, in patients with juvenile hypertrophy, the tissue is not normal and creation of a mobile pedicle may not be possible. Free nipple grafting may be the only viable option for these extremely large breasts. The amount of skin resection usually requires an inverted-T pattern. The nipple and areola are removed at the beginning of the procedure and replaced as a graft after the parenchyma is resected and the skin has been re-draped over the remaining breast tissue. Conversion to the free nipple graft technique may be required during the initial procedure if nipple appears significantly compromised.

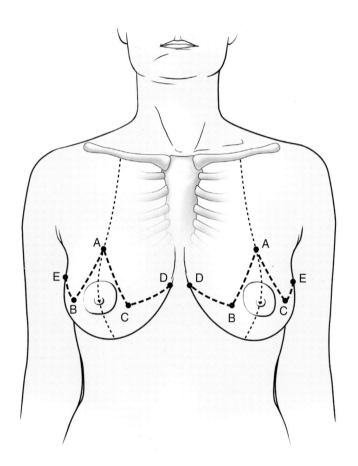

Figure 30-1 Markings for inverted T, or Wise, pattern skin resection.

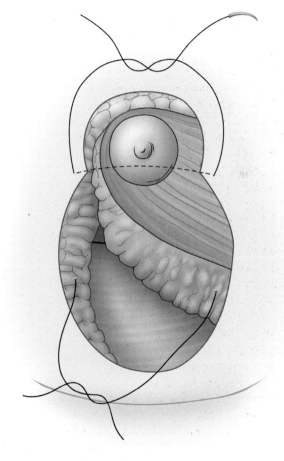

Figure 30-2 Closure of a breast reduction performed using a vertical skin resection and medial pedicle.

6. Potential problems with breast reduction include unsightly scarring, loss of sensation in the nipple and/or the breast skin, as well as possible inability to breast-feed. Sensation is equivalent for all pedicles with about 85% of patients recovering normal to near-normal sensation. Patients also need to realize that complete symmetry is never possible.

- Early surgical complications would include **hematoma** formation and impending **nipple compromise**. If a pedicle has been used and the nipple is dusky and engorged, the problem may be venous congestion and removal of some sutures may be indicated. Otherwise it is controversial whether intervention (e.g., removal and conversion to free nipple grafts) actually compromises the results. A significant hematoma needs to be evacuated surgically. Free nipple grafts are usually compressed with a bolster type of dressing.

- Later complications include **infection, poor wound healing**, and **seroma** formation. Tension on the skin may lead to wound healing problems. If nipple necrosis is evident at a follow-up appointment, it may be best to allow it to declare itself before debriding the dead tissue. Free nipple grafts often look as if some loss may occur but they should be left untouched after the bolster is removed. The patient should use some form of antibiotic ointment daily to keep the areolae moist during the healing process and activities should be restricted so that there are no shearing forces on the grafts. Seromas can be aspirated but are usually best left to resolve spontaneously.

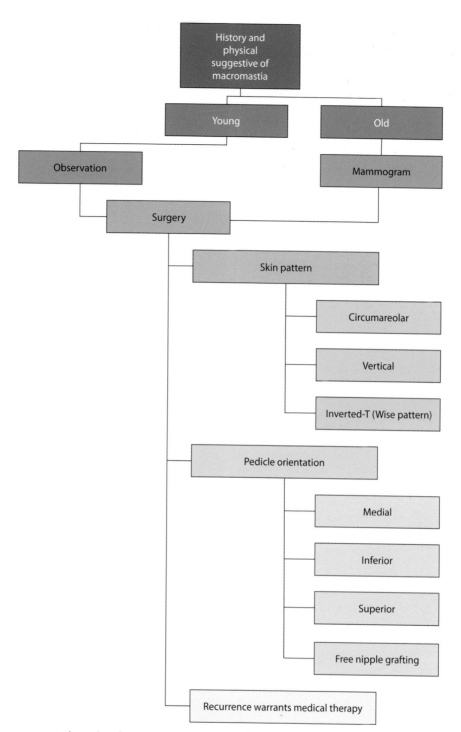

Algorithm 30-1 Management algorithm for patients with juvenile virginal macromastia.

PRACTICAL PEARLS

1. The approach to breast reduction in all ages should begin with a good history and physical examination since true pathology may be uncovered. The extent of the problem in a younger patient along with her maturity and acceptance of the limitations are key to making a good choice for treatment. Conservative management is always one of the options. Surgery may be indicated on an urgent basis in cases of juvenile breast hypertrophy. Any surgical approach will depend on the experience of the surgeon, the size of the breasts, and the patient's wishes.

2. Marking the new position of the nipple must be carefully determined using key landmarks. These include the inframammary fold and the upper breast border, both of which should be marked along the breast meridian with the patient standing. With the latter option, the nipple will lie 8 to 10 cm beneath this level It is better to make the new nipple position too low because it is almost impossible to correct a nipple which is too high.

3. A circumareolar reduction is best used with the very small reductions or with mastopexies, which do not require much nipple elevation. Otherwise the breast will look flattened and the areola will stretch. A vertical reduction works well for smaller reductions and those with adequate skin elasticity. These are rarely an option for patients with true juvenile hypertrophy—most of those patients will require an inverted-T skin resection pattern.

4. It is best when closing the incision in the vertical technique not to gather the skin. Redundant skin at the bottom will eventually flatten if there is minimal excess subcutaneous tissue left behind.

5. With any technique, it is best not to put the skin under excessive tension. Skin under tension stretches over time and skin under tension does not heal well. A small dart of inferiorly based skin may be included in the inverted-T pattern to enhance healing in the area where the suture lines meet along the inframammary fold. Traditionally, this is the area of most tension and most frequent wound dehiscence.

References

1. Psillakis JM, Cardoso de Oliveira M. History of reduction mammaplasty. In: *Reduction Mammaplasty.* Boston, MA: Little, Brown and Company, Boston; 1990:1-15.

2. Ribeiro L. Creation and evolution of 30 years of the inferior pedicle in reduction mammaplasties. *Plast Reconstr Surg.* 2002;110(3):960-970.

3. Spear SL, Howard MA. Evolution of the vertical reduction mammaplasty. *Plast Reconstr Surg.* 2003;112:855-868.

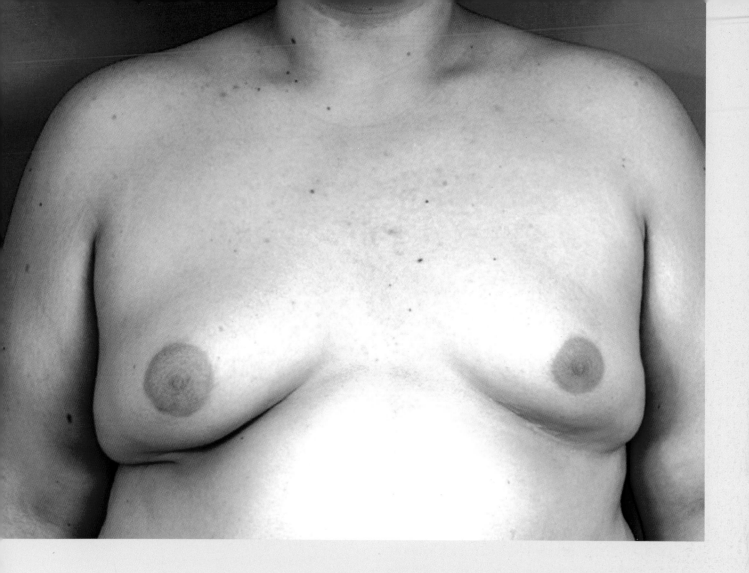

A local pediatrician refers you a 13-year-old

boy with familial concerns regarding his

appearance when not wearing his shirt.

CHAPTER 31

Gynecomastia

Dennis C. Hammond

1. The patient in question has bilateral enlargement of the breasts. In males, breast enlargement usually implies gynecomastia, but malignancy should be considered and ruled out. There is no relationship between gynecomastia and breast cancer in adult males. To some extent, gynecomastia is fairly common. It is caused by an increase in ductal tissue and stroma; true acinar lobules are not seen. Gynecomastia may be caused by any of the following: (1) an increase in estrogens, (2) a decrease in androgens, and/or (3) a deficit in androgen receptors. The condition is benign and usually reversible (e.g., during puberty), but may also be idiopathic. Pseuedogynecomastia is an increase in breast size seen in weight gain. The etiology is often ascertained by history, physical, and laboratory studies. In 25% of patients, the cause is unknown. Specific questions to ask when obtaining a detailed history include:

- **How old is the patient and when did the breast development begin?** Gynecomastia occurs at times of male hormonal change: infancy, adolescence, and old age. It is seen in approximately 60% of all newborns as a result of transplacental passage of estrogens. Although often appearing transiently at birth, most cases of gynecomastia present at puberty, with an incidence as high as 65% in boys in the 14- to 15-year age group and lasting an average duration of 1 to 2 years. The condition disappears during the late teens with less than 10% remaining by age 17. It is important to remember that the condition is often a normal finding, even though it may be associated with a more serious disease in occasional cases. In middle-aged men, the incidence drops to 30% and then rises again in the seventh decade to more than >60%.

- **How large are the breasts?** Some have suggested that the breast be enlarged more than 2 cm for a diagnosis of gynecomastia.

- **Are there any isolated and enlarging masses in breast?** Male breast cancer, which accounts for approximately 1% of all breast cancer patients, should be considered in the patient with asymmetric enlargement, a discrete lesion, or symptoms of pain and tenderness.

- **Is the condition painful?** Gynecomastia is generally not painful and most patients are asymptomatic. In addition to raising the suspicion of conditions other than gynecomastia, breast pain has important implications for insurance coverage. Often, the condition is deemed solely cosmetic and thus not covered by certain carriers.

- **Is the condition stable?** When considering when to intervene surgically, it is best to wait until some relatively stable point is reached.

- **Is the patient overweight or has the patient's weight changed of late?** Rapid weight gain can present with breast enlargement but may not be true gynecomastia but rather "pseudogynecomastia".

- **Does the patient have coexisting medical conditions?** Systemic causes related to the development of gynecomastia need to be excluded. These include:
  — Liver disease such as hepatitis or cirrhosis
  — Lung carcinoma
  — Decreased testosterone levels can occur in patients with **carcinoma or malfunction of the testes.**
  — Certain **adrenal tumors** produce androstenedione, which is converted into a form of estrogen by the enzyme aromatase.
  — **Pituitary tumors** can also lead to diminished production of testosterone.
  — **Carcinoma of the colon or prostate**
  — **Thyroid disease**
  — **Testosterone imbalance**
  — Congenital syndromes such as **Klinefelter syndrome**
  — Familial and idiopathic causes
  — Debilitating diseases, such as severe burns.

- **Does the patient take any medication or use illicit drugs?** Both legal and illegal drugs can cause gynecomastia. The common ones include spironolactone, marijuana, cimetidine, digoxin, reserpine, estrogens, theophylline, diazepam (listed in order of the pneumonic "some men can develop rather excessive thoracic diameters.") Others include androstenedione—used as a performance enhancer in food supplements—and certain antipsychotics. Medications are responsible for 10% to 20% of cases in postadolescent adults.

Some act directly on breast tissue while others increase secretion of prolactin from the pituitary.

- **Does the patient have social problems related to his appearance?** Frequently, patients are upset with their appearance and have related problems with social interaction. This should be explored and noted.

- **Does the patient experience problem with libido?** Sexual dysfunction, including impotence, decreased libido and strength, are associated with hypogonadism and may present with gynecomastia.

- A thorough review of systems is directed toward the functions of the liver, testes, prostate, adrenal, pituitary, lungs, and thyroid.

2. The physical examination should focus on the breast and chest wall but in such instances, an almost complete examination from head to toe is required since an underlying etiology may be encountered in a variety of organ systems.

- **What is the patient's body habitus?** As mentioned, pseudogynecomastia is an increase in breast size seen with weight gain.

- **A thorough breast examination** should be performed to determine the relative fibrous and fatty components of breast tissue, the presence of excess skin, the size of areola, any discrete masses, any asymmetry, any nipple discharge, and/or any areas of tenderness.

- **Is there any axillary adenopathy?** Gynecomastia is not associated with lymphadenopathy, therefore its presence should question whether a malignant or infectious process is present.

- **Are there signs of feminization?** Testosterone/estrogen imbalance will often produce physical findings in addition to the breast enlargement. These may include changes in hair distribution, body habitus, or vocal quality.

- **Are there any stigmata of thyroid, kidney, or liver disease?** All may lead to hormone imbalance and resultant gynecomastia.

- **Does the patient have any visual field deficits?** Prolactin producing tumors of the pituitary can impinge on the optic chiasm if they grow large enough and cause a bilateral hemianopsia, in which the patient loses the lateral visual field of each eye.

- **Does the patient have any masses in the neck?** Tumors or disease of the thyroid can cause hyperthyroidism and a resultant decrease in the production of testosterone.

- **Does the patient have any abdominal masses?** Certain abdominal (and other) malignancies produce serum human chorionic gonadotropin (sHCG) Productive tumors of the adrenal, if large enough, can be palpable on thorough physical examination.

- **Are there any testicular masses?** In patients with gynecomastia, a genital examination should be performed to identify whether any testicular masses are present that would act as a source of hormone production.

3. Several laboratory studies are important to obtain as a means of ruling out causative factors in the development of gynecomastia:

- Serum laboratory values of the following should be requested:
  — Complete blood count, basic chemistry panel, and liver function tests should be obtained.
  — **Estradiol**, which if elevated should warrant a CT scan of the abdomen to rule out a tumor of the adrenal gland.
  — Luteinizing hormone (**LH**) and follicle stimulating hormone (**FSH**). A low level of **testosterone** in the presence of high levels of FSH and LH would warrant a karyotype analysis to rule out Klinefelter syndrome. Here, the incidence of carcinoma of the breast is 20 to 60 times that in idiopathic cases and therefore a **breast biopsy**, especially in unilateral cases, is also indicated.
  — Human chorionic gonadotropin (**HCG**), which if elevated should warrant an ultrasound of the testes.
  — In older patients, thyroid, liver, and renal function tests should be ordered along with a chest X-ray.

- **Urine studies** for the presence of 17-ketosteroids, androgens, and gonadotropic hormones.

- Mammography is not commonly used because the tissue is easily palpable and will be removed at the time of surgery for pathologic examination.

4. Preoperatively, consultation with an **endocrinologist** is indicated to coordinate and evaluate the various tests that may need to be obtained. For overweight patients, a **dietary** consult should also be arranged.

5. If puberty is the cause of the gynecomastia, it is best to follow the patient as long as 2 years to allow for spontaneous regression to occur.

- Medical therapies are indicated to treat cases in which there is an identifiable underlying cause.

    — **Testosterone** replacement may be used for cases of testicular failure.

    — **Tamoxifen** may be used for middle-aged men in which surgery is not an option.

    — **Danazol**, a gonadotropin inhibitor, may be used to reduce any pain associated with the gynecomastia.

- There are various surgical options, which are chosen based on the individual characteristics of the patient. The two factors which must be addressed are the glandular tissue and the overlying skin envelope. The glandular tissue may be removed with either suctioning or direct excision or combination of the two.

    — In younger patients, **direct excision** of the glandular tissue through a periareolar incision may be preferable and any needed skin correction may be performed at a later date. The skin will often shrink to an acceptable condition postoperatively and growth may further correct this problem.

    — When there is a small enlargement of breast tissue with *no skin excess*, **direct excision** is similarly recommended. The major concern is leaving enough tissue under the nipple to prevent retraction. The surgical plane is distinct and adequate subcutaneous tissue can be left on the thin skin of the chest wall so that it does not stick down.

    — When there is a more significant amount of breast tissue with or without excess skin, the correction is more difficult and presents several problems. The nipple button may be difficult to leave because much of it is fat rather than fibrous tissue. The plane is more indistinct and contour irregularities of the chest wall can occur with healing. Here, feathering the dissection at the edges is important and a **combination of direct excision and suction lipectomy** may produce the best results.

    — In cases where there is marked enlargement of the breast along with excess skin, some amount of skin excision is generally required. Often, the dissection in these cases is easier because of the needed exposure, especially if the nipple is moved at the same time. A headlight or fiberoptic retractor is utilized to facilitate hemostasis. Drains (Penrose or suction) should be used and brought out through the periareolar incision rather than a separate stab incision in the chest where they might leave a hypertrophic scar. A pressure dressing will help get the flaps to adhere and may reduce seroma formation.

6. There are several specific and nonspecific surgical complications that must be addressed with the patient preoperatively and managed postoperatively if they appear. All may be minimized by specific perioperative maneuvers.

- Clinically significant postoperative **asymmetry** is inevitable since all patients are asymmetric preoperatively. Measuring the amount of tissue resected and gauging which, if either, breast should be reduced more, may minimize significant postoperative asymmetry.

- **Incomplete volume reduction** results from fears of hollowing the chest from overresection of tissue. Except for a roughly 1-cm thick skin flap above the pectoralis fascia, the majority of tissue in the region of the breast may be resected. Slightly more tissue should be left beneath the nipple-areola complex to avoid retraction.

- Postoperative **irregularity** is difficult to avoid. Intraoperatively, the edges of the resection should be feathered to avoid abrupt changes in contour and a healthy skin flap should be left above the pectoralis to avoid skin adhering to fascia. A compression garment may be prescribed postoperatively to minimize localized fluid accumulation.

- **Recurrence** is less common if the cause of the gynecomastia is identified and removed. In addition, the wide tissue planes and scant remaining tissue make this less likely.

- **Hematoma** and **infection** are not unique to breast surgery but should be considered and addressed. Adequate intraoperative hemostasis and a postoperative compressive dressing help to minimize hematoma and seroma formation. A short course of perioperative antibiotics is prudent since surgery involves potentially contaminating lactiferous ducts.

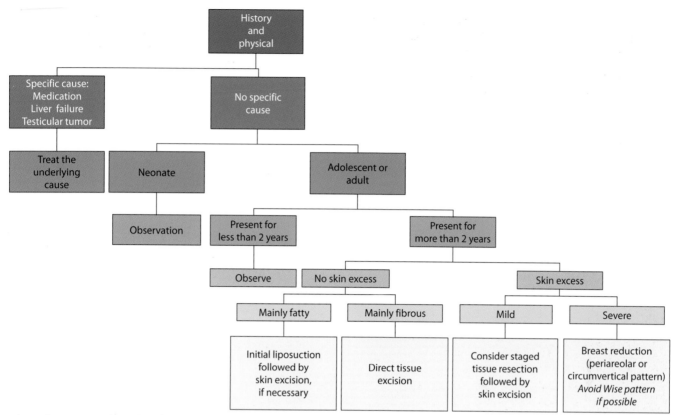

Algorithm 31-1 Algorithm for management of patients with gynecomastia.

PRACTICAL PEARLS

1. Do not hesitate to combine direct fibrous bud excision using the pull through technique with peripheral liposuction as the first line treatment as this will adequately treat most of the boys who present with gynecomastia.

2. For mild enlargement, stage skin excision as the ability of the skin to retract is great and might obviate the need for skin excision.

3. In cases of severe skin excess, do not hesitate to combine skin excision with volume reduction.

4. Make sure to leave at least 1 cm of glandular tissue beneath the areola to prevent nipple inversion. Leave adequate layer of subcutaneous fat over pectoralis fascia to prevent a concave breast. Use liposuction to optimize contouring.

5. Sit the patient up during surgery to be certain that excision is both adequate and symmetrical.

References

1. Hammond DC, Arnold JF, Simon AM, Capraro PA. Combined use of ultrasonic liposuction with the pull-through technique for the treatment of gynecomastia. *Plast Reconstr Surg.* 2003;112(3):891-895.

2. Morselli PG. Pull-through: A new technique for breast reduction in gynecomastia. *Plast Reconstr Surg.* 1996;97(2):450-454.

3. Rohrich RJ, Ha RY, Kenkel JM, Adams WP Jr. Classification and management of gynecomastia: Defining the role of ultrasound-assisted liposuction. *Plast Reconstr Surg.* 111(2): 909-23, 2003.

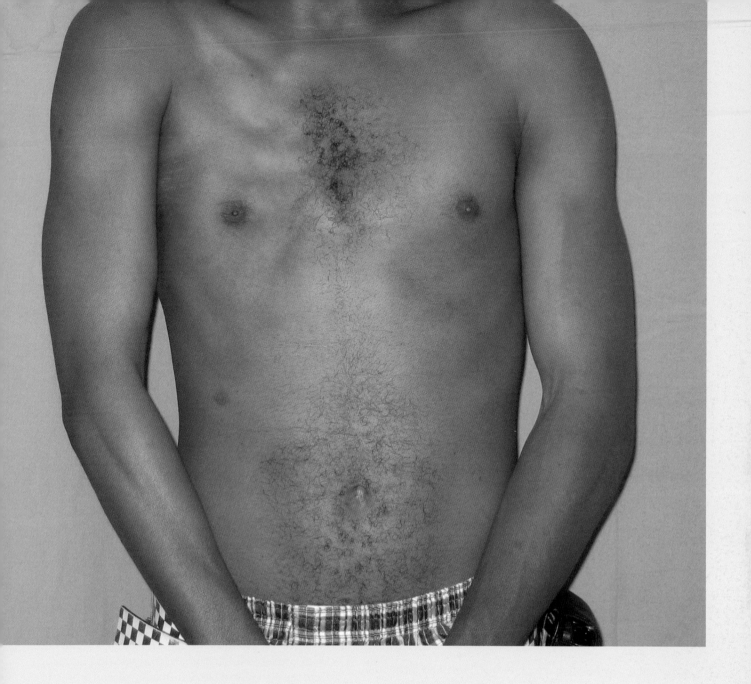

A 30-year-old man presents with asymmetry of the chest wall.

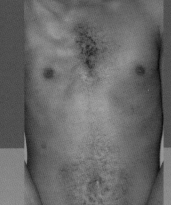

CHAPTER 32

Poland Syndrome

Nicolas Guay, MD

1. The patient in question has asymmetry of the chest wall. While most cases are iatrogenic in nature—following surgical intervention for breast lesions—some are congenital. Poland syndrome is a congenital asymmetry of the thorax which may involve the structural components of the chest and/or the breast. Poland syndrome occurs in approximately 1:30,000 births. It is mostly sporadic, almost strictly unilateral, and seen more commonly on the right. It is also referred to as Poland sequence since all of the anomalies of the hemithorax originate from a congenital hypoplasia of the subclavian artery. The more proximal the occlusion, the more the flow is decreased, and the more severe are the findings. Associated anomalies include Moebius syndrome (CN VI and CN VII), leukemia, and non-Hodgkin's lymphoma. Patients usually present in the teenage years. The most significant consideration when evaluating such patients is to perform a careful history and physical examination.

- **When did the deformity appear?** Poland syndrome is congenital anomaly that is present at birth but may not be noticeable until the patient reaches puberty. It should be noted that most young women presenting with chest wall asymmetry do not have Poland syndrome.

- **Are there any functional limitations?** These should be identified as they relate to each of the affected structures. Hypoplasia of the muscles may influence the choice of reconstruction.

- **What is the patient's occupation and avocations?** The use of certain muscles for reconstruction may be contraindicated in patients with specific occupations or interests. The mountain climbing instructor may not tolerate sacrifice of the latissimus muscle for breast reconstruction.

- **Does the patient have any coexisting medical conditions, take any medications, or have any allergies?** These are important as they relate to the suitability of the patient for one or more surgical procedures to reconstruct the breast and/or chest.

- **Is there any family history of breast disease?** Poland syndrome is not a precursor to malignant change. However, breast disease is always a concern and should be addressed with the patient at the time of presentation and as it relates to the various treatment options and techniques for cancer surveillance.

- **Does the patient smoke?** While not a contraindication to reconstruction, it is advisable that presurgical patients (and patients in general) discontinue smoking as it relates to a higher complication rate.

- **Does the patient have psychosocial concerns?** It is important to note what affect the asymmetry has on the patient's self-esteem and interaction with his or her peers. Some patients report unwillingness to participate in athletics for fear of having to change clothes in the company of others.

2. The physical examination should look for specific chest wall asymmetries, including anomalies of each structural layer of the thorax and upper extremity. Most female patients are referred for breast asymmetry, while most male patients present with hand anomalies.

- **Is there asymmetry of the breast?** Underdevelopment of the breast on one side of the chest is one of the hallmarks of Poland syndrome and the most common reason for consultation in older patients. Those entering puberty note asymmetric growth which may cause psychosocial problems. Breast development occurs in three phases. The first phase is nipple development from the ectodermal band during the second month of gestation. The second phase occurs at the fifth month of gestation when primitive mammary ducts develop. The final phase is the development of lobules under hormonal influence during puberty. The volume of the affected breast, the position of the inframammary fold, the asymmetry in position and volume of the nipple-areolar complex, and the discrepancy with the opposite breast must be carefully assessed and measured prior to treatment. Usually, the breast is hypoplastic but the nipple and/or areolar complex are formed. Bilateral cases are rare and an alternative diagnosis should be sought in such instances. Other congenital causes of chest wall asymmetry should be considered including amastia, athelia, tuberous breast, polymastia, and polythelia.

- **What is the status of the thoracic muscles?** An essential feature of Poland syndrome is the absence of the sternal head of the pectoralis major muscle. There may also be absence or hypoplasia of the pectoralis minor, serratus, infraspinatus, supraspinatus, external oblique muscle, and latissimus dorsi muscles. Involvement of the latter should specifically be noted since it affects the various treatment options. Some muscles are difficult to assess on examination.

- **Is the skin appropriate?** The surgeon must evaluate the quantity and quality of the affected thoracic skin, which affects treatment options. Hypoplasia of the skin, absence of subcutaneous fat, or absence of axillary hair are associated cutaneous anomalies.

- **Are there anomalies of the thoracic skeleton?** Abnormalities of the costal cartilages and anterior ribs are essential findings. A spectrum of rib cage abnormalities can be present, ranging from depression to hypoplasia to complete aplasia. Sternal deformity and a winged scapular (termed a "Sprengel deformity") can be present. The absence of the anterolateral ribs may cause herniation of the lung parenchyma. This is more common on the right chest wall than on the left.

- **Are there vascular anomalies of the chest or upper extremity?** Proximal anomalies, such as those of the subclavian vessels, are difficult to assess on physical examination, but the more distal vessels in the upper extremity should be evaluated. It is important to note that vessels potentially involved in reconstruction, such as thoracodorsal and internal mammary vessels can be affected.

- **Are there other findings in the upper extremity?** Concomitant findings of the ipsilateral extremity include shortening of the limb and brachysyndactyly. Also, there may be symphalangism with syndactyly and hypoplasia or complete absence of the middle phalanges.

3. In patients with Poland syndrome, **additional studies** may be required.

- Preoperative **mammograms** are not typically necessary in this population of patients. Most patients are young with dense breast parenchyma.

- Chest X-ray, CT scan, or MRI can assess the anomalies of the skeleton and help decide on reconstruction options or design a customized implant.

- Preoperative arteriogram may be required if a pedicled latissimus dorsi (thoracodorsal vessels) or free flap (internal mammary vessels) is considered as a reconstruction option.

4. Patients with Poland syndrome should be seen by a geneticist but specific consultations are generally not required since there is no underlying physiologic derangement.

- The severity of the combined anomalies may be classified as follows:
  - **Class I**: chest asymmetry as a result of a hypoplastic breast, small elevated nipple, hypoplastic pectoralis muscle, and normal thoracic skeleton.
  - **Class II**: chest asymmetry as a result of a hypoplastic breast, hypoplastic or absent nipple, absent sternal head of the pectoralis muscle, and minor anomalies of the thoracic skeleton.
  - **Class III**: chest asymmetry as a result of a hypoplastic breast, hypoplastic or absent nipple, absent sternal head of the pectoralis muscle, and marked anomalies of the thoracic skeleton.

5. **Treatment** is primarily for cosmetic purposes. Patient education and careful assessment is the key to a successful reconstruction. The patient's goals must be discussed and the different treatment options reviewed in detail.

- The indications and timing of surgery are important. Surgery may be postponed until after breast maturity, around 18 or 19 years of age, to improve symmetry. Earlier correction may be indicated for psychosocial reasons. If indicated, tissue expansion may be performed beginning in childhood through puberty to keep pace with contralateral breast development.

- The chest wall is the foundation of the reconstruction. Customized chest wall implants, autogenous rib grafts, marlex or Prolene mesh, and sternal wedge osteotomy are used to replace severe deficits of the chest wall structures.

- The simplest form of breast reconstruction is with **tissue expanders and/or implants**. The expander option may be advantageous in developing patients to mirror growth of the contralateral side.

- The **latissimus dorsi muscle flap** covering an implant is the most popular technique. A versatile selection of implant sizes are available to match any sized contralateral breast mound (independent of autologous tissue volume option); it offers appropriate implant

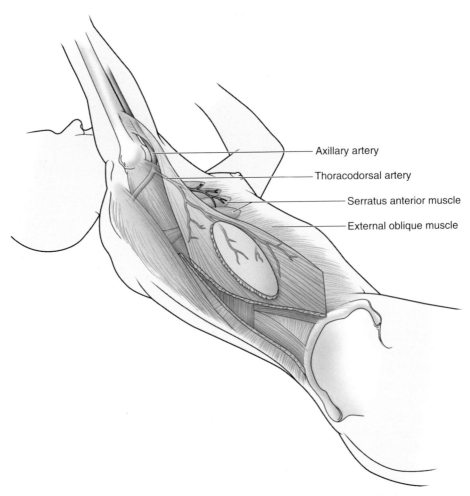

Axillary artery
Thoracodorsal artery
Serratus anterior muscle
External oblique muscle

Figure 32-1 Schematic drawing highlighting latissimus dorsi musculocutaneous flap for breast or chest wall reconstruction.

coverage lacking in this syndrome; and can recreate an appropriate axillary line.

• Other autologous tissue reconstruction options may be required if the patient's skin is hypoplastic, the muscle coverage is inappropriate, and the thoracodorsal vessels are not viable to support latissimus muscle transfer.

— A **superior or inferior artery gluteal artery flap** may be preferred in younger, nulliparous women with a paucity of abdominal skin and soft tissue. A **rectus abdominis flap** is more often used in older patients in whom the internal mammary vessels are intact.

6. Surgical results may be affected by the development of **complications**, particularly in those patients with severe chest wall deformity who were treated at a young age with customized chest wall implants. Potential complications include:

• **The development of infection** and/or **hematoma** are not specific to the type of reconstruction performed but are always a concern and should be uncommonly encountered.

• **Asymmetry** is assured after any reconstruction since no two breasts are completely identical. This should be noted to the patient and family while symmetry should be sought both of the nipple-areolar complex and of the breast mound size. Primary expanders will allow increases or decreases in size to match the contralateral breast before a final implant is inserted.

• Implant **capsular contracture** is a possibility with all augmentation cases and is certainly possible in this setting as well.

• Partial or total **flap loss** is the most feared complication following reconstruction. Prior to transfer, the adequacy of the pedicle should be ascertained and the flap transferred so as not to kink or compromise the circulation. Frequent postoperative observation should seek to identify and emergently correct any problems with vessel patency and flap viability.

• Autologous tissue **donor site morbidity** is specific to the muscle chosen. With latissimus transfer, injury to the long thoracic nerve (C_5-C_7), which runs along the lateral chest wall and innervates the serratus muscle,

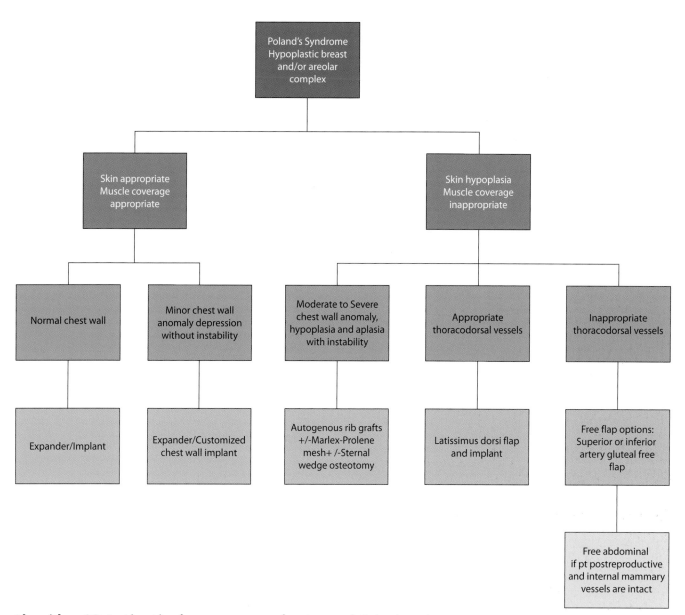

Algorithm 32-1 Algorithm for management of patients with Poland syndrome.

will produce winging of the scapula. This will be most prominent when the patient pushes the outstretched arm against a wall. With rectus transfer, weakness of the anterior abdominal wall can lead to ventral hernia formation.

- The presence of added soft tissue and potentially an implant may **interfere with cancer surveillance**. Baseline mammography should be obtained following healing and surveillance should utilize techniques to displace the implant from the remaining breast parenchyma.

PRACTICAL PEARLS

1. The initial patient assessment is crucial to establish an accurate diagnosis.

2. It is essential that preoperative assessment includes all structural layers of the thorax (skin, muscle, chest wall, and vasculature).

3. Additional studies, thoracic CT scan, and arteriogram may be necessary to complete the assessment of all layers of the thorax.

4. Patient education about the nature and potential outcomes and complications of each procedure is the key to successful reconstruction.

5. The surgeon must offer a surgical option related to the severity of the thoracic anomalies to minimize patient morbidity.

References

1. Freire-Maia N, Chutard EA, Opitz JM, Freire-Maia A, and Quelce-Salgado-A. The Poland syndrome. Clinical and genealogical data, dermatolyphic analysis, and incidence. *Hum Hered.* 1973;23:97.

2. David TJ. Familial Poland anomaly. *J Med Genet.* 1982;19:293.

3. Bouvet JP, et al. Vascular origin of Poland's syndrome. *Eur J Pediatr.* 1978;128:17.

4. Merlob P, et al. Real-time echo-Doppler duplex scanner in the evaluation of patients with Poland sequence. *Eur J Obstet Gynecol Reprod Biol.* 1989;32:103.

5. Herrman J, et al. Studies of malformation syndromes of man. Nosologic studies in the Hanhart and the Mobius syndrome. *Eur J Pediatr.* 1976;122:19.

6. Sackey K, et al. Poland's syndrome associated with childhood non-Hodgkin's lymphoma. *Am J Dis Child.* 1984;138:600.

7. Shamberger RC, Welch KJ, Upton J III. Surgical treatment of thoracic deformity in Poland's syndrome. *J Pediatr Surg.* 1989;24:760.

8. Clarkson P. Poland's syndactyly. *Guy's Hosp Rep.* 1962;111:335.

9. Ravitch MM. Poland's syndrome: A study of an eponym. *Plast Reconst Surg.* 1977;59:508.

10. Ohmori K, Takada H. Correction of Poland's pectoralis major muscle anomaly with latissimus dorsi musculocutaneous flaps. *Plast Reconst Surg.* 1980;65:400.

11. Hester TR, Bostwick J III, Poland's syndrome: Correction with latissimus dorsi tansposition. *Plast Reconst Surg.* 1982;69:226.

12. Argenta LC, et al. Refinements in reconstruction of congenital breast deformities. *Plast Reconstr Surg.* 1985;76:73.

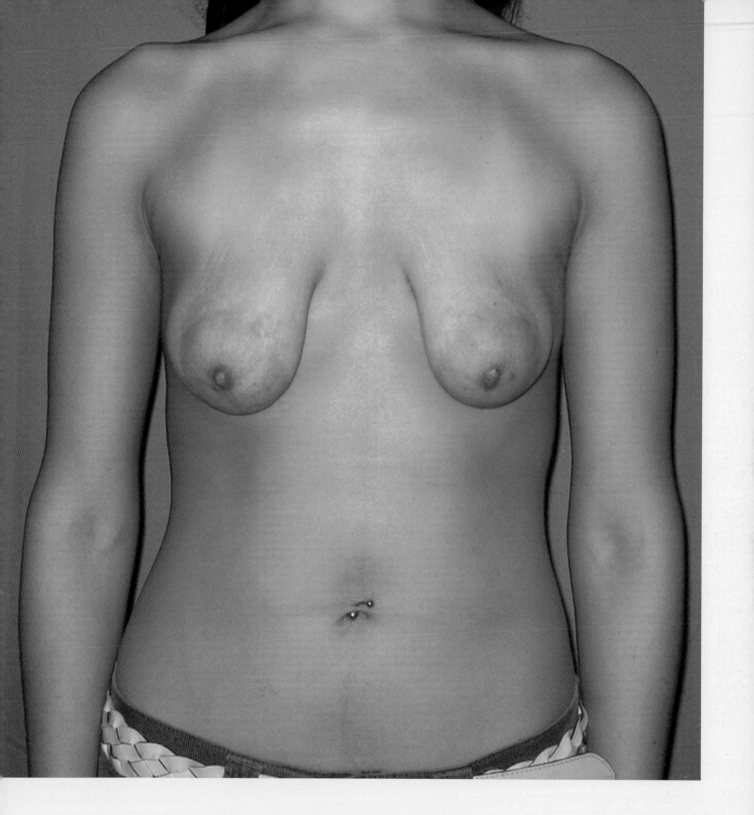

A 22-year-old woman presents with concerns

about the appearance of her breasts.

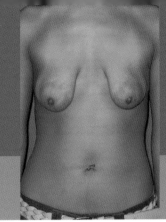

CHAPTER 33

Tuberous Breast Deformity

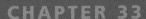

R. Michael Koch

1. The patient in question has a deformity of the breasts characterized by a narrow, constricted base and a large areola. In the absence of prior trauma or surgery, several congenital conditions should be considered. Breast development occurs in three phases. In the first phase, the nipple develops from a band of ectoderm during the second month of gestation. The second phase occurs at the fifth month of gestation when primitive mammary ducts develop. Finally, the lobules develop under the influence of increased hormone levels during puberty. Several terms should be understood when discussing congenital anomalies of the chest and breast. "Amastia" is the absence of development of one or more breasts, with or without the nipple/areola complex. "Athelia" is the absence of development of the nipple alone. "Polymastia" and "polythelia" describe the development of more than one area of breast tissue and more than one nipple (usually along the milk line), respectively. Poland syndrome is a congenital asymmetry of the thorax, which may involve the chest and/or breast. Breasts with a narrow, constricted base and parenchyma that seem to herniate into a large areola are characteristic of a tuberous breast deformity. The exact etiology of the tuberous breast deformity is currently unknown, but is likely an error during breast development or the result of limited growth of the investing fascia. Clinically, it represents a more extreme manifestation of the constricted breast deformity. The most significant consideration when evaluating a woman with aesthetic concerns is to perform a careful history and physical examination so as to establish an accurate diagnosis.

- **How old is the patient and when did the deformity become noticeable and/or concerning?** Patients with concerns regarding breast development are often seen in their late teens and early 20 years. Often, they will not change clothes in front of their peers and shy away from athletics.

- **What was the patient's birth history?** Iatrogenic trauma can lead to an arrest of breast development. Anterior placement of chest tubes in the neonatal period, for example, can lead to breast tissue hypoplasia.

- **Does the patient have any coexisting medical conditions, take any medications, or have any allergies?**

A history of prior surgery of the fingers to release a syndactyly, for example, points to a diagnosis of Poland syndrome, rather than a tuberous breast deformity. A concomitant Moebius syndrome (CN VI and CN VII palsy) is similarly seen with Poland syndrome. These are also important as they highlight the suitability of the patient for surgery.

- **Does the patient have any psychological concerns regarding the appearance of her breasts?** The deformity typically becomes evident during breast development in the teenage years. As such, the emotional squeal of the condition can be enormous.

2. The key findings in patients with tuberous breast deformity are limited to the breasts themselves. Following items need to be identified during careful physical examination:

- **What is the shape of the breast?** The tuberous breast is usually narrow, typically associated with inferior and medial parenchymal deficiency.

- **What is the appearance of the nipple/areola complex?** There is a characteristic herniation of breast tissue through an areola, which has a widened diameter.

- **Where is the inframammary fold?** In these patients, the inframammary fold is usually high and more lateral than normal. In addition, the nipple-to-inframammary fold distance is shortened.

- **Is the deformity uni- or bilateral?** Tuberous breast deformity is commonly bilateral, often with symmetric amounts of parenchymal constriction and hypoplasia as well as areolar herniation. Of patients presenting for augmentation to correct the deformity, roughly 90% have asymmetric involvement while the remainder are symmetric. Differences in breast volumes and dimensions as well as the degree of breast ptosis should be noted and recorded preoperatively.

- **Are there any chest wall findings?** Chest wall asymmetry might indicate an alternative diagnosis of Poland syndrome, which includes absence of the sternal head of the pectoralis major muscle as well as absence or hypoplasia of the pectoralis minor, serratus, infraspinatus, supraspinatus, external oblique muscle, and/or latissimus dorsi muscles.

- **Are there any additional findings?** With a tuberous breast deformity, there are no associated musculoskeletal abnormalities. The presence of associated findings should suggest an alternate diagnosis.

3. **Preoperative mammography** is not typically necessary in these patients. The condition is benign and often presents for consultation at an age when mammography in general is not recommended on account of normally dense breast tissue. Other studies, such as ultrasonography or MRI, are of little benefit.

4. No specific consultations are required in managing patients with this deformity. In the presence of more significant psychosocial concerns, a **psychological** consultation is helpful.

5. Surgical intervention is best performed when breast growth is complete. The optimal strategy is determined by the degree and severity of the deformity. Moderate-to-severe deformity in which there is a paucity of overlying skin as well as parenchymal tissue might require a two-stage approach utilizing primary tissue expansion followed by secondary augmentation. The most common surgical approaches address different facets of the problem. Some or all may be employed in any given case depending upon the specific findings identified:

- Simple augmentation (subglandular)—For many patients, the tuberous breast is hypoplastic and augmentation with an implant is important to achieve symmetry. Smooth, round, silicone gel-filled implants are placed in a subglandular pocket; however, other options such as textured or anatomically shaped, saline implants may be used with similar results. The implants may be placed through a periaerolar or inframammary approach.

- Circumareolar mastopexy—Typically, the tuberous breast has a NAC diameter of 7 to 8 cm. A new NAC of 3 to 4 cm may be chosen and a cuff of dermis 2 to 3 cm in width around the new NAC will need to be deepithelialized prior to closure.

- Radial parenchymal incisional release—Performed on the deeper aspect of the gland, this addresses the constricting ring of tissue at the base of the breast.

- Internal, glandular flaps—Additional incisions perpendicular to the radial ones may be performed to produce multiple flaps that can be rotated to compensate for the lack of parenchyma in hypoplastic areas.

- Lowering of the inframammary fold—Usually the fold is higher in the affected breast and needs to be lowered to produce symmetry at the base.

- Enlargement of the lower pole skin envelope with tissue expansion—This would be the first step in a two-stage approach that would later employ placement of a permanent implant.

6. Complications from reconstruction of the tuberous breast are most likely related to the postoperative appearance of the breasts; however, more common postoperative problems may also occur.

- More than slight **asymmetry** is concerning and should be discussed preoperatively with the patient and family. It is debatable whether or not bilateral involvement affords greater or lesser ease in creating a symmetrical appearance.

- Augmentation alone can create an unnatural "**double bubble**" appearance. Subpectoral placement creates a similar double IMF if the implant is large and continued ptosis of the glandular tissue if small. Following adequate expansion, a permanent implant may be substituted in a two-stage approach.

- **Infection** and **hematoma** are not specific to reconstruction of the tuberous breast but are always a concern and should be uncommonly encountered. Infection may require removal of the implant and delayed replacement when clinically stable.

- **Contracture** of the implant capsule is always a possibility and may be more noticeable with subglandular placement.

- The presence of an implant may **interfere with cancer surveillance**. Baseline mammography should be obtained following healing and surveillance should utilize techniques to displace the implant from the remaining breast parenchyma.

PRACTICAL PEARLS

1. The initial patient assessment is crucial to establish an accurate diagnosis and plan treatment options.

2. The preoperative assessment should evaluate all components of the deformity (inframammary fold, breast parenchyma, nipple/areolar complex, etc.) so that the optimal combination of techniques is utilized.

3. In unilateral cases, careful examination of the contralateral breast is important. The opposite side may be larger and more ptotic than normal with a tight inframammary fold, which may need to be addressed.

4. For patients with a normal contralateral breast, the volume of the implant should be selected to allow the tuberous breast to match the size of the normal breast. To facilitate this, it may be easier to perform the augmentation *prior* to the mastopexy.

5. Tuberous breast deformity is a significant malformation that can negatively influence one's psychosocial state. In general, treatment has a positive effect on the patient's emotional well-being even though the results are sometimes less than perfect.

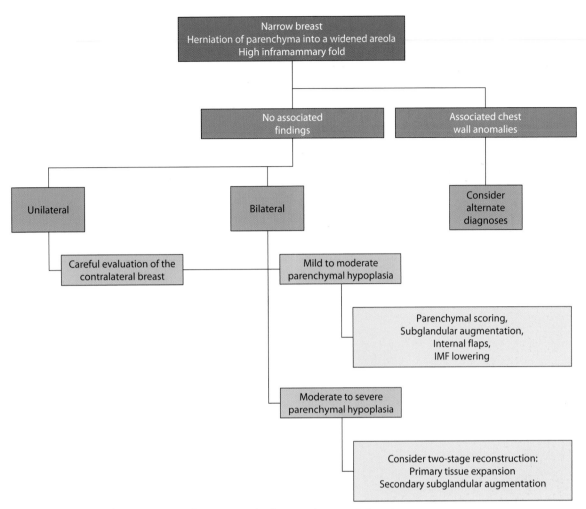

Algorithm 33-1 Algorithm for patients with suspected tuberous breast deformity.

References

1. Rees TD, Aston SJ. The tuberous breast. *Clin Plast Surg.* 1976;3:339–347.

2. Hoffman S. Correction of tuberous breasts. *Plast Reconstr Surg.* 1998;102(3):920–921.

3. Hammond DC. Augmentation mammaplasty in the patient with tuberous breasts and other complex anomalies. In: Spear SL, ed. *Surgery of the Breast: Principles and Art.* Philadelphia, PA: Lippincott Williams & Wilkins; 2006:1367–1376.

4. DeLuca-Pytell DM, Piazza RC, Holding JC, Snyder N, Hunsicker LM, Phillips LG. The incidence of tuberous breast deformity in asymmetric and symmetric mammaplasty patients. *Plast Reconstr Surg.* 2005;116(7):1894–1899.

5. Muti E. Personal approach to surgical correction of the extremely hypoplastic tuberous breast. *Aesthetic Plast Surg.* 1996;20:385–390.

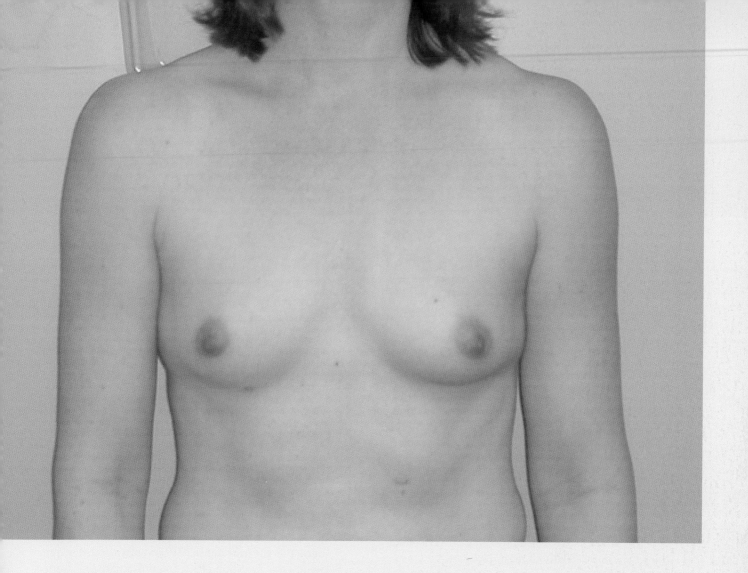

A 39-year-old woman presents to your office with concerns about the size of her breasts.

CHAPTER 34

Subjective Hypomastia

Paul D. Smith

1. The most significant consideration when evaluating a woman for breast augmentation is to understand her motives for the procedure and to ensure that she has reasonable expectations. Patients are most often seen either in their early twenties with subjective hypomastia or later, usually after pregnancy when they frequently present with glandular ptosis. When such a patient is seen for consultation, several concerns are paramount.

   - **What are the indications for augmentation mammaplasty?** Indications consist of hypomastia, glandular ptosis or grade 1 ptosis, and congenital issues such as tuberous breast deformity, Poland syndrome, or volumetric asymmetry.

   - **What are the contraindications for augmentation mammaplasty?** Unrealistic expectations, body dysmorphic disorder, presence of untreated breast oncologic disease, unstable weight, ongoing breast feeding, grade 2 or 3 ptosis without mastopexy.

   - **Is there a personal or family history of breast disease or cancer?**

   - **Are there associated congenital anomalies?** Congenital anomalies of the breast tissue should be identified since they may warrant alternative management options. It is critical to obtain a history of breast disease with a concentration on breast cancer in both the patient and her family. The current guidelines by the American Cancer Society recommend a baseline mammogram at 40 years of age and yearly after that.

2. The physical examination should look for chest wall asymmetries, differences in breast volumes and dimensions as well as the degree of breast ptosis. It is essential that preoperative measurements be as accurate as possible.

   - **Are there any suspicious physical findings?** Unusual masses in the breast or axilla, the skin dimpling, and/or nipple discharge are all worrisome signs. The presence of chest wall asymmetry and shoulder and spine conditions could affect overall symmetry. Sternal width and inframammary fold locations are critical landmarks that play a role in operative planning and may affect postoperative appearance. It is imperative to identify and communicate all preoperative asymmetries to the patient prior to the procedure.

   - **What is the quality of the breast skin?** Evaluate the skin tone, elasticity, and presence or absence of striae.

   - **What are the breast measurements?** Breast measurements are typically used to determine implant size and shape consist of the following:
     — Sternal notch to nipple distance.
     — Nipple to inframammary fold distance.
     — Base diameter of the breast.
     — Intranipple distance.
     — Amount of forward mobility of the nipple when traction is applied anteriorly.

   - **How much parenchymal coverage is there?** The greater the projection and parenchymal coverage of the breast, the less projection will be needed in the underlying implant.

   - **How does the preoperative shape of the breast influence the surgical approach?** In patients that require significant dissection of the inframammary fold caused by a constricted base, a periareolar or transaxillary approach may be more beneficial. Patients with small areolas are not candidates for silicone breast implants placed through a periareolar approach. Rather, an inframammary approach will allow the greater width required.

3. Preoperative mammograms are not necessary in a young patient (twenties) with no family history of breast cancer. However, as the patient approaches her forties, a baseline mammogram prior to surgical intervention is a prudent approach to this question. Mammograms are necessary, if the patient is more than 40 years of age or there is a strong family history of breast cancer.

4. In the healthy patient, there are no specific consultations required before proceeding with breast augmentation. Specific medical consultations may be obtained based upon each individual patient's medical history.

5. Preoperatively, the patient's desired breast size should be discussed and the types of implants available should be reviewed in detail.

   - **Implant type:** The number of implants on the market are too numerous to adequately describe in this forum; however, the three variables that must be considered are the surface (smooth or textured), the shape (round

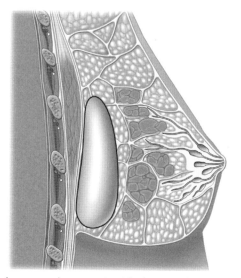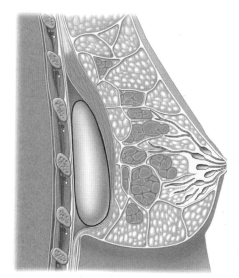

Figure 34-1 Schematic drawing highlighting subglandular and submuscular placement of breast implants.

or anatomic), and the filler (silicone or saline). Each of these options has their benefits and limitations. A short list of these differences are:

— **Smooth versus textured:** Smooth implants are less palpable than are textured implants. Textured implants have greater propensity to show dimpling or waviness. They also have lower capsular contracture rates than smooth (especially with first- and second-generation silicone implants).

— **Round versus anatomic:** Round implants will not preferentially treat the superior pole deficiencies that anatomic implants address. Anatomic implants have the potential to rotate and therefore cause asymmetries.

— **Saline versus silicone:** Saline implants have lower capsular contracture rates than silicone. They also can be placed through much smaller incisions. Silicone implants feel more natural than saline implants. Rupture from silicone however is more difficult to diagnose, requiring mammograms, ultrasounds, and MRIs. Silicone implants also do not adjust to the patient's body temperature as quickly and can feel cold after swimming in cool water.

- There are four potential access incisions commonly used and advantages and disadvantages to each. Most notably, a disadvantage of the last two access incisions is the requirement of additional specialized equipment for visualizing the dissection planes:
  — Inframammary
  — Periareolar
  — Transaxillary
  — Transumbilical

- There are four possible tissue planes ("pockets") in which the implant may be placed with advantages and disadvantages to each:
  — Subglandular
  — Subfascial
  — Submuscular: Lies beneath the pectoralis major muscle.
  — Dual plane: A combination of the implant lying below the muscle superiorly, and below the breast parenchyma inferiorly.

6. Finally, the patient needs to understand the potential complications that may occur with augmentation mam-

maplasty and the postoperative care. Reoperation is the rule, not the exception. Implants are not meant to be permanent. They will eventually need to be replaced, therefore, ongoing clinical evaluation is important.

- **Capsular contracture** will occur naturally over time. There are varying degrees of contracture. Baker classifies these from I to IV; graduating from soft and natural (I), to firm (II), to firm with visible deformity (III), to hard, visible deformity, and pain (IV). This may ultimately result in the need to remove the implant, remove the capsule, and place a new implant.

- **Leak or rupture** occurs in less than 1% of implants. If a saline implant leaks, it usually does so slowly over the course of a few days to weeks. The diagnosis is usually made by the patient. Silicone implants require more extensive diagnostic tests, the best being an MRI which is 98% sensitive and 96% specific.

- **Implant migration and asymmetry.** The normal patient has some asymmetry and augmentation may enhance this. The implant may migrate inferiorly with the weight of the implant and the stretch of the overlying soft tissues; it may also rotate which is a concern for anatomic implants.

- **Change in nipple sensation address nipple size.** Five percent of patients may lose some nipple sensation on one of the breasts. To some patients, nipple sensation is of paramount importance, in these instances, augmentation may be contraindicated because there is no way to guarantee the preservation of normal nipple sensation. It is normal to have increased sensitivity of the nipple for 6 to 9 weeks following a breast augmentation. Areolar diameter may become more pronounced following an augmentation. This can be corrected with a periareolar mastopexy, but scarring may be a problem if not adequately purse stringed with a permanent suture.

- **Hematoma** can occur in less than 1% of cases, early diagnosis and evacuation will limit the long-term sequelae, namely, scarring and contracture.

- **Infection** is best treated with early recognition, washout of the pocket, culturing the fluid, and removal of the implant. Some recent studies suggest immediate replacement with a new implant after aggressive washout may improve the likelihood of salvage up to 70%.

- Postoperatively, standard mammograms may require an additional view called an Ecklund view that displaces the breast away from the implant to be able to adequately assess the entire breast. **Interference with cancer surveillance** is of concern but there are no reports that cancer stage at the time of diagnosis is greater in patients with breast implants than in those without.

PRACTICAL PEARLS

1. Preoperative patient education and guiding the patient's expectations are critical aspects of the surgical process. Assess and describe all preoperative asymmetries to the patient at the initial consultation and document these photographically as well as in writing. Breast implants are not permanent; reoperations are the rule, not the exception.

2. Explain that the patient's own anatomy, specifically the base diameter, determines the upper limit of the implant volume. Going beyond this upper limit can lead to untoward consequences such as visible rippling; overstretch of the skin envelope, and ultimately a poorer aesthetic outcome.

3. Two borders are dependent on the surgeon's dissection, regardless of the implant size or shape. These are the medial border of the pocket and the inframammary fold. The medial border helps determine the cleavage definition, and the inferior or inframammary border determines the immediate implant location on the chest. Unfortunately this latter border may change based on the patient's tissue characteristics and the weight of the implant. The lateral dissection should depend on the diameter of the implant, and the superior dissection along with the lateral dissection is especially pertinent in patients with anatomic implants to minimize the chance of implant rotation. Minimizing the lateral dissection helps limit postoperative lateral migration of the implant.

4. When placing an implant in the subpectoral pocket, complete release of the muscle inferiorly along with the overlying pectoralis fascia is essential.

5. Focus on the ability to use every approach and every variation of implant. Don't limit your or your patient's options.

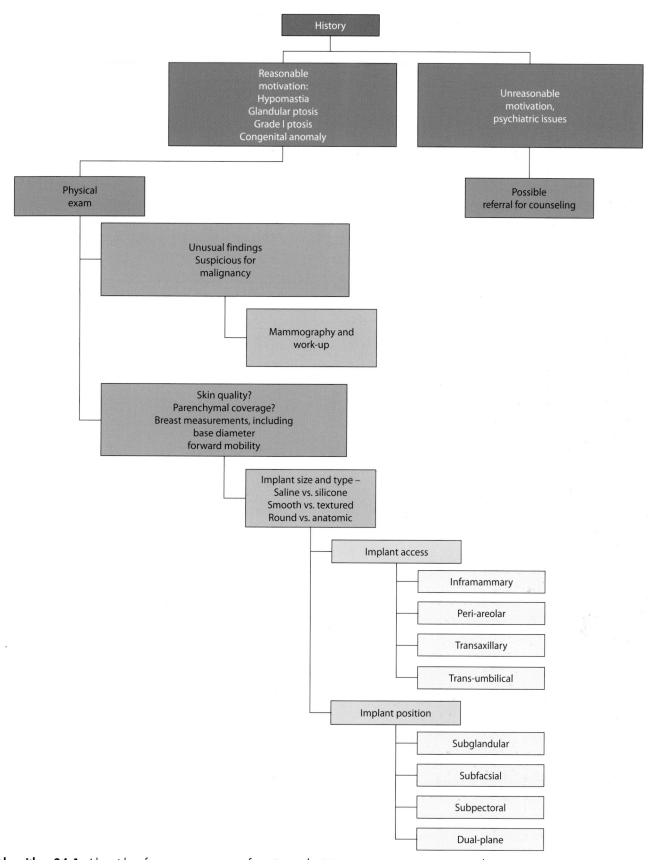

Algorithm 34-1 Algorithm for management of patients desiring augmentation mammoplasty.

References

1. Tebbetts JB, Adams WP. Five critical decisions in breast augmentation using 5 measurements in 5 minutes: The high five decision support process. *Plast Reconstr Surg.* 2005;116:2005.

2. Spear SL, Bulan Erwin J, Venturi ML. Breast augmentation. *Plast Reconstr Surg.* 2006;(7S Suppl):188S-196S.

3. Nahabedian M, Hidalgo DA, Maxwell GP, Young VL. Panel discussion—Management of complications in augmentation mamma-plasty. *Plast Reconstr Surg.* 2006;118(4 Suppl) 57.

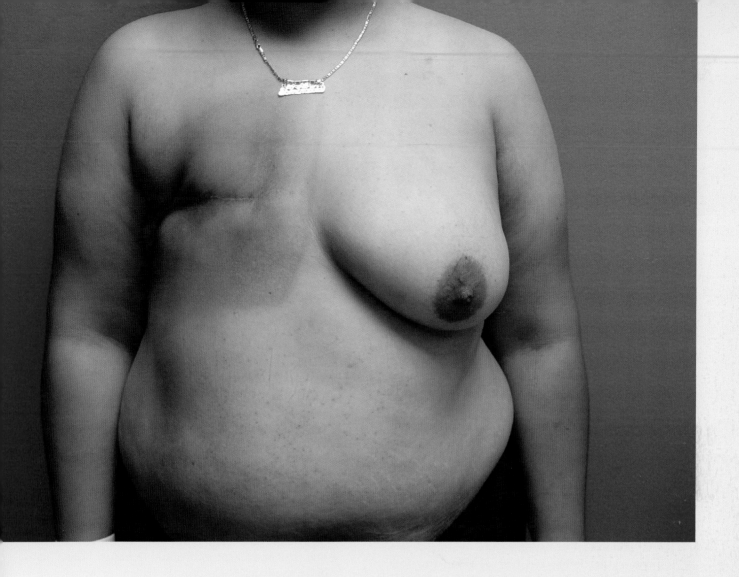

A 30-year-old woman presents to your office requesting a consultation for breast reconstruction.

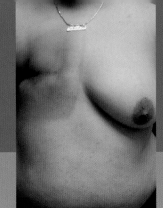

Breast Cancer

Charles E. Butler

1. The patient in question has a history of right breast cancer and an acquired right breast deformity caused by her prior surgery. Patients are frequently seen for consultation regarding breast reconstruction either before or after mastectomy. Some have had additional nonsurgical treatment, others have not. A thorough history and physical is important to determine the reconstructive options and avoid potential complications.

- **How old is the patient and when was her initial and subsequent surgeries?** Patients may undergo a combined excision and immediate reconstruction or present sometime following initial excision for secondary reconstruction.

- **Did the patient receive adjuvant therapy in the form of either chemotherapy and/or radiation therapy?** It is essential to determine whether or not neoadjuvant radiation therapy was given or is planning on being given. The use of radiation in the treatment plan influences the timing and type of reconstruction. Most surgeons advocate the use of autologous tissue for breast reconstruction in the setting of radiation. Similarly, if radiation therapy is expected, most surgeons will opt to wait until after the radiation therapy is completed before performing a delayed reconstruction with autologous tissue.

- **How long ago did the patient complete radiation?** If the patient's radiation course has been completed, most surgeons will wait at least 6 months after the completion of radiation before performing a delayed reconstruction. The decision to operate depends on the quality of the radiated tissues.

- **What are the patient's expectations for the size of her reconstructed breast?** Often, the contralateral breast is the goal for the size of the reconstructed breast. However, if the contralateral breast is excessively large or ptotic, as determined by the patient, then the new goal of the reconstructed breast is the size selected by the patient. In this situation, a second procedure will be required to improve symmetry. A reduction mammoplasty, mastopexy, or augmentation can be performed either at the same time as the contralateral reconstruction or after.

- **What other surgeries has the patient had?** Previous abdominal or pelvic surgery can alter the blood supply to the tissues of the abdominal wall making breast reconstruction with abdominal tissue transfer more complicated. Previous surgery is not a contraindication, but must be taken into consideration when planning an abdominal tissue transfer for breast reconstruction. Similar considerations must be made when using tissue from other sources as well.

- **What medical conditions does the patient have?** Healthy patients may be candidates for any type of reconstruction, whereas older patients or those in compromised health are probably best suited for the simpler procedures, submuscular implantation, or tissue expansion. Diseases that affect wound healing such as diabetes, scleroderma, or lupus can increase the risk of complications following breast reconstruction. It is important to obtain a thorough history in order to adequately inform the patient of the risks of the procedure.

- **Is the patient a smoker?** Active smoking can compromise both the reconstructed breast as well as the donor site and mastectomy flaps. All patients should be encouraged to stop smoking prior to surgery. The decision to offer certain reconstructive options and withhold others is surgeon-dependent and often based on experience.

2. The physical examination should focus on the contralateral breast and its dimensions as well as the degree of ptosis. All possible donor sites should be examined for adequacy of tissue volume and the presence of scars. An overall assessment of the patient's health should also be made.

- **Is there evidence of residual or recurrent breast disease?** Prior to beginning a course of reconstruction, the presence of residual or recurrent disease should be ruled out. This is best done with careful palpation of the existing suture line and skin flaps as well as areas of suspected lymphatic spread.

- **Does the skin of the ipsilateral breast have changes consistent with radiation injury?** Because of the soft tissue injury from radiation therapy, most surgeons prefer using autologous tissue for breast reconstruction. Unlike nonradiated skin, tissue subjected to radiation therapy is frequently indurated, less pliable, and more likely to heal with complications. If radiation therapy is planned, most surgeons will opt to wait until after the radiation therapy is completed before performing a delayed reconstruction with autologous tissue to avoid damage to the transferred tissue.

- **What are the dimensions of the contralateral breast?** When selecting a tissue expander or implant, it is imperative to know the width of the contralateral breast as well as the approximate volume and projection.

- **Does the patient have adequate abdominal tissue for reconstruction?** Using abdominal skin and soft tissue requires that there be an adequate volume to meet the size requirements of the reconstructed breast and be able to close the abdomen primarily. Athletes with little body fat have smaller recipient site requirements but may also have scant donor tissue with which to reconstruct the breast.

- **Does the patient have a diastasis of the rectus abdominis muscles or palpable abdominal hernias?** When planning breast reconstruction based on abdominal tissue, the patient must be examined for any fascial laxity between the rectus abdominis muscles or any overt hernias. Rectus diastasis will result in a more lateral position of rectus abdominis muscles and the abdominal contents remain intraperitoneal. Similarly, the presence of an abdominal or umbilical hernia is important to know prior to raising an abdominal flap to avoid injuring any herniated organs, usually bowel.

- **Does the patient have functional latissimus dorsi muscles?** Examination of the latissimus dorsi muscles should be performed in all patients undergoing breast reconstruction but is of particular importance in those patients who have had an axillary node dissection. The patient is asked to press inwards with her hands on her hips. If the latissimus dorsi muscle is not functional on the side where a patient has had an axillary node dissection, then the nerve and possibly the blood supply may have been compromised, rendering the muscle not suitable for pedicle breast reconstruction.

3. The type of breast pathology is important and should be sought from the pathology report. Most cancers arise from the ductal elements of the breast after passing, presumably, through a sequence of premalignant stages.

- Ductal carcinoma in situ (DCIS) is confined by the basement membrane of the breast ducts. It most commonly presents on mammography as microcalcifications and occurs in several histologic patterns including comedo and noncomedo.

  — Comedo DCIS is characterized by pleomorphic cells, high grade nuclei, and central areas of necrosis.

  — Noncomedo DCIS itself occurs in several subtypes that are generally not as cytologically malignant as comedo DCIS and may be difficult to distinguish from atypical hyperplasia. Although technically in situ, DCIS is treated as a malignant process.

- Infiltrating ductal carcinoma accounts for over 75% of all cases of breast cancer. Grossly, it appears as a gray-white, irregular, spiculated mass that is hard and gritty on cut section. It has no specific microscopic features but can be recognized histologically as an invasive adenocarcinoma involving the ductal elements. A number of histologic variants arise from ductal epithelium.

  — **Medullary carcinoma** (6% of invasive cancers) tends to grow to a large size and is well circumscribed. Medullary carcinoma has a favorable prognosis even in the presence of nodal metastases.

  — **Tubular carcinoma** is a rare histologic variant in its pure form and accounts for 2% of breast cancer. It is characteristically small and is usually found on mammography. It tends to be highly differentiated and has an excellent prognosis.

  — **Mucinous or colloid carcinoma** is another well-differentiated variant, which tends to form a well-circumscribed soft, gelatinous mass.

- Lobular carcinoma in situ (LCIS) has no radiologic or physical manifestations and has traditionally not been regarded as a malignancy. It is usually an incidental finding after a biopsy of a mass or mammographic abnormality. Current evidence suggests that LCIS is a marker for an increased risk of developing cancer in either breast.

- Invasive lobular carcinoma accounts for 5% to 10% of infiltrating cancers. Once it has become invasive, lobular carcinoma has a similar prognosis to the ductal type. It tends to be extensively infiltrative without a distinct tumor mass. Histologically, the cells demonstrate a characteristic single-file pattern. The tumor does not form microcalcifications and mammographic detection may be difficult.

There are no specific studies recommended for breast reconstruction.

- A recent **mammogram** (within 1 year) should be obtained for any breast prior to surgical intervention. This is relevant for procedures performed on the contralateral breast for symmetry.

- If a patient has had previous abdominal surgery then it is reasonable to get a **Doppler** study of the patient's abdominal blood supply prior to performing an autologous tissue transfer based on the rectus abdominis perforators.

4. The management of breast cancer is best addressed via a multidisciplinary approach that involves an oncologist, a breast surgeon, a plastic surgeon, and a radiation oncologist. Thoughtful coordination between these teams will facilitate the highest level of comprehensive care.

5. With regards to the surgical options for breast reconstruction, there are three broad categories: tissue expanders and implants, autologous tissue, and a combined approach using both an implant with autologous tissue. The amount of skin needed to replace the skin removed in the mastectomy is an important consideration. If the skin requirement is such that the wound will not close without new skin, then skin will need to be brought in from somewhere else, typically the back or the abdomen in the form of a flap. The quality of the mastectomy flap tissues is also the key. If the tissues are of such poor quality that expansion is not an option then replacing the tissues with healthy nonradiated flap tissue is preferred. The size and shape of the contralateral breast must be evaluated and a determination made as to which reconstructive procedure can best match it or the ultimate goal for the patient's desired breast reconstruction. A reduction mammoplasty, mastopexy, or augmentation to the contralateral breast can also be considered, if indicated.

- **Implant reconstruction**
  - **Implant (single stage):** This technique provides a breast mound of acceptable shape and volume in women with small to moderate-sized breasts. Placement beneath the pectoralis major muscle provides an added layer of healthy tissue between the implant and the mastectomy flaps, diminishes visibility, and improves the shape and contour of the reconstructed breast. The single-stage technique is rarely performed and requires ample skin and soft tissue coverage in the mastectomy flaps. One technique employs acellular dermal matrix sutured to the inferior edge of the muscle and then to the chest wall as a means achieving complete implant coverage.

  - **Expander then implant (two stage):** This is the most common form of breast reconstruction in the United States. At the time of the mastectomy, a tissue expander is placed in a submuscular position and partially filled with sterile saline. After approximately a 2-week period, weekly expansions are performed until the desired volume is achieved. Typically, each expansion is 50 to 100 cc per week over a 4 to 6-month expansion period. Use of tissue expanders allows for safe stretching (or expansion) of the mastectomy flap skin to a sufficient volume for insertion of an implant. The advantages of this technique are that it combines smaller operative procedures that have a faster recuperation time. The results of this technique are typically better for bilateral reconstructions. It is easier to match two implant-based breast reconstructions to each other than to a normal breast. The short-term disadvantages of this technique include more frequent office visits for percutaneous expansion and mild discomfort (caused by the pressure) after expansions. Long-term disadvantages are related to the device. These include capsular contracture, device failure, infection, exposure, and implant migration.

- **Autologous reconstruction**

  - **Abdominal tissue:** There are several techniques to transfer abdominal tissue to the chest for breast reconstruction. The **pedicled transverse rectus abdominis myocutaneous (TRAM)** is the most common type of abdominal tissue transfer for breast reconstruction. Abdominal skin and fat beneath the umbilicus are transferred to the chest based on a blood supply from the superior epigastric system which runs inferiorly on the undersurface of the rectus abdominis muscle. Healthy patients with an adequate volume of abdominal soft tissue may be good candidates for pedicled TRAM flap reconstruction. However, previous abdominal surgery may have compromised the blood supply by dividing the rectus muscle. Most surgeons consider heavy smoking and diabetes to be relative contraindications to a pedicled TRAM flap procedure. "Delaying" the pedicled TRAM by dividing the deep inferior epigastric vessels at a preliminary procedure may decrease the complication rate in smokers and diabetics. The advantages of the TRAM flap technique are the absence of any foreign body implant, the additional body contouring abdominal lipectomy, and the excellent long-term results that can be achieved. The disadvantages are that it is an operation of greater magnitude and has a longer postoperative recuperation time. The **free TRAM** differs from the pedicled TRAM by utilizing the dominant deep inferior epigastric system blood supply to the rectus abdominis. Since these vessels must be divided from the external iliac vessels prior to transfer, successful reconstruction requires the microvascular anastomosis of at least one artery and one vein. The internal mammary vessels in the chest are typically the recipient vessels of choice for this procedure; however, the thoraco-dorsal vessels in the axilla may also be used. The advantage of the free TRAM flap is that it utilizes the dominant blood supply to the tissue allowing for maximum perfusion and minimal fat necrosis, as opposed to the pedicled TRAM, which is based on the nondominant blood supply to the flap. The main disadvantage is the risk of thrombosis of the microvascular anastomoses and subsequent total flap loss, something that is not a problem with a pedicled TRAM. For the free TRAM to be accept-able, the flap failure rate needs to be lower than the overall 5% figure that is cited in the literature for most free flaps. Several published series show a 1% failure rate for the free TRAM flap making it as reliable as a pedicled TRAM. The only abso-lute indication for the free TRAM is previous upper abdominal surgery that has divided the superior muscle pedicle, so that a pedicled TRAM cannot be performed. The only contraindication is previous lower abdominal surgery that has interrupted the inferior epigastric blood supply. Most abdominal scars, either upper or lower, do not preclude use of the free TRAM flap, but may limit how much flap is available by crossing scar lines. **The muscle-spar-ing TRAM** is a refinement of the free TRAM tech-nique that leaves much of the rectus abdominis muscle intact. The goal of this surgery is to provide adequate blood supply to the flap while minimiz-ing donor site complications such as hernia for-mation and abdominal wall weakness that result from complete muscle harvest.

— The latest generation of TRAM flaps is the **abdomi-nal perforator flap.** This technique is different from the prior types of abdominal tissue transfer because it lacks a muscular component. The flap is supplied by perforators branching off of their respective pedicle and perfuse the skin and fat of the abdomi-nal wall. The deep inferior epigastric artery perfo-rator (DIEaP) flap is the most common one used for breast reconstruction. The rectus abdominis fascia and muscle are split to allow for the dissec-tion of the perforators and the pedicle. The advan-tage of this flap is that it maximally preserves rec-tus abdominis muscle, which has been shown to minimize abdominal wall donor site morbidity in bilateral breast reconstruction. The disadvantage is that this flap has less perfusion because it typi-cally incorporates fewer perforators than a mus-cle-sparing or free TRAM flap. Also, the dissection of this flap can be quite tedious if the perforators travel within the muscle for an extended course. The superficial inferior epigastric artery (SIEa) flap is another perforator flap used for breast recon-struction. It is based on the superficial inferior

epigastric vessels and does not involve the rectus abdominis muscle or fascia. The main advantage of this flap is that the dissection has no impact on the abdominal wall fascia or muscle, thereby eliminat-ing the possibility of weakness, bulge, or hernias related to the flap harvest. The main disadvantage of this flap is that it is not readily available in most patients. Often the vessels are deemed too small for safe microvascular transfer. Even when the vessels are present, they are usually much smaller than the deep inferior epigastric vessels. This makes for a more technically challenging procedure.

— **Gluteus flap** is usually reserved for patients who require autologous tissue but are not candidates for abdominal tissue transfer. The two main flaps used are the superior gluteal artery perforator (SGAP) flap and the inferior gluteal artery perforator (IGAP) flap. The advantages are that in the right patient these flaps can provide shapely autologous breast reconstruction with an almost unnoticeable scar on anterior inspection. The disadvantages are the potential for donor site deformity in the buttock and the need for revision, the small size of the vessels, and the difficulty in flap dissection, usually requir-ing multiple changes in the patient's position.

— **Thigh tissue** is only used in unique patients with thigh adiposity that are not candidates for other types of autologous reconstruction. The transverse upper gracilis (TUG) flap and the anterior lateral thigh (ALT) flap are examples of thigh-based breast reconstruction.

— **Latissimus dorsi flap** is an extremely versatile flap. It can be used alone but is much more commonly used in conjunction with an implant for breast reconstruction. The latissimus dorsi is a pedicled myocutaneous flap based on the thoracodorsal ves-sels and rotated from the back to the chest usually to cover an implant. This is a reliable method for breast reconstruction in both the immediate and the delayed setting. It can be used following radiation to bring healthy vascularized tissue into a radiated bed and cover an implant or tissue expander. The latissimus dorsi flap can also be used in nonradiated patients to replace a large skin deficit created by the mastectomy or in segmental mastectomy patients to fill in a partial defect. The main disadvantages to this flap are related to its posterior location. Dur-ing surgery, the patient must be repositioned at least once. The donor site tends to have a high seroma rate and although many strategies have been devel-oped to prevent this, it remains as a problem.

• **Reconstruction of the nipple** is usually performed with a second operative procedure, although it can be deferred to a third procedure. Local or general anesthesia can be used on an in- or outpatient basis. The method selected depends on the size and color of the opposite nipple and areola, the type of breast

225

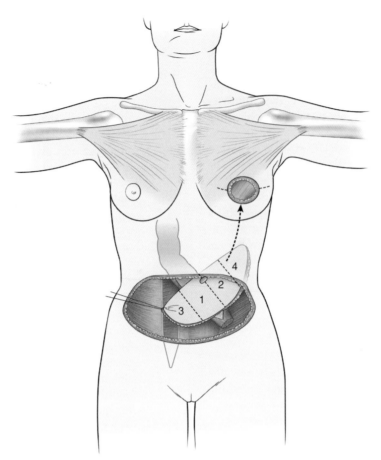

Figure 35-1 Schematic drawing highlighting transverse rectus abdominis musculocutaneous flap for breast reconstruction.

mound on which it is placed, and the patient's and surgeon's preference. Techniques for nipple reconstruction include:

— When the contralateral nipple is of **adequate size** and the patient is accepting, a **composite graft** can be taken from the opposite nipple. It comes from the lower one-half of the nipple or the tip, depending on its shape. This graft is sutured to the central portion of the de-epithelialized areola site and generally "takes" well. Other composite graft donor sites, such as ear lobule and toe pulp, have been reported, but they are generally not as satisfactory.

— Local flaps may also be used for nipple reconstruction. The most popular technique is perhaps the "skate" flap, which is designed in a linear configuration radiating from the central base with large wings on each side. The wings are elevated at the level of the deep dermis, and the linear portion includes deep fat held at a 90-degree angle and wrapped with the wings themselves. Other flaps have also been described that are similar in principle.

- The areola is usually created by either a grafting technique or by intradermal tattooing.

— The graft donor site is based on the color required to match the opposite areola. When a tan areola

is needed (as is generally the case in Caucasian patients), the upper inner thigh is the most frequent donor site (closed primarily and hidden in the perineal crease). Axillary dog ears, abdominal redundant skin, or any other easily accessible area can be used regardless of color if another tattooing is to be done. The graft is defatted to a thick split-thickness and sutured to the de-epithelialized area on the breast mound. A small hole is made in the center through which the nipple is pulled. A bolster dressing is generally placed over the graft for several days.

— Tattooing, as an alternative technique, is also popular. Intradermal pigmentation placed by traditional tattoo methods and equipment can be used for nipple coloration, for areola adjustments and coloration over previously placed grafts, or for areola creation directly on the breast mound without using a grafting technique as described above.

6. The complications of breast reconstruction are related to the specific type of reconstruction performed. However, there are certain complications that can occur regardless of the reconstruction.

- Mastectomy **flap necrosis** is a common complication that is unrelated to the type of reconstruction, but ultimately can negatively influence the outcome. Skin

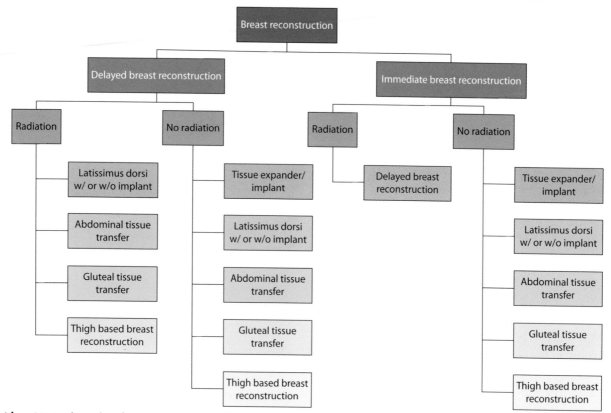

Algorithm 35-1 Algorithm for management of postmastectomy breast reconstruction.

erosion with expander extrusion may result if this occurs. Careful evaluation of the mastectomy skin flaps and appropriate debridement at the time of breast reconstruction will minimize this problem.

- **Hematoma** and **seroma** are two other common complications that can occur. Donor site complications are specific to the type of flap harvested and are more commonly seen with latissimus flap harvest.

- **Fat necrosis** is another complication that is believed to be related to inadequate circulation to the flap. This complication is seen more commonly when large flap are raised on a tenuous blood supply.

- **Infection** in either the autologous tissue or an implant may occur. Infection in the presence of an implant may require removal of the device until the infection clears followed by delayed replacement. Some surgeons have been successful with administering parenteral antibiotics and close observation in early cases of infection in hopes of avoiding implant removal.

- **Expander malfunction** may occur, including deflation, malposition, or malfunction of the inflation port.

- The soft tissues around the implant may create a **capsular contracture.** If significant, correction involves excision of the capsule and the replacement of the implant.

- Healing of the abdominal wound may occur following harvest of abdominal wall tissue. Flap slough, **abdominal wall weakness, or hernia** formation are all potential complications. Closure under minimal tension will minimize wound healing problems in healthy patients. Preservation of the rectus muscles, as with perforator flaps, will minimize hernia formation.

- With latissimus reconstruction, involuntary flexion of the transposed muscle can occur. Shoulder and arm donor morbidity is minimal but may also be present, as is some depression in the back donor area.

PRACTICAL PEARLS

1. Breast reconstruction is an elective procedure that can be performed at any time or not at all.

2. Each patient is unique and no one type of breast reconstruction is appropriate for every patient.

3. The goal of breast reconstruction is to have the patient appear symmetrical in clothing.

4. A history of or plan for neoadjuvant radiation is a major factor in determining the optimal type of breast reconstruction being performed.

5. It often takes a minimum of two, and usually three, procedures to complete a fully reconstructed breast. The entire process often takes 1 year to complete.

References

1. Alderman AK, Wilkin EG, Kim HM, et al. Complications in postmastectomy breast reconstruction: Two-year results of the Michigan Breast Reconstruction Outcome Study. *Plast Reconstr Surg.* 2002109:2265.

2. Kronowitz SJ, Robb GL. Breast reconstruction with postmastectomy radiation therapy: Current issues. *Plast Reconstr Surg.* 2004;114:950.

3. Spear SL, Onyewu C. Staged breast reconstruction with saline-filled implants in the irradiated breast: recent trends and therapeutic implications. *Plast Reconstr Surg.* 2000;105:930.

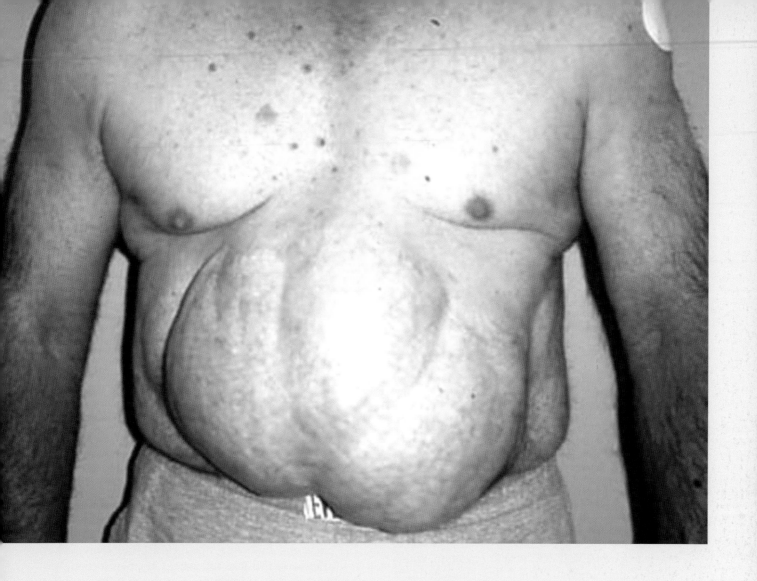

The patient in the photograph is a
55-year-old man who presented to the office
with complaints about the appearance of
abdomen following prior surgery.

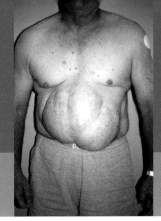

CHAPTER 36

Abdominal Wall Defect

Henry C. Vasconez

1. Defects of the anterior abdominal wall are most often the result of prior trauma or surgery. There is usually not a diagnostic dilemma but rather a therapeutic one. There may be skin loss and/or fascial/muscle loss. Information needs to be obtained that will assist in the reconstruction. Important questions in a detailed history include:

- **What was the nature of the original injury?** The history of the injury, as well as other attempts at reconstruction, can avoid serious complications. For example, a wound resulting from prior repair of an abdominal aortic aneurysm might have sacrificed important lumbar perforators making skin flap elevation prone to necrosis.

- **Have there been prior attempts at reconstruction?** Aside from simple skin grafting, other local or remote reconstructive procedures may have been attempted. Choices include a groin flap, which is limited to lower abdominal wall defects, and omentum, which requires more intra-abdominal dissection and little wall strength.

- **Was alloplastic material, such as mesh used in the repair?** Reconstruction of the tough fascia requires similar durable options. Textured mesh tends to become imbedded in the surrounding tissues and is frequently difficult to remove. Knowing this before surgery is important. Additionally, polypropylene mesh tends to fragment. Gore-Tex produces fewer adhesions, is more easily removed, and is slower to induce fibrosis, but may have lower wound strength.

- **Is there a history of radiation to the abdomen?** In the face of prior radiation, tissues have poor vascularity and heal less reliably. In this case, local tissue transfer may not be a reasonable alternative.

- **Does the patient have normal bowel habits?** Evidence of intermittent obstructive symptoms should be addressed by the general surgeon prior to embarking on reconstruction of the abdominal wall. History of drainage from the wound would suggest the presence of an enterocutaneous fistula and might change the immediate treatment options.

- **Is the patient embarrassed by his appearance?** The presence of a wide, closed abdominal wall hernia is not an emergency since there is little risk for strangulation. Most patients present to improve the appearance of their abdomen.

- **Does the patient have comorbid conditions?** Many patients have other comorbid conditions that preclude major preoperative surgery. In such cases, deferring surgery may be a more prudent strategy.

- **Does the patient smoke?** Wide elevation of abdominal wall skin and muscle flaps in an active smoker has an increased incidence of wound healing problems.

2. A thorough physical examination focusing on the chest and abdomen will help identify any pitfalls one might encounter in proceeding with surgery.

- **Are there any scars/incisions on the abdomen and medial thighs?** Extensive undermining of the abdominal wall may compromise areas that have already been traumatized. Common scars include right subcostal incisions following open cholecystectomy, lower transverse incisions following Caesarian section, vertical midline laparotomy wounds, and various other incisions. All should be noted in the context of future reconstructive efforts.

- **Where are the fascial margins?** Examining the patient in a supine position with their legs bent relaxes the abdominal muscles and makes palpation of the intra-abdominal contents easier. Asking the patient to subsequently sit up tenses the muscles, especially the rectus muscles, making the fascial margins more taut and easier to palpate.

- **Is there loss of domain?** Chronic herniation of intra-abdominal contents into an extra-abdominal hernia sac leads to a loss of domain. The abdominal space which was previously sufficient to house all of the intra-abdominal contents becomes too small. This may be as a result of the swelling of the intestines and/or constriction of the abdominal cavity.

- **Are the edges of the wound intact?** Areas of persistent wound dehiscence might indicate the presence of a fistula or predict future problems with wound healing.

- **Can you pinch the skin graft between the fingers?** Often it is possible to determine preoperatively how adherent underlying bowel is to a skin graft. The less adherent a graft, the easier it is to remove it, lyse adhesions, and return the abdominal contents to the abdomen.

- **Are there any other previously unrecognized masses or lesions?** These should be addressed before proceeding to abdominal wall reconstruction. Reconstructive efforts maybe done concomitant with other procedures or be delayed further.

3. The preoperative workup for patients needing abdominal wall reconstruction should include imaging studies and an assessment of the nutritional status.

- A **CT scan** of the abdomen and pelvis with intravenous contrast will identify any loops of bowel or other intra-abdominal contents adherent to the existing abdominal wall. It will also evaluate masses or lesions.

- A separate contrast study with injection of dye into a draining wound may be helpful to identify the course of fistula.

- Laboratory values include basic hematologic and chemistry values as well as albumin and prealbumin levels. Coagulation studies may be added if concerns exist.

4. All of the patient's medical conditions should be controlled and the nutritional status optimized prior to undergoing abdominal wall reconstruction. Management in concert with a **gastroenterologist** and **general surgeon** is prudent. Usually, the surgeon will assist with exposure of the fascial edges and lysis of intestinal adhesions.

5. While aesthetic units are not an issue in the abdomen, reconstruction of the anterior abdominal wall does imply repairing the fascia rather than simply the skin and subcutaneous tissues. For the case in question, an adequate reconstruction was performed using a skin graft. At the time of the initial surgery, it may be assumed that there was vascularized underlying tissue to support the graft. The technique is fairly easy to perform but leaves the patient with little support and a large ventral hernia. It is often performed when direct approximation is not possible or the patient cannot tolerate major surgery.

- Bowel preparation is advisable in the case of inadvertent enterotomy. It is advised that the general surgeon be in the operating room or available, if this occurs. Sutures to bury denuded serosa or formal bowel

resection may be required. The approach should be from the uninvolved margins. Healthy lateral fascia should be sought and old mesh either left alone or removed if there is concern.

- As with other areas of the body, expansion of neighboring soft tissue can be used to close large wounds of the abdomen. The expanders may be placed through a vertical incision in the posterior leaf of the internal oblique aponeurosis and between the internal oblique and the transversus abdominis. Some have described insufflation of the peritoneal cavity with 5 to 10 L of gas via a 19-gauge needle as a means of creating space for displaced contents and increasing the stretch of existing tissues.

- In many cases, the preferred option is the technique of "**components separation**." Here, the anterior rectus sheath and rectus abdominis muscle are peeled off the posterior sheath and the more lateral external oblique muscle is separated from the internal oblique. The resultant compound flap of anterior fascia/rectus muscle/internal oblique muscle/transversus abdominis muscle can be advanced medially. The amount of advancement varies by location: 5 cm at the epigastrium (10 cm, if bilateral), 10 cm at the waist (20), and 3 cm at the suprapubic region (6).

- In the rarer case where there is a true absence of adequate lateral tissue, local flaps may be used.

  — The **anterolateral thigh flap** is based on perforators from the lateral circumflex femoral artery. The skin territory runs from the greater trochanter to the region above the patella. It pivots 2 cm below the inguinal ligament and may reach up to 8 cm above the umbilicus.

  — Pedicled muscle flaps include the **rectus abdominis** muscle, which if available may be widely mobilized, turned over, and covered in mesh anteriorly.

  — Other options include the **latissimus dorsi** and **tensor fascia lata** muscles, which are both fairly large and possessing a reliable blood supply, and the **rectus femoris** and **gracilis** muscles, which are better suited for smaller defects.

- Free flaps utilizing any of the above muscles are less commonly used. Recipient vessels include the superior and inferior epigastric and the gastroepiploic vessels.

6. Postoperative complications should be anticipated and alternative strategies be planned prior to beginning reconstruction.

- Manipulation of the bowel and lysis of adhesions often results in **postoperative ileus**. For this reason, patients are admitted postoperatively for observation and slow advancement of the diet.

- **Wound healing problems** may result from elevation and devascularization of skin flaps.

- Inadvertent injury to the bowel may lead to the formation of an **enterocutaneous fistula**. Of note, negative pressure therapy (i.e., vacuum-assisted closure [VAC] device) is not recommended by the manufacturer.

PRACTICAL PEARLS

1. Preoperative preparation of the patient is very important and oftentimes underestimated. This is more important, if the reconstruction needs to done sooner rather than later. Smoking curtailment, bowel preparation and preoperative CT scan are key. Nutritional status should be optimized to improve wound healing but as intra-abdominal pressure is raised in closing large defects of the abdomen, the patient can better be weaned from the ventilator.

2. If possible, reconstruction should wait until active infection or inflammation has been cleared. This is not always an option and consequently will markedly raise the incidence of postoperative infectious complications, dehiscence and ultimate failure of the repair. Appropriate antibiotic therapy, removal of infected mesh, drainage of pockets of fluid or abscess is useful for a successful reconstruction.

3. The decision whether to perform acute or delayed reconstruction is a determining factor in the final outcome. Immediate reconstruction after trauma or oncologic resection is best. However, other factors such as: the stability of the patient, limited reconstructive options or large loss of tissue, significant infection or contamination, the need to perform other procedures, the presence of an enterostomy will argue strongly for delay.

4. The use of autologous or nonautologous materials for reconstruction depends on many factors. Certainly, the status of the wound and the overall health of the patient are very important. Many times, we will see patients referred to us because they have already failed prosthetic or simple local flap closure attempts. Unless, no other options are available, or conditions have changed markedly, these failed methods should not be reattempted. An autologous, components sliding technique, or major flap coverage should be considered.

5. In very large, chronic, scarred defects of the abdomen with loss of domain and scarcity of tissue as in the case presented, a delayed reconstruction is preferred after the colostomy has been closed and the patient optimized. A components separation consisting of major lateral relaxing incisions in the external oblique musculature and internal (peritoneal/preperitoneal) relaxing incisions as well are necessary. These defects may require the placement of mesh to control for future possible herniation. Acellular human dermis has been shown to be effective in these situations.

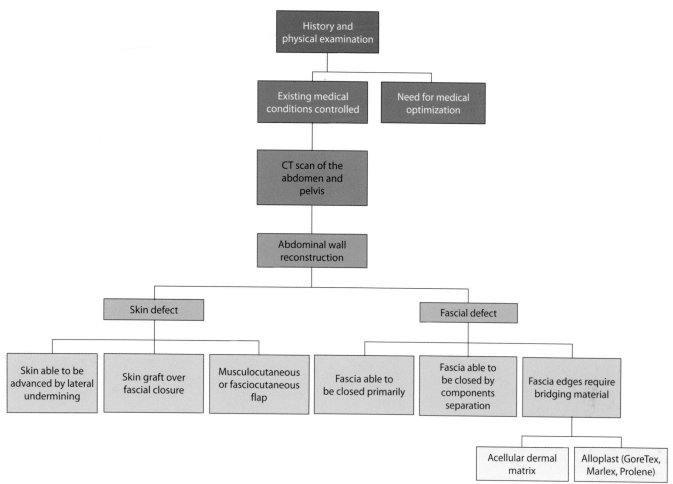

Algorithm 36-1 Algorithm for management of patients with large ventral hernias.

References

1. Ramirez OM, Ruas E, Dellon AL. "Components separation" method for closure of abdominal wall defects: An anatomic and clinical study. *Plast Reconstr Surg.* 1990;86:519.

2. Rohrich RJ, Lowe JB, Hackney FL, et al. An algorithm for abdominal wall reconstruction. *Plast Reconstr Surg.* 2000;105:202.

3. Grevious MA, Cohen M, Jean-Pierre F, et al. The use of prosthetics in abdominal wall reconstruction. *Clin Plastic Surg.* 2006;33:181–197.

4. Lowe JB. Updated algorithm for abdominal wall reconstruction. *Clin Plastic Surg.* 2006;33:225–240.

5. Nozaki M, Sasaki K, Huang TT. Reconstruction of the abdominal wall. In: Mathes SJ. Vol. VI. 2nd ed. *Plastic Surgery.* 1175–1195, Philadelphia, PA: Saunders Elsevier; 2006.

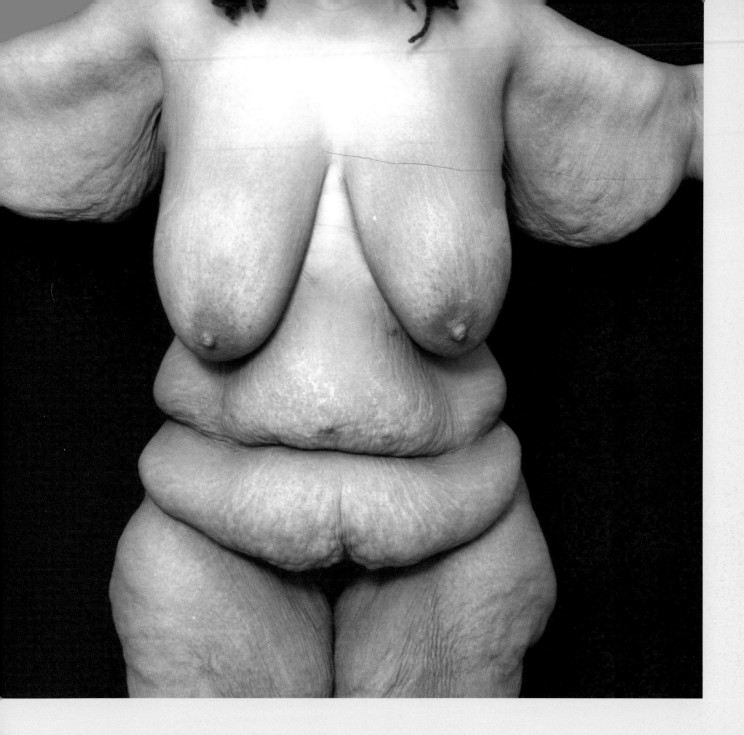

A participant at a local health fair approaches you about improving the appearance of her body after surgery to improve weight loss.

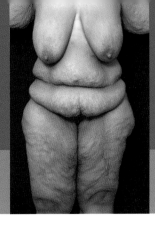

CHAPTER 37

Postbariatric Reconstruction

Thomas P. Sterry

1. When treating patients with excessive weight loss following bariatric surgery—either gastric bypass or gastric banding—one must determine the overall health of the patient and his/her ability to recover from body contouring surgery. It is important to recognize that obesity is often associated with a variety of other medical problems (e.g., diabetes mellitus) which can encumber a patient's recovery. Therefore, the plastic surgeon must begin with some basic questions.

- **Which bariatric procedure have you had?** It is helpful to have some basic understanding about the various bariatric procedures that are available. Modern bariatric procedures commonly performed include laparoscopic gastric banding, Roux-en-Y gastric bypass, and biliopancreatic diversion with duodenal switch (BPD).

  — The gastric band procedure is a purely obstructive technique that makes it physically difficult for patients to consume large amounts of food. It can produce slow but steady weight loss, if the patient is monitored appropriately and the band is adjusted on a regular basis.

  — The gastric bypass procedure involves the creation of a Roux-en-Y anastomosis as well as reducing the size of the gastric pouch. This is considered to be both an obstructive and a malabsorptive technique. Adjustments are not typically performed (and may be contraindicated) but patients need to follow-up with their bariatric surgeon on a regular basis for monitoring purposes. It is also worth noting that this is the group of patients at risk for the dumping syndrome with the ingestion of very rich foods. Their diet is therefore somewhat limited postoperatively and favors weight loss.

  — The BPD operation is essentially a sleeve gastrectomy that is combined with bypassing a significant length of absorptive small bowel. This operation is typically reserved for patients who are "superobese" and can produce more dramatic weight loss than the other two procedures described. Long-term follow-up care is critical in these patients who are prone to a variety of malnutrition issues such as hypoproteinemia, hypocalcemia, and prolonged bleeding times.

- **When was your weight loss surgery?** The timing of bariatric surgery with relation to plastic surgery is critical. Every effort should be made to be sure that the patient's weight loss has been maximized prior to performing any body contouring operations. The development of skin laxity after a body lift, for instance, can be quite vexing for both the patient and surgeon. Contouring procedures should be delayed until the patient stops losing weight for three consecutive months. This typically requires approximately 18 months for Roux-en-Y patients, and two years for gastric banding or duodenal switch patients.

- **How much weight have you lost?** The change in body mass index (BMI), as well as the current BMI can be indicative of how well the patient will do with plastic surgery. For instance, a patient who has had a major bariatric operation (e.g., gastric bypass) will typically lose approximately 70% of their excess body weight. If they have not, this may be an indication that they have not altered their lifestyle significantly enough to give them an optimal outcome. It can be very difficult for an individual to change their eating habits and many patients continue on a high carbohydrate, high fat regimen which can impede their weight loss progress. Outcomes after body contouring procedures tend to parallel those with bariatric surgery. Compliance after a procedure such as a lower body lift is as important as good surgical technique. Patients need to wear their compressive garments, avoid heavy lifting or excessive stretching, and care for their wounds appropriately. If the patient has not participated in their own recovery after bariatric surgery, then they may not be optimal candidates for plastic surgery either. Furthermore, the BMI at the time of body contouring may be correlated with the incidence of postoperative complications. That is, patients who are overweight have an increased incidence of a variety of complications with body contouring surgery as opposed to normal weight counterparts.

- **Do you take nutritional supplements?** Many excessive weight loss patients achieve their goals through malabsorptive procedures which necessitate the prescription of a variety of dietary supplements including iron, calcium, and vitamins A, D,

E, and K. Well-run bariatric programs require regular monitoring of a variety of physiologic parameters in order to ensure the health of their patients. However, compliance with these regimens can be difficult to maintain. Many patients are able to live their lives quite happily without taking their supplements and do not comprehend the danger that they are in should they have a major body contouring operation or some other unplanned physiologic stress. Whereas in an otherwise healthy young patient it is typically acceptable to proceed to surgery without the need for laboratory work being performed, a complete blood count, electrolytes, coagulation parameters, and protein levels should be reviewed by the plastic surgeon prior to taking bariatric patients to the operating room. A variety of potential problems can be avoided in this way. For instance, iron deficiency, or macrocytic (Vitamin B_{12} deficiency) anemia with hematocrit levels in the 20s are not uncommon in this population. Body contouring procedures can require several hours of operating time with large undermined areas and can lead to significant blood loss. The use of blood transfusions can be avoided if patients are properly optimized for surgery. Asking about the patient's compliance with their supplement regimen also helps the plastic surgeon to understand how willing the patient may be to partner with the surgeon postoperatively. It should be emphasized that surgeon and patient must work as a team during the recovery period in order to achieve the best outcome possible.

- **Does the patient have any other medical conditions?** Many patients will present after excessive weight loss and appear to be perfectly healthy at first glance. The plastic surgeon must remain diligent in pursuit of a complete history in this population. These patients may have led unhealthy lifestyles, which contributed to their obesity and may have a variety of occult ailments. Many patients will not volunteer or may even deny a history of disease such as diabetes or hypertension because their symptoms have improved, but this does not change the fact that they had a given pathological entity. The impact that a long history of, for instance diabetes, may have on a patient who does not presently require any medications in order to control blood sugar will have on recovery is questionable at best. Certainly, it is believed that patients are improving their risk with surgery, but this does not mean that it is decreased to that of the rest of the population. As a result, of these issues, the plastic surgeon needs to ask specific questions regarding the following.

— **Diabetes mellitus:** Is there a history of insulin dependence? If yes, for how long? Which health care professional is currently managing their care? It is incumbent upon the plastic surgeon to determine the extent to which the patient is at risk for wound healing issues prior to the creation of a variety of flaps used in body contouring techniques.

— **Hypertension:** Does the patient still require medications? The risk of hematoma is significant in these patients and the blood pressure must be tightly controlled. Moreover, the history of hypertension, even in the face of a patient who is normotensive at the time of surgery may leave the patient at risk for other morbidities such as stroke or myocardial infarction. Risk after weight loss is improved, but remains higher than in it would be if the patient had no history of hypertension.

— **Sleep apnea:** Does the patient require a continuous positive airway pressure (CPAP) machine? One might want to reconsider performing major body contouring surgery if the answer is "yes." Persistent sleep apnea can confuse the postoperative picture and prompt the surgeon to initiate an unnecessary pulmonary workup in an attempt to rule out morbidity such as a pulmonary embolus or pneumonia. Furthermore, operations such as abdominoplasty will tend to aggravate the problems associated with sleep apnea thereby exacerbating the confusion. Patients with sleep apnea significant enough to require the use of c-pap should be referred to the appropriate sleep specialist or internist for optimization prior to undergoing plastic surgery.

— **Deep venous thrombosis:** Has the patient had a deep vein thrombus (DVT) in the past? Many plastic surgeons are surprised to find that the answer is "yes." Their excess weight puts them at increased risk, especially at the time of the bariatric surgery. Even without a history of DVT, many bariatric surgeons will require placement of a vena cava filter before performing weight loss procedures. This information can be very helpful when caring for patients after extended body contouring procedures. It is also helpful in deciding whether or not to operate on the patient in the first place.

- **Has the patient ever smoked?** A complete history including all the periods when the patient tried to stop, but returned to tobacco should be obtained. The patient should be informed that smokers, regardless of the number of cigarettes consumed each day, bore a 46% complication rate as opposed to nonsmokers whose rate has been estimated at approximately 14% in the same study. Clearly, one would wish to operate on a patient who has never used tobacco, but a more distant history of smoking seems intuitively more favorable, if not quantifiably so, than a more recent one. Furthermore, every patient should be asked to sign a declaration regarding their smoking history as a standard part of their informed consent.

2. Patients desiring body contouring are most concerned with several keys areas, each of which should be evaluated and addressed. Areas most affected by weight gain and subsequent loss include the abdomen, the breasts, the arms, the thighs, and posterior torso, among others.

- The defining physical characteristic in this population of patients is usually the abdominal panniculus, which may present in a myriad of shapes and sizes. A grading system to help establish a universal nomenclature for use in describing the magnitude of the panniculus has been described by health professionals working with this population (see Table 37-1).

- **What is the shape of the torso?** Some patients present with a "double" panniculus in which there are large folds of excess skin laxity both above and below the level of the umbilicus. Impressive results have been noted in these patients following complete abdominoplasty (Table 37-1).

- **What is the size and shape of the mons pubis?** The mons may hang pendulously in a manner similar to the abdominal panniculus and some patients and may require a "monsplasty." These findings underscore the need to photograph all patients completely undressed,

Table 37-1 Classification of Panniculus Grade

GRADE 1	Panniculus barely covers the pubic hairline, but not the entire mons pubis
GRADE 2	Extends to cover the entire mons pubis
GRADE 3	Extends to cover the upper thigh
GRADE 4	Extends to cover the midthigh
GRADE 5	Extends to cover the knees or beyond

without the use of typical paper garments for the sake of modesty. These are true medical findings that must be documented in a manner that can be referred to at a later date if necessary.

- **Are there rashes or other dermatologic concerns beneath the folds of the panniculus?** Many patients will complain about a variety of boils, panniculitis, folliculitis, and frank purulent accumulation beneath the folds of these large sheets of tissue. These claims must be confirmed by the physician with photographic evidence whenever possible in order to assure proper cooperation of third-party payers. Frank lymphedema of the abdominal panniculus as well as purulent drainage emerging from the umbilicus may be noted.

- **Are there surgical scars?** One must note the placement of old surgical scars as well as their appearance (e.g., hypertrophic or keloid). Furthermore, careful palpation of the abdomen should be performed in search of ventral fascial defects. Many of these patients have occult hernias in the tissues underlying old surgical scars. It is better to search for these preoperatively than to discover them after the creation of a major abdominal catastrophe in the operating room. In patients with a severely hanging panniculus (grade 4 or 5) the umbilical stalk is often extraordinarily long with a tenuous blood supply. The patient must be informed of the possibility that the umbilicus may not survive in these cases. Lastly, it should be pointed out that for many patients who are trying to achieve a slender waistline, a rotund body habitus preoperatively can pose a real challenge to the plastic surgeon. Patients may require extensive liposuction of the flanks, and perhaps a fleur-de-lis abdominoplasty in order to create an appreciable waistline. Patients with a "pinched" midsection laterally can be sculpted into an hourglass postoperatively with much more ease than can an amorphous or round-shaped torso.

- **Does the patient have breast ptosis?** The breast tissue of patients following excessive weight loss tend to be ptotic due to the dramatic loss of volume. Several grades of ptosis have been described (Table 37-2).

- **Does the patient have ptosis of the upper arm skin/soft tissue?** With the popularity of bariatric surgery, there has been a resurgence of interest in brachioplasty procedures. These had lost favor with the advent of liposuction in the 1980s.

- **Does the patient have ptosis of the thigh skin/soft tissue?**

3. A complete set of hematology and chemistry laboratory values is advisable as part of the preoperative plan for all bariatric patients. While performing surgery on an otherwise healthy young patient would not necessitate such measures, the bariatric population is, oftentimes, malnourished. They rely on a range of supplements in order to maintain their health and should be constantly monitored by a physician familiar with their physiology on a regular basis. It has been documented that these

patients (especially BPD patients) are at risk for prolonged PT and bleeding times independent of PT.

- At minimum, clotting studies including a **prothrombin time** (PT) and a **partial thromboplastin time** (PTT) should be noted.

- A **complete blood count** (CBC) as well as iron studies (e.g., transferrin, TIBC, ferritin) should be performed in order to rule out the possibility of iron deficiency or macrocytic (vitamin B12 deficiency) anemia.

- Protein levels (including **albumin** and **prealbumin**) are a rough indication of the patient's nutritional health and ability to heal wounds following surgery.

- **Lymphoscintigraphy** is recommended if there is any indication of swelling in the lower limbs before attempting any form of thigh lift operation in these individuals. The lymphatic and venous outflow for patients who have been more than 100 lbs overweight is not uncommonly compromised. Operations such as these could be the last insult required to create a lifetime of suffering with lymphedema.

4. Laboratory tests combined with a thorough medical history should guide the surgeon to the necessary preoperative consultations. On occasion, one or more medical specialists may offer significant input into the management of these cases.

- A **hematologist** may be helpful with the management of various anemias or in control of clotting factors.

- A **cardiologist** is obviously required from time to time in patients who are at increased risk.

- An **endocrinologist** is occasionally helpful in caring for patients with diabetes mellitus, is hyper- or hypothyroid, and for patients with polycystic ovary disease.

5. Treatment options as per a reconstructive ladder

- While it may initially seem not to matter where one begins the reconstruction of the massive weight loss patient, many prefer to begin with the **torso** and move to other areas from this new fixed starting point. Once the midsection is fixed in place, it is easier to know how and where to affix the thighs, breasts, and arms. For patients with severe panniculitis, or who are at increased risk of complications, a panniculectomy may be more appropriate. However, for the vast majority of patients who have lost more than 100 lbs, a lower body lift (LBL), or at least an extended abdominoplasty is more optimal. By treating the anterior and posterior aspects of the torso as one aesthetic unit, and therefore, operating on both areas at the same time, it is believed that the patients entire "body suit" can be tightened in a single operation. It has been proposed that the fascial system acts like a finger trap, and that by performing a lower body lift, one can create an overall better body contour horizontally as well as vertically. It should be noted that the latest version of this technique involves an abdominoplasty with an outer thigh and buttock lift

and without intervention on the medial thighs. Most surgeons do not advocate addition of an inner thigh lift at the time as the torsoplasty for fear of complications. For those patients who are particularly amorphous and lack a definable waistline, one may consider performing a Fleur-de-Lys abdominoplasty in an attempt to enhance the horizontal component of the operation. Many surgeons reserve this approach for patients who already have a midline abdominal scar.

- Any number of techniques may be used to reconstruct the ptotic breast, in this population. The Wise pattern technique is able to remove a large amount of excess skin tissue that tends to accumulate laterally. On occasion, an upper torsoplasty may be performed with a scar extending posteriorly toward the patient's back in order to eliminate excess upper back skin, which is contiguous with the excess breast skin laterally.

— Surgeons with less experience should beware the temptation to perform an augmentation/mastopexy operation at one sitting. This operation is quite challenging and should be performed for weight loss patients on only rare occasions. Amongst the challenges is development of a "double bubble" breast denoted by excess breast tissue drooping over well-placed implants. Since revisions are common, it is highly recommended to perform a mastopexy first and, when satisfied with the result, contemplate placement of implants for augmentation.

— Many male weight loss patients are diagnosed with grade III gynecomastia (see Table 37-2). However, the term "gynecomastia" implies that the patient has breast tissue present on the chest wall when in fact they have excess skin laxity and not excessive breast tissue. This condition may therefore be referred to as pseudogynecomastia after weight loss surgery (PAWLS). Men with PAWLS may require mastopexy, but the techniques used are significantly different for men as compared to women.

Table 37-2 Classification of Breast Ptosis

First degree	Mild ptosis; the nipple lies at the level of the inframammary fold
Second degree	Moderate ptosis; the nipple lies below the level of the fold, but remains above the most projecting portion of the breast.
Third degree	Severe ptosis; nipple lies below the inframammary fold at the lower contour of the breast and skin brassiere.
Pseudoptosis	The inferior pole of the breast droops, but the nipple lies above the level of the inframammary fold. The areola to inframammary fold distance is increased.

- To address the ptosis of the upper arm skin and soft tissue, liposuction is of little use in patients with true skin laxity. Several techniques have been described to excise the redundant tissue while placing the scar along the bicipital groove. The pattern is an L-shape that courses from the elbow medially and includes excess axillary skin. The addition of a Z-plasty in the axilla has been advocated by some but may lead to tissue breakdown more frequently than not.

  — It should be noted that scarring from this procedure is not only more visible than others, but also seems to take longer to mature. These wounds tend to remain erythematous for a much longer period of time than most others and it should be emphasized to the patient that 12 to 18 months will be necessary before the final result will be apparent.

  — When performing brachioplasty one must be familiar with the anatomy of the medial antebrachial cutaneous nerve. This sensory nerve emerges from the inner aspect of the midhumerus from a subfascial plane and runs more superficially inferiorly around the elbow. Injury to this nerve can be quite irritating to the patient manifesting as neuroma, numbness, or paresthesias, to the medial half of the forearm. Superficial dissection in the lower portion of the arm is crucial in avoiding its injury.

- As mentioned earlier, the medial thighs are typically addressed well after (3 months minimum) the torso has been addressed with abdominoplasty, or lower body lift. This is to allow the other wounds to become fixed in scar and relatively immobile before placing tension on the pubic region once again. Liposuction may be performed to the entire thigh along with a crescent-shaped skin excision superiorly within the groin. The superficial fascial suspension system (SFS) of the thigh soft tissue is then sutured to firm tissue above including Coopers ligament, periosteum of the ischium, or the thickened tendinous portions of the adductor muscle group. Sutures in these areas are clearly uncomfortable and the patient must be aware that sitting during the postoperative period can be challenging.

  — A longitudinal scar down the inner aspect of the thighs is not created unless absolutely necessary. While this method is clearly effective in terms of creating a favorable contour, it is also associated with a more prolonged recovery time, increased pain, and leaves the patient prone to lymphedema if too much vasculature is removed or damaged in the process. If this approach is taken, incisions should be restricted to the area above the knee.

6. The potential for surgical complications in this population of patients is not trivial and must be addressed with the patient in its entirety on one or more occasions preoperatively.

- Without question, the most common complication while working with excessive weight loss patients is **seroma** formation, which may be seen in up to a third of patients. The placement of "progressive tension sutures" has become more common and may decrease the likelihood of seroma formation. Techniques have been described to perform these cases without the use of drains; however, this is not considered to be the standard of care. The treatment of a seroma is controversial and may vary from observation, to serial aspiration, to reinsertion of a drain, or even to insertion of a sclerosing agent. Serial aspiration combined with the use of a snug fitting compression garment may be the most effective.

- Whether because of the unusually large undermined area or some other physiologic change after bariatric surgery, the risk of **hematoma** appears to be elevated in these patients. Meticulous hemostasis must be achieved prior to wound closure. Furthermore, the surgeon must maintain a high index of suspicion during the postoperative period because detection of hematoma can be challenging. A careful physical examination and the monitoring of vital signs are the best indicators of hematoma whereas serial hematocrit levels only seem to confuse the surgeon. Fluid shifts typically create a falsely lowered hemoglobin level during the first few days postoperatively, while an increased pulse rate in the absence of hypertension is still indicative of bleeding. A CT scan may be helpful in making the diagnosis, but clinical examination remains the gold standard in determining whether or not to return to the operating room for exploration and evacuation.

- Every patient being considered for an operation must discuss with their surgeon the potential for **unfavorable scars**. This is particularly important when performing brachioplasty because these wounds are not necessarily covered by everyday garments. Hypertrophic scarring may be managed with frequent massage, silicone sheets, and the application of local steroids.

- With the performance of several operations in the groin region (e.g., abdominoplasty, medial thigh lift, longitudinal thigh lift) the potential for **lymphatic interruption** is significant, particularly when dealing with patients whose vascular system may already be challenged by their history of morbid obesity. When performing any of these operations, the surgeon should preserve all the major components of drainage from the lower extremities. The inguinal lymph nodes should be swept aside, but maintained intact and unharmed with every operation and the saphenous vein should be preserved during thigh-lift surgery.

- **Wound dehiscence** is a recognized complication after each of these procedures. This may be because of the aggressive surgery, a history of smoking, diabetes mellitus, or simply to the fact that fatty tissue has a relatively poor blood supply. Undermining should be limited to only those areas that are absolutely necessary.

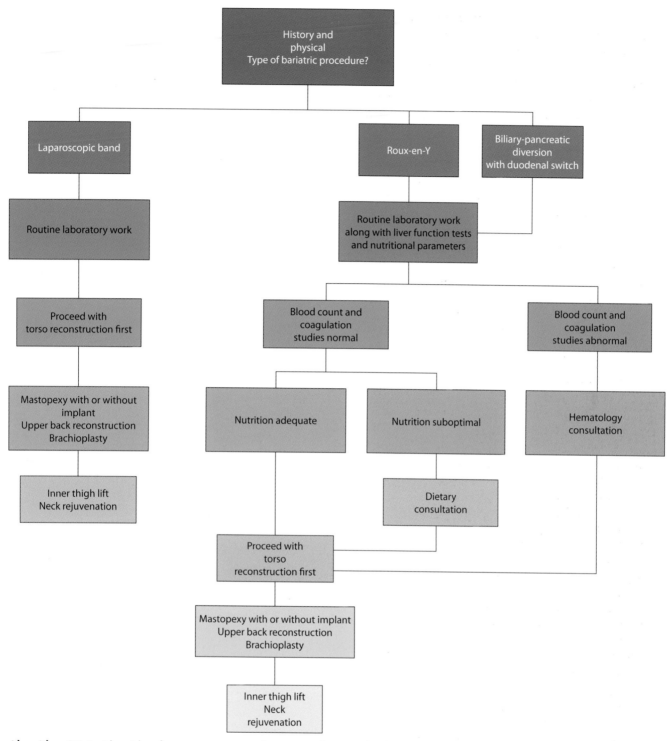

Algorithm 37-1 Algorithm for management of patients desiring body contouring following bariatric surgery.

PRACTICAL PEARLS

1. With abdominoplasty, the use of three-way sutures during closure from the superior fascia of the abdominal flap to that of the inferior wound, to the underlying abdominal fascia will help to both decrease the likelihood of seroma, and to control scar placement.

2. With a lower body lift, the surgeon should resist the temptation to remove fatty tissue from the buttock region, when working posteriorly. This will lead to a flatted buttock and a loss of naturally occurring lordosis in the lower back. On the other hand, liposuction to the flank area and lower back will assist in the creation of a full and aesthetically pleasing buttocks region.

3. With brachioplasty, the core tissue (e.g., humerus and muscle) is relatively noncompressible while the soft tissues surrounding it (e.g., fat and skin) are elastic and swell tremendously during surgery. Arm swelling during brachioplasty can be a nuisance, but must be addressed. Elevating the arms during surgery, working swiftly, and performing progressive tension suture maneuvers will all help to prevent unfavorable results or the inability to close wounds. Closure from the most distal areas progressively towards the axilla will also assist in the elimination of a "dog ear" problem.

4. The thigh lift is best performed with the patient prone and the table in a jack knife position and then be completed with the patient turned supine. This will improve visualization of the posterior groin and allow for a better result with less operating time.

References

1. Manassa EH, Hertl CH, Olbrisch RR. Wound healing problems in smokers and nonsmokers after 132 abdominoplasties. *Plast Reconstr Surg.* 2003;111(6):2082-2087.

2. Igwe D, Malgorzata S, Lee H, Felahy B, Tambi J, Fobi M. Panniculectomy adjuvant to obesity surgery. *Obesity Surgery.* 2000;10:530-539.

3. Lockwood T. Superficial fascial system (SFS) of the trunk and extremities: A new concept. *Plast Reconstr Surg.* 1991;87:1009-1018.

4. Sterry T, Sacks J. Plastic surgery after excessive weight loss. *Laparoscopic Bariatric Surgery.* Philadelphia: Lippincott; 2005:314-324.

5. Aly AS, Cram AE, Chao M, Pang J, McKeon M. Belt lipectomy for circumferential truncal excess: The University of Iowa experience. *Plast Reconstr Surg.* 2003;111(1):398-413.

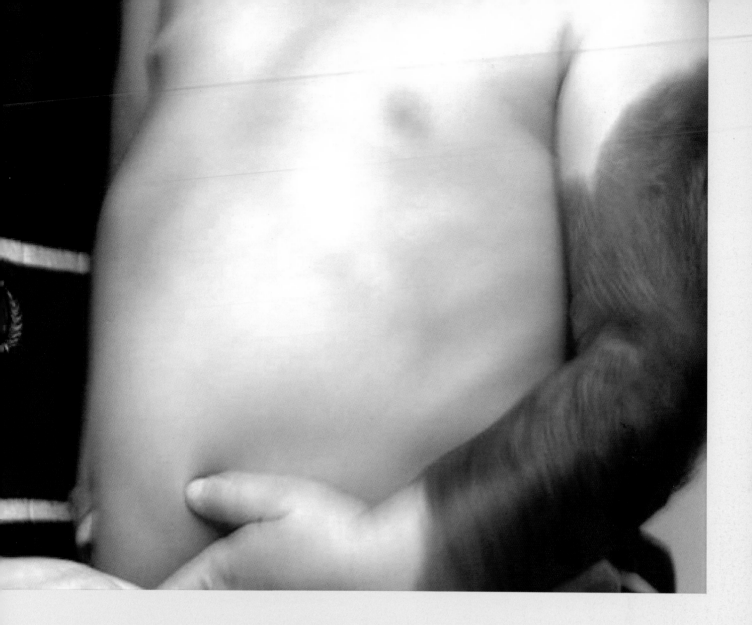

Patient is a 1-year-old girl who presents to

the plastic surgery clinic with an isolated

lesion of the left upper extremity.

(Photograph Courtesy of Steven J. Kasten, MD.)

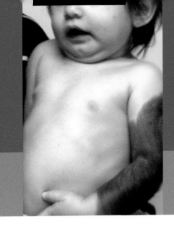

CHAPTER 38

Congenital Melanocytic Nevi

Rafael J. Diaz-Garcia and Paul S. Cederna

1. The initial step in managing any cutaneous lesion is to establish the appropriate diagnosis prior to planning any therapeutic intervention. A thorough, directed history should be obtained from either the patient, or more commonly the parents, to reduce the differential diagnosis. The lesion shown above is a pigmented and hair-bearing lesion in an otherwise healthy infant. Based on its appearance, the lesion is most likely a giant, hairy nevus. This type of lesion is a subset of congenital nevi that are either noticed at birth or develop within a few months thereafter. They are also commonly referred to as congenital melanocytic nevi (CMN) and carry descriptive designations based upon their anatomic distribution: bathing suit nevus, vest-like nevus, garment nevus, and cape-like nevus.

   - **Was the lesion present at birth?** By definition, CMN are present at birth. They develop *in utero* between the 5th and 24th weeks of gestation, when melanoblasts migrate from the neural crest to various regions of the body. However, some smaller CMN may not be apparent at birth because they lack visible pigment. The incidence of CMN is approximately 1% to 6%. These lesions are less common in children from Latin America and slightly more common in children from Japan. Giant congenital hairy nevi are much less common with an incidence estimated as one in 20,000 newborns.

   - **Has the lesion changed/increased in size?** The natural history of CMN is one of growth in proportion to the rest of the body. With time, they may undergo changes in size, color, nodularity, and hair growth. Such changes usually stabilize in adulthood, but this is not always the case. Patients may also complain of symptoms of pruritus within the CMN.

   - **Is there a family history of similar lesions?** Although there are reports of familial clusters of CMN, the vast majority of cases occur sporadically. In review of the literature, Danarti et al. described 14 reports of familial large CMN, and they proposed an inheritance pattern where the trait manifests itself in heterozygous individuals at an early developmental stage. This is concordant with the mosaic distribution of lesions and sporadic nature of the majority of cases.

2. A careful physical examination with careful measurements of the dimensions of the lesions and photographic documentation should be performed when the patient is initially evaluated. These early records will allow the clinician to identify clinically significant changes in the lesion over time. In addition, suspicious areas in the lesion can be carefully monitored with these techniques to determine if biopsy is necessary to rule out malignant transformation (i.e., melanoma). In addition, when warranted, biopsies should be taken from several locations since histology can vary in different regions of the same lesion.

   - **How does the lesion appear?** CMNs are larger on average than acquired nevi. They are usually round or oval in shape with a smooth or lobular surface. The adnexal structures of the skin and texture are usually accentuated overlying the CMN. Pigmented lesions also typically have a fine, speckled pattern. They may be hairless or contain large, coarse hairs. Very dark pigmentation is rare in white infants but relatively common in darkly pigmented infants. Giant congenital nevi are divided into:

     — Superficial, well-differentiated lesions confined to the epidermis and upper dermis. These are lighter in color as the mature melanocytes are confined to the epidermis. They are found on the face, torso, and extremities.

     — Thicker, irregular lesions that extend into deeper structures, including nerves, vessels, muscle, and bone. These are darker lesions that appear most often on the back, scalp, and buttocks.

   - **How many lesions are there? How large are they?** Most CMNs are small and singular. However, larger lesions may have multiple satellite nevi. Giant congenital hairy nevi are present in approximately 1 in 20,000 newborns. CMNs are most often classified by size, although this classification is arbitrary and is not based on any epidemiological evidence; small lesions are less than 1.5 cm in diameter, medium lesions are between 1.5 and 19.9 cm in diameter, and large or giant lesions are 20 cm in diameter or 2% of the total body surface area. CMNs have also been classified based on the surgical options available for treatment; small lesions may be easily resected and closed primarily, while giant lesions require tissue expansion or skin grafts for reconstruction.

- **Are there associated lesions?** Larger CMNs may be associated with other abnormalities, such as ocular manifestations, spina bifida occulta, neurofibromatosis, and neurocutaneous melanosis (NCM). In addition, there have been a number of associated tumors which arise in conjunction with CMNs include schwannomas, neurofibromas, hemangiomas, and Wilms' tumors.

- **Are there any suspicious concerns?** Malignant change should be suspected with growth of the lesion, pain, bleeding, ulceration, change in color, or pruritus.

3. The differential diagnosis for CMN is quite extensive and includes both benign and malignant lesions. It is critical to make the correct diagnosis, as this will have a direct impact on the treatment plan.

- Simple examination of the lesion may not provide sufficient information, and in these circumstances, **biopsy** of the lesion may be warranted. It is possible for areas of the same lesion to have different histologies, so it is prudent to take multiple punch biopsies of characteristic and questionable areas.

- The differential diagnosis for a CMN includes:

  — *Epidermal nevus*—These are usually linear lesions that may have a somewhat verrucous appearance, but lack hair. These lesions may also be pruritic. Occasionally, epidermal nevi are seen at birth, but most appear later in childhood.

  — *Café au Lait spot*—These are hyperpigmented lesions that can vary in color from light brown to dark brown, and typically do not distort the skin and do not display speckling. Numerous CAL spots warrant a workup for a neurocutaneous syndrome, most commonly neurofibromatosis type 1 (NF1). There are other medical conditions associated with CAL spots including McCune-Albright syndrome, tuberous sclerosis, and Fanconi anemia.

  — *Mongolian spot*—Mongolian spots typically present on the lumbosacral region of healthy infants and have a macular blue-gray pigmentation. Mongolian spots do not distort the skin surface and usually disappear spontaneously in early childhood, but

can persist for life. These lesions can be associated with a cleft lip, spinal meningeal tumor, melanoma, or inborn errors of metabolism.

— *Congenital Baker's melanosis*—These are large unilateral lesions usually located on the shoulders of males and appear as irregularly demarcated areas demonstrating hyperpigmentation and hypertrichosis. These lesions appear later in childhood than giant congenital nevi.

— *Nevus sebaceous*—Nevus sebaceous lesions usually present as a solitary, hairless, velvety, tan plaque on the scalp at birth or in early childhood. They may also present on other areas of the head and the neck. These lesions may develop into basal cell or squamous cell cancers over time.

— *Pigmented arrector pili hamartoma*—These are slightly pigmented lesions which are associated with prominent hair. One interesting characteristic is that they may become indurated and more prominent with massage.

— *Melanoma*—With any pigmented lesion, the greatest concern for both the patient and the physician is malignant transformation into a melanoma. There is much debate about the exact risk of melanoma in patients with giant congenital nevi, with reports ranging from 2% to 40%. A systematic review of the literature by Watt et al. concluded that the incidence of melanoma in <u>large</u> CMN patients was 2599 times greater than in the general population. Approximately half of the malignancies that occur in giant nevi patients develop in the first 3 years of life, 60% by childhood, and 70% by puberty. The diagnosis of melanoma is a devastating one, with a very poor prognosis once metastasis has occurred.

- Histologically, CMN lesions are distinguished from acquired nevi by the following criteria:

  — CMN cells extend into the lower two-thirds of the dermis and into the subcutaneous tissue.

  — CMN cells extend between collagen bundles of the reticular dermis as single cells or cords.

  — CMN cells extend around and into hair follicles, sweat glands, sebaceous glands, blood vessels, and nerves.

— CMN cells can infiltrate arrector pili muscles.

— CMN cells can simulate an inflammatory reaction with perivascular and perifollicular distribution.

4. The plastic surgeon should be involved with these patients early in the treatment course, particularly if the lesion is large and will need a multimodal reconstructive approach. Several additional services should be consulted to manage these patients not only acutely but also long-term.

- A thorough examination by a **dermatologist** and regular follow-ups should be arranged. Oftentimes, the dermatologist becomes the responsible physician for all other consultations.

- A **neurological** examination may be warranted, particularly in patients with axial lesions—cephalic, posterior cervical, and paravertebral. The greatest concern is NCM, and patients with lesions along the midline or head/neck should undergo a screening MRI of the brain and spine.

- A **neurosurgery** consultation should be arranged for in the presence of NCM, signs/symptoms of hydrocephalus or concerns for meningeal melanoma.

- For any lesions involving V1 or V2 dermatomal distribution, **ophthalmology** should be involved. They should also be consulted if concerned for neurofibromatosis, as Lisch nodules are the most common sign.

5. The goal of treatment is to remove the lesion with as few operative procedures as possible, while still obtaining negative margins. However, that is not always possible given that giant congenital nevi can have cells that extend past the subcutaneous tissue into fascia or bone. It has been well described that the depth of penetration of the lesion is positively correlated with the size of the lesion. Early biopsy should be performed on any/all questionable areas. Any lesion which has been identified as atypical requires immediate excision. Prophylactic excision of smaller lesions should be considered prior to 12 years of age. Giant congenital nevi should be evaluated before the age of 1 year since many will need multiple procedures before complete excision and reconstruction can be accomplished. Patients and parents should be warned that resection does not completely eliminate the risk of melanoma.

- The principles of the "reconstructive ladder" should be adhered to when developing a treatment plan for a patient with a CMN. The treatment should begin with **simple serial excisions**, if complete excision of the lesion can be accomplished within three procedures. Some surgeons would argue, however, that since a tissue expander reconstruction can be done in two stages, serial excision should be reserved for lesions that can be removed in one or two procedures. Resection is carried down through the dermis and into the subcutaneous tissue to maximize the chances of complete excision. Giant congenital nevi can sometimes involve the underlying muscle or bone, making negative margins difficult, if not impossible to achieve.

- **Skin grafts**, both split-thickness and full-thickness, have been the traditional mainstay for the reconstruction of large excisional defects. Split-thickness grafts have fallen out of favor, particularly in the extremities, because of their propensity for secondary contraction. Full-thickness grafts traditionally were limited by the availability of donor skin, but have become much more versatile in conjunction with tissue expansion. In addition, full-thickness skin grafts do not undergo as much secondary contracture as split-thickness skin grafts and are ideally suited for reconstructions across joint surfaces or on the face.

- **Tissue expansion** has become the workhorse for large CMN reconstruction, allowing for reconstruction of large excisional defects. Tissue expansion can be used for reconstruction in the following situations:

  — Can be placed in neighboring tissue for advancement flaps.

  — Can be used to increase the amount of tissue for full-thickness skin grafts.

  — Can be used to increase the amount of skin for free flaps.

- **Free flaps**—Microvascular free tissue transfers, particularly free TRAM and ALT flaps, have been described for reconstruction of large circumferential extremity defects following CMN excision. Free tissue transfer is a more challenging operative procedure but may provide tissue of better quality that matches the color and characteristics of the surrounding tissue. In addition, secondary scar contracture of muscle, skin, or fasciocutaneous flaps is very uncommon.

- **Cultured keratinocytes** are a recent advance which may be useful in cases where there is a paucity of native donor skin. Skin is harvested from uninvolved, normal skin, the keratinocytes are isolated and then grown in culture over a period of weeks. Unfortunately, there are a number of issues which prevent this technique from achieving widespread clinical applicability; the technique is very expensive, it requires substantial cell culture expertise, it requires a number of weeks to achieve a sufficient number of cells to be clinically useful, and the cultured keratinocytes are not very durable, once they are applied to the wound.

- **Dermal substitutes** have been used for decades in burn patients, but have only recently been described in CMN reconstruction. When the dermal substitutes are used in conjunction with split-thickness skin grafts, they can add thickness and durability to the graft. However, the dermal substitutes are very expensive, require several weeks between stages, and have a higher risk of infection.

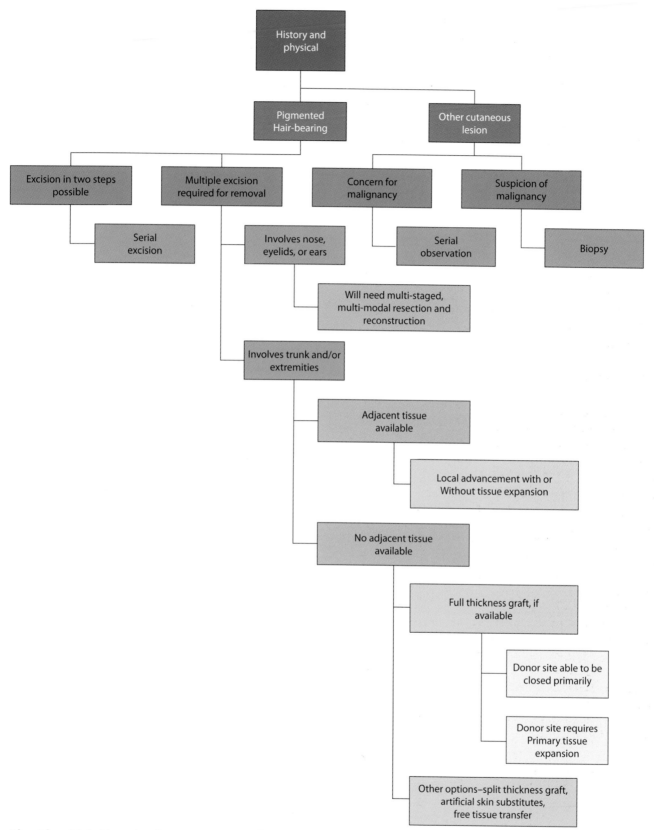

Algorithm 38-1 Algorithm for management of patients with a giant hairy nevus.

- **Dermabrasion, chemical peels, and lasers** can be used to lighten unresectable lesions and make them aesthetically more pleasing. However, the patient/family must be aware that the risk of malignant transformation is not reduced, and clinical observation of the lesion may be impaired with these techniques.

6. Complications may arise from the presence of the lesion as well as from any reconstruction procedures attempted.

   - CNS involvement should be suspected in patients with CMN who present with lethargy, seizures, vomiting, or signs of raised intracranial pressure from hydrocephalus. The risk for **NCM** in patients with giant nevi is unknown, but in a review of 289 cases demonstrated that all patients with large CMN who developed NCM had their nevi in axial locations (DeDavid et al.). Signs and symptoms of NCM usually manifests by 5 years of age. Symptomatic NCM has a grave prognosis, with death within 2 to 3 years of diagnosis.

   - As stated previously, **malignancy and malignant degeneration** is the greatest concern with any pigmented lesion. Many large CMN cannot be fully excised and thus pose a persistent risk. A priori, surgical resection should reduce the risk of malignant degeneration. However, nevi may maintain malignant potential after excision, and as a result, all patients require long-term close follow-up.

   - The rate of **graft or flap loss** is no greater in patients who have undergone excision and reconstruction of a congenital melanocytic nevus than any other reconstruction. Similarly, the complications associated with tissue expander reconstruction are also no different in this patient population and includes the typical

problems related to infection, implant exposure, dermal thinning, and skin necrosis. However, the psychological impact of a complication may be greater given the patient population.

PRACTICAL PEARLS

1. Tissue expanders are the mainstay of reconstruction, useful for both expanded skin flaps and expanded full-thickness skin grafts.

2. Serial excision should be used for lesions that can be removed in two or less operations.

3. Biopsy or remove any lesion that undergoes significant changes in size, color, or border irregularity.

4. Dermabrasion, chemical peels, and lasers can be used to lighten unresectable lesions. However, the patient/family must be aware that the risk of malignant transformation is not reduced, and clinical observation of the lesion may be impaired with these techniques.

References

1. Arneja, J.S., Gosain, A.K. Giant Congenital Melanocytic Nevi. Plast. Reconstr. Surg. 120: 26e, 2007.

2. Castilla, E.E. Da Graca Dutra, M., Orioli-Parreiras, I.M. Epidemiology of Congenital Pigmented Naevi: Incidence Rates and Relative Frequencies. Br. J. Dermatol. 104: 307, 1981.

3. Corcoran, J., Bauer, B.S. Management of Large Melanocytic Nevi in the Extremities. Jour. Craniofac. Surg. 16: 877, 2005.

4. Danarti, R., Konig, A., Happle, R. Large congenital melanocytic nevi may reflect paradominant inheritance implying allelic loss. Eur. J. Dermatol. 13: 430, 2003.

5. DeDavid, M., Orlow, S.J., Provost, N. et al. Neurocutaneous Melanosis: Clinical Features of Large Congenital Melanocytic Nevi in Patients with Manifest CNS Melanosis. J. Am. Acad. Dermatol. 35: 529, 1996.

6. Earle, S.A., Marshall, D.M. Management of Giant Congenital Nevi With Artificial Skin Substitutes in Children. Jour. Craniofac. Surg. 16: 904, 2005.

7. Ferguson, R.E.H., Vasconez, H.C. Laser Treatment of Congenital Nevi. Jour. Craniofac. Surg. 16: 908, 2005.

8. Gosain, A.K., Santoro, T.D., Larson, D.L., et al. Giant Congenital Nevi: A 20-Year Experience and an Algorithm for Their Management. Plast. Reconstr. Surg. 108: 622, 2001.

9. Jensen, J.N., Gosain, A.K. Congenital Melanocytic Nevi. In C.H. Thorne, R.W. Beasley, S.J. Aston, et al. (Eds.), Grabb & Smith's Plastic Surgery. Philadelphia: Lippincott, 2007. Pp. 120-123.

10. Marghoob, A.A. Congenital Melanocytic Nevi: Evaluation and Management. Dermatol. Clin. 20: 607, 2002.

11. Pearson, G.D., Goodman, M., Sadove, A.M. Congenital Nevus: The Indiana University's Approach to Treatment. Jour. Craniofac. Surg. 16: 915, 2005.

12. Quaba, A.A., Wallace, A.F. The Incidence of Malignant Melanoma (0 to 15 years of age) Arising in "Large" Congenital Nevocellular Nevi. Plast. Reconstr. Surg. 78: 174, 1986.

13. Ruiz-Maldonado, R., Tamayo, L., Laterza, A.M., et al. Giant Pigmented Nevi: Clinical, histopathologic, and Therapeautic Considerations. J. Pediatr. 120: 906, 1992.

14. Thaller, S., et al. Special Section: Giant Congenital Nevus. Jour. Craniofac. Surg. 16: 869, 2005.

15. Watt, A.J., Kotsis, S.V., Chung, K.C. Risk of Melanoma Arising in Large Congenital Melanocytic Nevi: A Systematic Review. Plast. Reconstr. Surg. 113: 1968, 2004.

16. Yovino, J., Thaller, S. Potential for Development of Malignant Melanoma with Congenital Melanocytic Nevi. Jour. Craniofac. Surg. 16: 871, 2005.

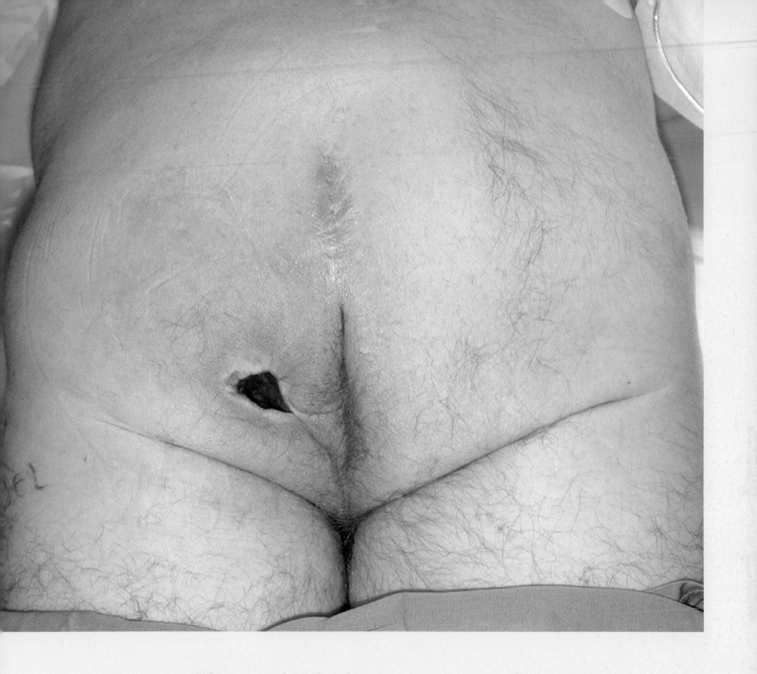

The rehabilitation medicine service requests your consult on a 45-year-old paraplegic male with a chronic draining wound on the posterior thigh.

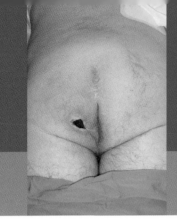

CHAPTER 39

Ischial Pressure Ulcer

Adam H. Hamawy and Jeffrey E. Janis

1. The patient in question appears to have a wound in the ischial region of the lower extremity. A thorough history of the pressure sore patient is paramount in order to understand the underlying etiologies so that these may be optimized or resolved prior to surgical reconstruction in order to ensure a successful long-term outcome. Without discovering and addressing the underlying cause behind the formation of the ulcer, any treatment is doomed to early failure. The causes of pressure sores are often multifactorial and involve one or more extrinsic (primary) and intrinsic (secondary) factors. The primary factors include unrelieved pressure, shear, and frictional forces exerting mechanical stress on the area. If the external compressive force exceeds the arterial capillary pressure (32 mm Hg) then perfusion is impaired and ischemia will ensue. In this sitting position, pressures are greatest near the ischial tuberosities, with measurements of up to 100 mm Hg. Over the last 25 years, several studies have been performed to determine the incidence of pressure sores in various environments. These tend to be highly variable, depending on the patient subpopulation and environmental factors. Generally, the prevalence of pressure sores range from 10% to 18% of patients in an acute care setting, 2.3% to 28% in long-term facilities, and 0% to 29% for those receiving home care. Those at highest risk are the older adults with femoral neck fractures, followed by quadriplegic patients, neurologically impaired young, and the chronically hospitalized. With pressure sores being so common, the cost for surgical and nonsurgical management is in the billions annually.

- **How long has the ulcer been present?** Ulcers of relatively new onset may respond to conservative measures, while more chronic ones tend to be more recalcitrant.

- **Is the patient ambulatory, wheelchair bound, or bed bound?** Ambulatory patients have better outcomes since ultimately they are less likely to return to the state that originally contributed to the ulcer. The location of the ulcer is also indicative of patient's current status. Ischial pressure sores are more likely to develop in patients that are able to sit and are wheelchair bound with most of the pressure being placed on the ischial tuberosities. Bed bound patients are more likely to get ulcers of their sacrum, heels, and occiput. The ambulatory status will also help guide with flap selection when it comes time for surgical repair.

- **What type of cushion is the patient sitting on and what training regimen is the patient using?** Why did this pressure sore occur in this location and what can we do to prevent it from recurring? Wheelchairs typically have a sling seat that leads to abnormal posture and cause asymmetric pressure distribution on both the ischium and trochanter. Specialized cushions are required for prevention. Cushions filled with gel, foam, air, or water are available to help distribute the weight onto the posterior thighs and decrease ischial pressure. However, although various wheelchair seats decrease pressures over the ischium, none will relieve them below the capillary pressure benchmark. Additional measures to relieve pressure are recommended to prevent ulcer formation such as the development of pressure consciousness in the patient. Seated patients must lift themselves or be lifted from their chairs for at least 10 seconds, every 10 minutes.

- **What type of mattress or bed is being used?** At least 4 inches of foam is required to provide modest protection. Normal mattresses offer little protection against ulcer formation. Alternating air cell (AAC) mattresses are composed of air cells oriented perpendicular to the patient and are available as overlays or as replacement mattresses. These air cells subsequently inflate and deflate and in doing so relieve pressure. Low air loss beds function by continuous loss of air from cells within the mattress that facilitate drying of the skin. These typically exert less then 25 mm Hg on any one point of the body. Air fluidized beds function by floating the patient on ceramic beads while warm regulated air is forced through. This also helps facilitate dry skin and maintain a pressure below 20 mm Hg.

- **What additional factors are associated with the etiology of this pressure sore?** In addition to unrelieved pressure, extrinsic mechanical factors include friction and/or shear forces. Friction causes loss of the outermost skin layer resulting in exposure of the underlying tissue and increased water loss. This most often occurs during patient transfers or movement. Shear forces are mechanical forces parallel to the tissue plane. This results in stretching or compression of the muscle perforators to the skin and can lead to ischemic necrosis. Other causes contributing to pressure sore formation include altered sensory perception, altered activity and mobility, ischemia and sepsis, infection, small vessel occlusive disease, anemia, malnutrition, and altered level of consciousness.

- **What other comorbidities and does the patient have?** Other commonly cited intrinsic factors associated with the development of pressure sores include diabetes, peripheral and cardiovascular disease, acute neurological disease, and orthopedic injury.

- **Does the patient smoke?** Smoking decreases tissue perfusion and predisposes to necrosis. Patients should not smoke for 4 to 6 weeks before any repair and at least 6 weeks after to optimize flap viability. Long-term cessation is encouraged to prevent additional ulcers from forming.

- **What options for closure, including surgical, have been tried?** What type of wound care has the patient received in the past? What types of surgical attempts at closure have been tried? If necessary, prior medical records and operative reports should be sought out.

2. Ischial, trochanteric, and sacral regions are the most common sites for pressure sores. Characteristically the overlying skin defect only represents a small portion of the overall affected tissue. Muscle is more sensitive to pressure and begins to necrose after 4 hours of ischemia while skin can tolerate up to 12 hours before showing signs of necrosis. This results in the typical inverted cone geometry of pressure sores in areas where a substantial muscle is present.

- **How extensive is the pressure sore?** When an eschar is present, the ulcer cannot be staged accurately because of the incomplete information about the depth and extent of tissues involved. Limited bedside débridement may be useful to facilitate local wound care preoperatively and evaluate the extent of the defect. Sometimes it is difficult to determine the true boundaries of the ulcer. The staging system proposed by the National Pressure Sore Advisory Panel

Table 39-1 Staging for pressure ulcers

Stage	Description
I	Nonblanchable erythema of intact skin.
II	Partial thickness skin loss presenting clinically as a blister, abrasion, or shallow crater.
III	Full-thickness tissue loss down to, but not through, fascia.
IV	Full-thickness tissue loss with involvement of underlying muscle, bone, tendons, ligaments, or joint capsule.

Consensus Development Conference is similarly valid for ischial ulcers as it is for sacral ulcers.

- **Is there associated infection?** Wound healing will not occur in the presence of ischemia or infection. The presence of infection in pressure sore patients is not infrequent. In darkly pigmented individuals, redness may not be noticeable, in which case other signs of infection, such as warmth, edema, induration, or firmness must also be used as indicators.

— Indwelling bladder catheters or self-catheterization programs result in urinary sepsis in one-third of paraplegic patients. If left untreated, urinary infections can be a constant source of bacteremia.

— Patients with high spinal cord lesions are susceptible to pulmonary infections caused by diaphragmatic dysfunction. A program of pulmonary toilet including positioning, side-to-side rolling, incentive spirometry for deep breathing and coughing, chest physical therapy, and bronchodilators is recommended.

— Morbidity and cost of treating pressure sores are significantly increased because of the unrecognized osteomyelitis. The most common organisms include skin flora (*Staphylococcus*, *Streptococcus*, *corynebacterium*) as well as and enteric organisms (*Proteus*, *Escherichia coli*, and *pseudomonas*).

Topical antibiotics such as silver sulfadiazine can be applied to the wound to decrease bacterial colonization. This, however, can lead to opportunistic infections if overused.

- **How close to the rectum is the ulcer?** Fecal and urinary incontinence results in persistent moisture and contamination of the wound and may cause a significant problem in the postoperative period. While a dressing can temporarily cover the area, this often is not adequate to protect the site. In grossly contaminated wounds, it may be prudent to perform a temporary diverting ostomy preoperatively. This can be reversed after the patient has recovered. Urinary incontinence may be addressed with a suprapubic tube.

- **Does the patient demonstrate a spasm of the axial skeleton or limb contracture?** Spasm and limb contractures are common in patients with spinal cord injuries. Relief of spasticity and proper patient positioning is key in dispersing areas of high pressure on the body. In addition, spasms cause undue tension across an incision and may thus compromise the repair. It is believed that loss of super spinal inhibitory pathways is the mechanism of spasm in these patients. The incidence varies with the level of injury. The more proximal the lesion, the higher the incidence of spasm (100% near the cervical region, approximately 75% in the thoracic region, 50% in the thoracolumbar region). If a spasm is not eliminated prior to any surgical procedure, the pressure sore will most likely recur.

- **What is the patient's nutritional status?** This is a critical question to ask before proceeding with any surgical management. Malnutrition will delay wound healing and ultimately result in a poor outcome. If the patient is unable to take an adequate amount of daily nutrition, then supplemental means should be utilized. Tube feedings, either continuous or at night (delivered in a low residue form, since fecal incontinence and soiling of these wounds is a significant problem in many patients), are preferable to parenteral hyperalimentation. If malnutrition is severe, calorie counts should be started as soon as the patient is hospitalized to determine daily intake.

3. A number of valuable preoperative studies should be obtained preoperatively to minimize postoperative complications.

- Serum laboratory studies are always indicated but several important values should be noted:

  — The **white blood cell count** with differential—used to assess presence of infection. The hemoglobin and hematocrit- used to assess presence of potentially correctable forms of anemia

  — Glucose and HgbA$_1$C. Adequate control of serum glucose levels must be maintained preoperatively and continued during recovery for proper healing to occur.

— Optimal healing exists when serum **albumin** is maintained above the 3.0 gm/dL. **Prealbumin** normally ranges from 16 to 35 mg/dL. The prealbumin level is one of the markers that allow for earlier recognition of and intervention for malnutrition. Prealbumin production decreases after 14 days of consuming a diet that provides only 60% of required proteins. Synthesis of prealbumin increases above baseline levels within 48 hours of protein supplementation. A notable change of the prealbumin level can be significant as early as after 1 week. Be aware that serum prealbumin levels may also rise during prednisone therapy and in patients using progestational agents. Zinc deficiency may lower prealbumin levels, but vitamin deficiencies do not. Assuming there are no other stress factors, 25 to 35 cal/kg of nonprotein calories should be delivered daily. Daily protein requirements will be 1.5 to 3.0 cal/kg, depending on the size of the ulcer and starting protein and albumin levels.

— Note that although correction of vitamin deficiencies are important, supplementation of **vitamins and minerals** in the nondeficient patient has *not* been shown to have a positive effect on wound healing. Vitamin C is essential for the synthesis and maintenance of collagen during wound repair. Levels are often reduced in the older adults and patients with spinal cord injuries. Vitamin A deficiency may also impair wound healing and increase susceptibility to infection. Note that Vitamin A may also be used to counteract the effect of corticosteroids on wound healing. Zinc is specifically involved with epithelization and fibroblast proliferation and plays a role in wound healing as a cofactor for protein synthesis. Ferrous iron and copper are necessary for normal collagen metabolism. Blood levels should be assessed and supplemented as part of the nutritional care.

- A quantitative culture of any questionable wound is prudent prior to surgical intervention.

- Bone biopsies from the wound are ideally obtained for quantitative culture. The most useful single test is a core needle bone biopsy. Culture directed systemic antibiotics coverage should be initiated and continued for 6 weeks to eliminate osteomyelitis or reduce the amount of bone involved.

- Magnetic resonance imaging (MRI) is 97% sensitive and 89% specific in evaluating the extent of osteomyelitis and has proven to be more accurate than other imaging modalities. It is excellent in distinguishing between bone and soft tissue and detecting changes in the bony architecture. It also has the advantage of being multiplanar.

4. An aggressive program of **physical therapy** is important to avoid contracture, which occurs with the tightening of both muscles and joint capsules. Patients with significant hip and\or knee contractures should have every attempt

made to treat these contractures prior to surgery. If not, the pressure sores will most likely recur. If the patient is placed in an alternative position, then the pressure will only be redistributed, and a different area will be at risk for breakdown. If physical therapy is unsuccessful at relieving the contractures, tenotomies may be performed. In mobile patients, however, releasing the hip contractures may lead to a flail extremity, which will interfere with transferring. Numerous treatment modalities exist for the management of ischial pressure ulcers. Conservative treatment modalities include pressure dispersion, control of spasticity, control infection

- The initial goal is to avoid further progression of the sore by relieving the source of pressure. A simple program of turning the patient at regular intervals will allow for recirculation to the affected areas. In addition, various available mattress systems are designed to relieve pressure, including foam, static flotation, alternating air, low air loss, and air fluidized beds. Air fluidized beds are most effective at reducing the external pressure but are heavy and may cause pulmonary problems and\or electrolyte and water losses, especially in the older adults.

- In order to achieve proper positioning of the patient, spasticity must be relieved. This can be achieved pharmacologically or surgically.

  a. Diazepam, 10 to 40 mg, maybe given every 8 hours or in combination with Baclofen.

  b. Baclofen is usually started at 10 mg every 6 hours and may be increased to as much as 25 mg every 6 hours.

  c. Dantrolene, 50 to 800 mg every 12 hours. Some caution should be used because hepatotoxicity has been reported. Serum transaminases should be monitored.

- If patients fail to respond to medical therapy for their spasms, then surgical intervention may be indicated. The surgical management of spasms include peripheral nerve blocks, epidural stimulators, Baclofen pumps, neurosurgical ablation with cordotomy or rhizotomy, and/or amputation.

- Reduction of bacterial load by aggressive debridement of any necrotic tissue present and achieving healthy, viable wound edges is essential. If osteomyelitis is present, flap closure should be delayed 6 weeks for intravenous antibiotic therapy in order to attempt to downstage or eliminate underlying bony involvement.

- Negative pressure wound therapy may be employed that uses a polyurethane or polyvinyl alcohol foam sponge cut to fill the dimensions of the ulcer and covered with an adhesive drape to create an airtight seal. Negative pressure, commonly 125 mm Hg, is applied. This stimulates and accelerates the formation of granulation tissue by removing interstitial fluid containing cytokines, collagenases, and elastases that inhibit fibroblast formation and decrease tissue perfusion.

The negative pressure also stimulates cellular proliferation and protein synthesis which speed the reduction of wound dimension. Wounds treated in this way have also shown decreased number and variety of bacterial colonization.

- There will usually be a period of time in which the ulcers can be treated nonsurgically. If during this time the ulcer appears to be healing significantly, continuation of nonoperative treatment is indicated. Some patients may never be candidates for surgical correction because of significant medical problems. In these cases, avoidance of unrelieved pressure, control of infection (local and remote), controlled incontinence, and improved nutrition may lead to successful ulcer closure or at least may allow for a stable wound that does not progress.

- The most successful treatment of pressure sores is prevention. However, once ulcers have progressed to stage 3 or 4, conservative therapy is often protracted and unsuccessful. Surgical treatment is indicated for most of these cases. When planning a surgical strategy, the surgeon should consider not only the present surgery, but also the need for subsequent surgical procedures. In most cases, placing the patient in the jackknifed flexed position during surgery is best for accurately determining the size of the ulcer. The surgical management for pressure sores follows these main principles.

  — First, a complete excision of the ulcer bursa, and any heterotopic calcification must be performed. Débridement should be accomplished in the operating room, where adequate lights, assistance, and ability to control bleeding can be obtained. The use of wetting solution (1 liter of normal saline with 30 mL of 1% plain lidocaine, if sensate, plus 1 mL of 1:1000 concentration epinephrine) infiltrated around the bursa can help with hemostasis and assist by hydrodissecting the bursa from the surrounding tissue.

  — Second, ostectomy of all devitalized or infected bone to clinically hard, healthy, bleeding bone is important to remove any potential nidus for ulcer recurrence and/or future infection. To minimize the creation of new problems, only the minimum amount of necessary ischium should be removed at the time of débridement. It is important that specimens be sent for culture to aid in postoperative antibiotic coverage. Radical ostectomy is avoided since it may lead to excessive bleeding, skeletal instability, and redistribution of pressure points to adjacent areas. Some authors have advocated total ischiectomies for these ulcers. Although the recurrence rate was decreased from 38% to 3%, it was also associated with the formation of a contralateral ischial ulcer in almost one-third of the patients. Bilateral ischiectomies have also been proposed, but the redistribution of pressure has caused perineal ulceration, and this can be complicated by the formation of

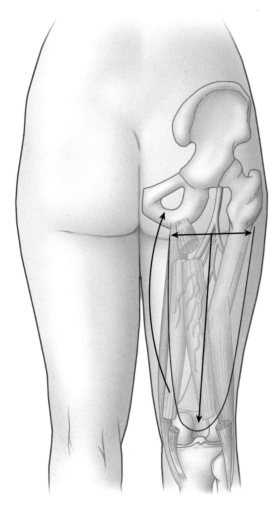

Figure 39-1 Schematic drawing highlighting posterior thigh flap reconstruction.

urethral fistulas. Meticulous hemostasis should be achieved after debridement of bone to avoid formation of hematomas that may compromise the overlying flap.

— Assessment of the three-dimensional defect and elimination of any gap of the soft tissues reduces potential fluid collection and must be taken into account and filled when choosing flaps for coverage. Primary closure may be tempting, but it should be kept in mind that these ulcers represent an absence of tissue, and primary closure almost always leaves a subcutaneous "dead space." In addition, adjacent tissues are usually less compliant as a result of chronic inflammation/induration. A flap of adequate bulk brings healthy compliant tissue to fill this gap. Primary closure of deep pressure sores, in general, is destined for failure.

— Finally, suitable closure of the defect is achieved by transferring in well-vascularized, durable tissue to achieve a tension free repair. Avoidance of incision lines on seating surfaces is also important

in helping to prevent recurrence. This is achieved by a flap designed to allow coverage of the ulcer but should not prevent the use of other, secondary flaps for pressure sore recurrence. As a general rule, the largest flap of the simplest design is the flap of choice as it allows rerotation if the ulcer recurs.

— Skin grafts are possible in the case of superficial ulceration. They tend, however, to provide unstable coverage with only a 30% success rate associated with this technique in the pressure sore patient.

— Fasciocutaneous flaps offer an axial blood supply with durable coverage and minimum potential for a functional deformity. The flap more closely reconstructs the normal anatomic arrangement over bony prominences. The disadvantages, however, include limited bulk for large ulcers that have a significant 3-dimensionality. Common fasciocutaneous flaps used to cover ischial pressure sores are the gluteal fasciocutaneous flap, the posterior thigh flap, and anterolateral thigh fasciocutaneous island flap.

— Musculocutaneous flaps also offer an excellent blood supply with bulky tissue. Like fasciocutaneous rotation flaps, they are also able to be rerotated or readvanced because of their excellent vascularity and the generous perfusion they bring to the wound. Disadvantages include atrophic muscles in the older adults and in spinal cord patients and creation of a functional impairment in ambulatory patients. Therefore, a patient's ambulatory status must always be taken into account when deciding on what type of coverage to use.

a. A superiorly based **gluteal musculocutaneous flap** may be rotated to fill the defect. However, the gluteus maximus is not considered expendable in ambulatory patients. In those cases where the ability to walk must be preserved, the muscle may be split and partially elevated as a segmental flap leaving the intact half for function.

b. The **posterior thigh musculocutaneous advancement flap** includes the biceps femoris, semimembranosus, and semitendinosus muscle and soft tissue overlying medial posterior thigh. They are adequate for small to moderate-sized defects. One advantage is the ability to readvance tissue as necessary on account of the segmental type blood supply that exists in this region off of the femoral artery. They are reliable and commonly designed as a V-Y advancement or V-Y-S advancement-rotation flap.

c. The **tensor fasciae latae (TFL) flap** is occasionally used to close the ischial ulcers. Unfortunately, the distal aspect of the flap, which is used to reach the ischial region, is usually too thin to offer adequate padding to be effective in this type of ulcer.

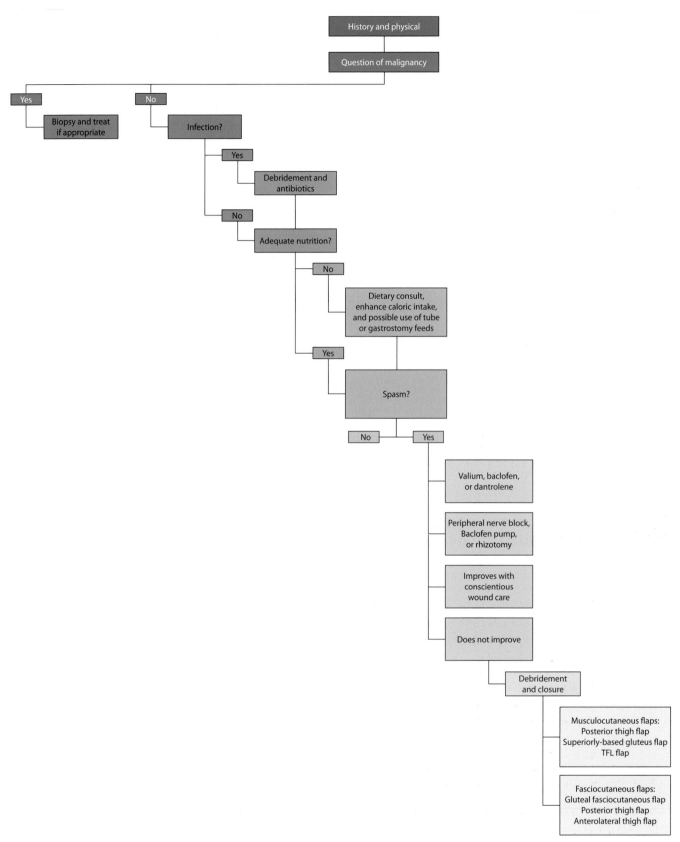

Algorithm 39-1 Algorithm for management of patients with ischial wounds.

1. A dilute solution of methylene blue and saline can be topically applied to the bursa at the start of the case to help define the bursal cavity and leave a visual guide prior to excision.

2. Infiltrate peribursal area with wetting solution using a liposuction infiltration cannula prior to excision to hydrodissect the bursa from surrounding tissue and minimize blood loss.

3. Design flaps as large as possible with suture lines away from area of direct pressure.

4. Ostectomize to clinically hard bone. Use of a micro-collagen fibrillar hemostat such as Avatene (C.R. Bard, Inc., Murray Hill, NJ, USA) for hemostasis instead of electrocautery to avoid creating new bone necrosis caused by thermal injury.

5. Dissect sharply to avoid thermal damage to flap.

6. Undermine only what is needed to mobilize the flap to fill the defect and avoid violating adjacent flap territories in order to allow for possible future flap coverage.

7. Use staples for skin closure to minimize ischemia.

- Postoperative care is as important as the preparation for ensuring the surgery's success. Any special beds must be ready before proceeding with the operation so that they are ready immediately postoperatively. A flap can fail in the recovery room while awaiting a bed ordered as an afterthought. The patients are kept flat, in a supine position, with no pressure allowed to the surgical site. Patients are usually kept in the hospital at least 1 week for the results of bone cultures obtained during ostectomy. Antibiotics should be continued for 3 to 6 weeks based on these results. At 5.5 weeks, seat mapping is performed by physical medicine and customized seats are fabricated to avoid continued pressure over vulnerable points. At 6 weeks, a seating protocol can begin and is supervised by physical medicine and rehabilitation physicians.

6. Complications following the closure of ischial wounds in complicated patients are not uncommon and their potential should be identified preoperatively so that they may be minimized postoperatively.

- The accumulation of fluid beneath the flap, either as a hematoma or a seroma, is not unlikely since many patients are managed with anticoagulants that may or may not be discontinued around the time of surgery. It is always prudent to leave one or more drains beneath a flap to collect any residual fluid.

- Persistent infection is certainly a concern and may be minimized by staging the initial debridement prior to the definitive closure and careful preoperative determination that any existing infection has been eradicated.

- The most common complication is **recurrence**, which occurs in up to 80% of patients. Prevention and avoidance of recurrence requires cooperation and motivation of the patients and those who provide the care for the patient. The reason for the high rate of recurrence is multifactorial. The underlying medical problems often still exist. There is continued altered mentation. Nursing care remains labor-intensive (turning, local wound care, avoidance of urine and fecal contamination). In short, unless the predisposing factors can be modified (e.g., altered behavior, alleviating spasm, release contractures), there is no reason to provide surgical treatment to an otherwise clean wound.

References

1. Lindon O, Greenway RM, Piazza JM. Pressure distributuion on the surface of the human body I. Evaluation in lying and sitting positions using a "bed of springs and nails." *Arch Phys Med Rehabil.* 1965;46:378-385.

2. Langemo D, Olson B, Hanson D, et al. Pressure ulcer research: Prevalence, incidence, and evaluation of effectiveness of protocols. *The Prairie Rose.* 1993;62:13-16.

3. Klitzman B, Kalinowski C, Glasofer SL, et al. Pressure ulcers and pressure relief surfaces. *Clin Plast Surg.* 1998;25:443-450.

4. Foster RD, Anthony JP, Mathes SJ, et al. Ischial pressure sore coverage: A rationale for flap selection. *Br J Plast Surg.* 1997;50:374-379.

5. Mathes SJ, Nahai F. Reconstructive surgery: Principles, anatomy and technique. New York, NY; St. Louis, MO: Churchill Livingstone; *Quality Medical Pub.* 1997.

6. Hurteau JE, Bostwick J, Nahai F, et al. V-Y advancement of hamstring musculocuataneous flap for coverage of ischial pressure sores. *Plast Reconstr Surgery.* 1981;68:539-542.

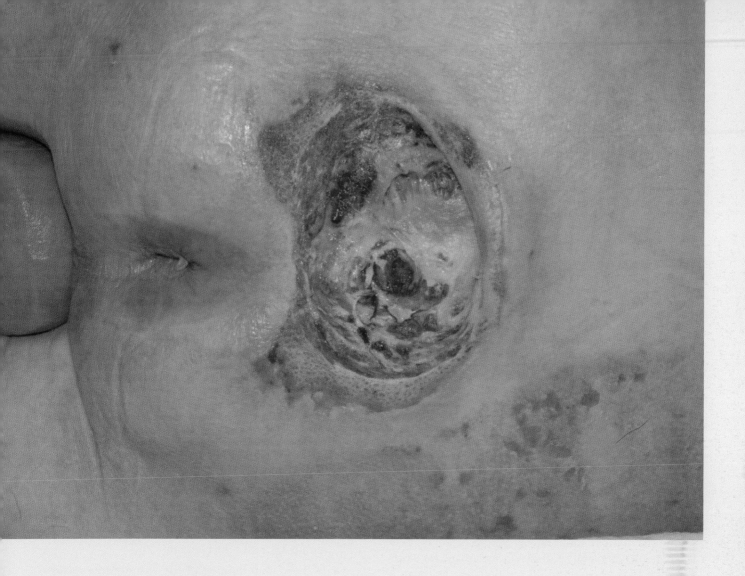

The intensive care unit requests your consult

on a 73-year-old critically ill patient with

open wound over the buttocks.

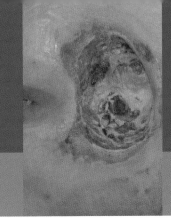

CHAPTER 40

Sacral Pressure Ulcer

C. Scott Hultman

1. Ulcers of the soft tissue overlying the sacrum are unfortunately common in chronically supine patients. In addition to unrelieved pressure, factors contributing to pressure sore formation include altered sensory perception, incontinence, exposure to moisture, altered activity and mobility, friction, and shear force. A thorough history is important to obtain in that it provides clues to the underlying etiologies that need to be addressed if treatment is to be successful. The common physiologic process is unrelieved pressure. Ulcers begin in the deeper tissues nearest to a bony prominence. If the external compressive force exceeds pressure in the capillary bed, perfusion is impaired and ischemia will ensue.

- **How long has the ulcer been present?** Ulcers of relatively new onset may respond to conservative measures, while more chronic ones tend to be more recalcitrant.

- **Is the patient ambulatory, wheelchair-, or bedbound?** Ambulatory patients do not usually get ulcers since they are able to shift positions on their feet. A period of inactivity, however, may predispose to the development of an ulcer if precautions are not taken and/or the patient's nutrition is less than adequate. For the patient with a sacral ulcer, chronic recumbence is likely to have been in the supine position.

- **What type of mattress and turning regimen is the patient using?** Normal mattresses offer little protection against ulcer formation. Airflow mattresses are better, while air and sand mattresses offer the least pressure.

- **What options for closure, including surgical, have been tried?** Prior attempts at closure should be sought since old incisions and atrophic surrounding muscle may limit the successive surgical options.

- **Does the patient have any medical comorbidities?** Commonly cited in many studies was the association with concomitant medical problems, including cardiovascular disease (41%), acute neurologic disease (27%), and orthopedic injury (15%). In addition to medical problems, age is an associated factor for pressure sore formation.

- **What is the patient's social history?** Patients with documented noncompliance, inadequate resources at home, unstable psychiatric illness, or a history of substance abuse are poor candidates for surgical intervention. A history of active or previous nicotine use increases the risk of poor wound healing.

2. The sacral, ischial, and trochanteric and regions are the most common sites for pressure sores. Characteristically, the overlying skin only represents a small portion of the overall affected tissue so a thorough physical examination should inspect not only the area in question, but also the surrounding soft tissues.

- **How large is the defect?** Small defects may be debrided and closed primarily with surrounding tissue, whereas larger wounds require flaps or grafts for reconstruction.

- **How deep is the defect?** Superficial defects may be protected and allowed to reepithelialize if nutrition is adequate. Deeper lesions will heal less rapidly and require operative intervention.

- **Is there undermining of the surrounding tissues?** Sometimes it is difficult to determine the true boundaries of the ulcer. A dilute solution of methylene blue and hydrogen peroxide can be instilled at the start of the case to help define the cavity and leave a visual guide prior to excision.

- **Which tissue types are involved?** When an eschar is present, the ulcer cannot be staged accurately because of the incomplete information about the depth and tissues involved. Limited bedside debridement may be useful to facilitate local wound care preoperatively. Involvement of bone is concerning since exposure usually leads to infection, which is then difficult to clear with antibiotics. The staging system most commonly accepted is that of the National Pressure Sore Advisory Panel Consensus Development Conference (1989): Stage 1 is defined as intact skin with non-blanchable redness. Stage 2 pressure sores have partial thickness loss of dermis, presenting as a shallow ulcer. A stage 3 pressure ulcer has full-thickness loss of skin with exposed fat. Stage 4 pressure sores have full-thickness loss with exposed muscle, tendon, or bone.

- **Are the surrounding tissues edematous?** The role of edema in promoting the infection process seen in pressure sores must not be overlooked. Compressed, denervated skin is known to become edematous by several processes.

- **Does the patient lack sensation in the region of the wound?** Compounding this process is the fact that the tissues are denervated. The loss of sympathetic tone of the blood vessels causes vasodilatation and leads to greater engorgement of the vessels and further, greater edema.

- **Is there associated infection?** Wound healing will not occur in the presence of ischemia or infection. The presence of infection in pressure sore patients is not infrequent. In darkly pigmented individuals, redness may not be noticeable, in which case other signs of infection, such as discoloration, warmth, edema, induration, or firmness must also be used as indicators. Bladder catheters, pulmonary sources, and bone involvement are all potential sources of infection.

- **How close is the anus to the ulcer?** Contamination of the wound with stool may be a problem in the postoperative period. Often, a dressing can temporarily protect the area. In grossly contaminated wounds, it may be prudent to perform a temporary diverting ostomy preoperatively. Urethrocutaneous and rectovaginal fistulas mandate diversion of the urinary and fecal streams, respectively.

- **Does the patient demonstrate spasm or contraction of the extremities?** Spasm is common in patients with spinal cord injuries. It is believed that loss of supraspinal inhibitory pathways is the mechanism of spasm in these patients. The incidence varies with the level of injury. The more proximal is the lesion, the higher the incidence of spasm (100% near the cervical region, approximately 75% in the thoracic region, 50% in the thoracolumbar region). If spasm is not eliminated prior to any surgical procedure, the pressure sore will inevitably recur. Contracture is seen with longstanding denervation and may complicate the reconstructive efforts. This may be present with sacral wounds but is usually less of a complicating factor.

3. Preoperative studies are important when considering the therapeutic options for a sacral pressure ulcer.

- **What is the patient's nutritional status?** A cursory physical examination should identify the overall nutritional status. Areas of wasting may be clues to malnutrition. Laboratory values, including albumin, prealbumin, and transferrin levels, among others, are useful to document the patient's nutritional status. Optimal healing exists when serum albumin is maintained above 2.0 gm/dL. Additional studies include total lymphocyte count, serum transthyretin, and a metabolic cart to determine caloric need and consumption.

- Culture of the questionable wound is prudent prior to surgical intervention. A bone biopsy obtained in the operating theater will provide the most sensitive and specific information regarding the presence of osteomyelitis.

- The preoperative workup should also include complete blood count to assess hematocrit, wound blood cell count, and platelet levels; serum electrolytes to rule out renal dysfunction and acid-base disorders; liver function tests to assess synthetic function; PT and PTT to screen for coagulopathy; urinalysis with culture and sensitivities; and chest X-ray and EKG in patients with cardiac disease.

4. Conservative treatment measures in conjunction with the primary service and rehabilitation service should always be instituted first and may certainly supplement any surgical interventions.

- The initial goal is to avoid any further progression of the sore by relieving the source of pressure. A simple program of turning the patient at intervals will allow for recirculation in the affected areas. In addition, various available mattress systems are designed to relieve pressure, including foam, static flotation, alternating air, low-air-loss, and air fluidized beds. The purpose of these beds is to more evenly distribute the patient's weight to minimize pressure in any one area. An air and sand bed can be most effective at reducing the external pressure but is heavy and may cause pulmonary problems and/or electrolyte and water losses, especially in the elderly.

— Assuming there are no other stress factors, 25 to 35 cal/kg of nonprotein calories should be delivered daily. Daily protein requirements will be 1.5 to 3.0 gm/kg, depending on the size of the ulcer and the starting protein and albumin levels.

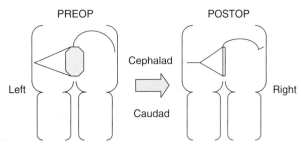

Figure 40-1 Closure of sacral pressure sore with left gluteal V-Y and right gluteal rotation-advancement flaps.

— Vitamins A and C are important in wound healing.

— Zinc is specifically involved with epithelization and fibroblast proliferation.

— Calcium is a cofactor for many enzymatic pathways.

— Ferrous iron and copper are necessary for normal collagen metabolism. Blood levels should be assessed and supplemented as part of the nutritional care.

- If the patient is unable to take an adequate amount of daily nutrition, supplemental means should be utilized. Tube feedings, either continuous or at night (delivered in a low residue form, since fecal incontinence and soiling of these wounds is a significant problem in many patients), are preferable to parenteral hyperalimentation. If malnutrition is severe, calorie counts should be started as soon as the patient is hospitalized to determine daily intake.

- Medications are available to reduce spasm.

— Valium (10 mg) may be given every 8 hours or in combination with baclofen.

— Baclofen is usually started at 10 mg every 6 hours and may be increased to as much as 25 mg every 6 hours.

— Dantrolene, 50 to 800 mg every 12 hours. Some caution should be used because hepatic toxicity has been reported, and serum transaminases should be monitored. If patients fail to respond to medical therapy, surgical intervention may be indicated.

— The surgical management of spasm includes peripheral nerve blocks, epidural stimulators, Baclofen pumps, and/or surgical or medical rhizotomy with phenol. Since clinical improvement can occur up to 18 months after injury, surgical rhizotomy is not performed during this period. In addition, some spinal cord lesions are not complete, and rhizotomy must be used with care to avoid exacerbating the injury.

- An aggressive program of physical therapy is important to avoid **contracture**, which occurs with tightening of both muscles and joint capsules.

- It is always prudent to attempt ulcer closure without surgical means. This may include standard dressing changes with wet-to-dry gauze or negative pressure wound therapy with a sponge and an occlusive dressing. There will usually be a period of time in which the ulcers can be observed. If during this time period the ulcer appears to be healing significantly, continuation of nonoperative treatment is indicated. Some patients may never be candidates for surgical correction because of significant medical problems. In these cases, avoidance of unrelieved pressure, control of infection (local and remote), control of incontinence, and improved nutrition may lead to successful ulcer closure or at least may allow for a stable wound that does not progress.

5. Primary closure usually results in a short-term solution with significant recurrence rates. The most successful treatment of pressure sores is prevention. However, when creating a surgical plan, the surgeon should consider not only the present surgery, but also the need for subsequent surgical procedures. The surgical management for pressure sores follows three main principles.

- First, **excisional debridement** of the ulcer, its pseudobursa, and any heterotopic calcification may be performed in a staged or immediate fashion, depending upon the clinical status of the patient and the wound. Debridement should be accomplished in the operating room, where adequate light, assistance, and ability to control bleeding can be obtained. With potential infection, it is important that specimens be sent for culture to aid in postoperative antibiotic coverage and in the selection of the most effective topical antimicrobial agent. At the end of the case, the wound can be lightly packed with gauze soaked in saline, silver sulfadiazine, mafenide acetate, dilute iodine, or 0.025% Dakin's solution. Regardless of which agent is used, dressings are changed every 6 to 8 hours, and it is the mechanical debridement associated with dressing changes, as much as the solution employed, that may be responsible for decreasing the bacterial count. A negative pressure wound dressing may also be used for wound care.

- Second, **ostectomy** should be performed to reduce any bony prominence and address any chronic osteomyelitis. To minimize the creation of new problems, only a minimum amount of ischium should be removed at the time of debridement. Radical ostectomy is avoided since it may lead to excessive bleeding, skeletal instability, and redistribution of pressure points to adjacent areas. Some authors have advocated total ischiectomies for these ulcers. Although the recurrence rate was decreased from 38% to 3%, it was also associated with the formation of a contralateral ischial ulcer in almost one-third of the patients. Bilateral ischiectomy has been proposed, but redistributed pressure has caused perineal ulceration, and this can be complicated by the formation of urethral fistulas.

- Finally, **closure** of the wound is achieved with healthy, durable tissue. Flap design should allow coverage of the ulcer but should not prevent the use of other, secondary flaps for pressure sore recurrence. As a general rule, the largest flap of simplest design is the flap of choice as it allows rerotation, if the lesion recurs.

  — Primary closure may be tempting, but it should be kept in mind that these ulcers represent an absence of tissue, and primary closure almost always leaves a subcutaneous "dead space." In addition, adjacent tissues are usually less compliant than would be necessary for a tensionless, primary closure.

  — Skin grafts are possible in the case of superficial ulceration. They tend however to provide unstable coverage with only a 30% success rate is associated with this technique.

  — The most commonly employed flaps to close sacral defects are **fasciocutaneous** flaps utilizing the gluteal fascia. These may be designed as rotational flaps—uni-or bilateral—or advancement flaps, usually V-Y flaps.

  — The most commonly described **musculocutaneous** flaps are based on the gluteus maximus muscle (see photograph). Depending on the size of the ulcer, previous operations, and ambulation of the patient, many different options are available. The gluteal flap can be based superiorly or inferiorly, part or all of the muscle or both muscles may be used, it can be constructed of muscle or muscle and skin, and it may be rotated, advanced, or turned over. Other flaps available include the transverse and vertical lumbosacral flap, which is based on lumbar perforating vessels. Perforator flaps based upon the superior gluteal vessels have also been recently described.

- As a general rule, the largest flap of simplest design is the flap of choice as it allows rerotation, if the lesion recurs.

6. Complications are not uncommon in such patients with significant comorbidities that will continue even following successful wound closure.

- The accumulation of fluid beneath the flap, either as a hematoma or a seroma, is not unlikely since many patients are managed with anticoagulants that may or may not be discontinued around the time of surgery. It is always prudent to leave one or more drains beneath a flap to collect any residual fluid. Management of the recurrence often begins with local wound care and readdressing the factors that caused the ulcer. When all have been addressed satisfactorily, a second attempt at closure—using either the same flap or a different flap—may be entertained.

- Persistent infection is certainly a concern and may be minimized by staging the initial debridement prior to the definitive closure and careful preoperative determination that any existing infection has been eradicated.

- The most common complication is **recurrence**. Prevention and avoidance of recurrence require cooperation and motivation of the patient and those who provide the care of the patient. The reasons for the high rates of recurrence are multifactorial. The underlying medical problems often still exist. There often continues to be alterations in the patient's mental faculties. Nursing care remains labor-intense (turning, local wound care, avoidance of urine and fecal contamination). In short, unless the predisposing factors can be modified (e.g., alter behavior, eliminate spasm, release contractures), there is no reason to provide surgical treatment for an otherwise clean wound.

PRACTICAL PEARLS

1. Successful surgical outcomes are dependent upon careful selection of patients who are motivated and cooperative, have reasonable resources and social support, have abstained from nicotine use, and who have developed a positive, longitudinal relationship with the health care team.

2. Strong consideration should be given to preoperative creation of a diverting colostomy to keep the wound clean and aggressive assessment and treatment of osteomyelitis to maximize the chances for successful closure.

3. Given the high probability of recurrence, flaps used to cover pressure sores should be designed so that tissue can be reharvested and readvanced. Always consider what the next procedure will be.

4. Postoperative care includes use of an air-fluidized bed for at least 2 weeks, pulmonary toilet and deep venous thrombosis prophylaxis, closed suction drains, and referral to physical medicine for rehabilitation.

5. Patients who are not operative candidates can be treated with local debridement and subatmospheric sponge dressing.

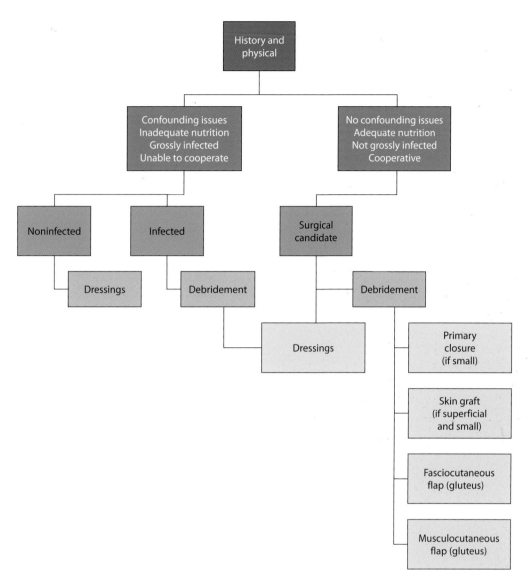

Algorithm 40-1 Algorithm for management of patients with sacral wounds.

References

1. Bass MJ, Phillips LG. Pressure sores. *Curr Probl in Surg.* 2007;44(2):101-143.

2. Scheufler O, Farhadi J, Kovach SJ, Kukies S, Pierer G, Levin LS, Erdmann D. Anatomical basis and clinical application of the infragluteal perforator flap. *Plast Reconstr Surg.* 2006;118(6):1389-1400.

3. Reddy M, Gill SS, Rochon PA. Preventing pressure ulcers: A systematic review. *JAMA.* 2006;296(8):974-984.

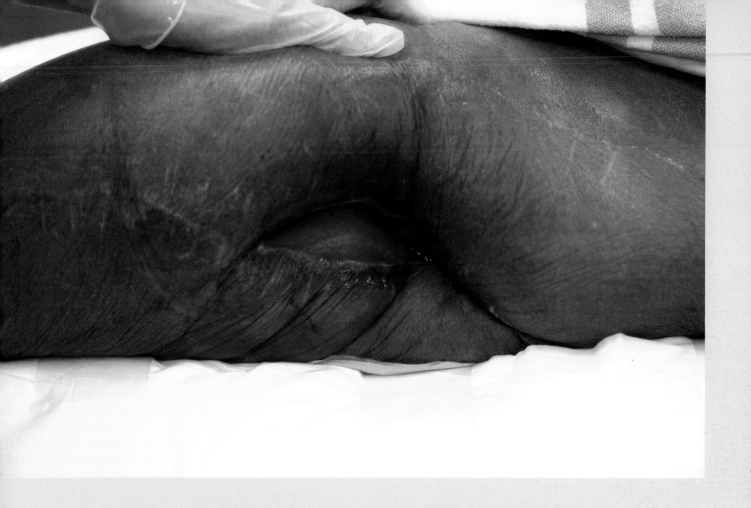

While rounding on the rehabilitation floor of your hospital, the internist asks to you consult on a patient recently admitted from another institution.

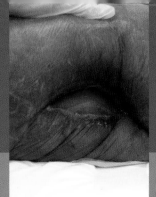

CHAPTER 41

Trochanteric Pressure Sore

Harvey Himel

1. The patient appears to have a wound in the region of the lateral hip. Often, these are caused by pressure over the greater trochanter of the femur in patients who lie in the lateral decubitus position for extended periods of time. In addition to unrelieved pressure, factors contributing to pressure sore formation include altered sensory perception, incontinence and other forms of excess moisture, altered activity and mobility, friction, and shear forces. A thorough history is important to obtain in that it provides clues to the underlying etiologies that need to be addressed if treatment is to be successful. The common pathophysiologic mechanism for deep ulcers is unrelieved pressure. These ulcers begin in the deeper tissues nearest to a bony prominence, where cutaneous perfusion originates in the deep soft tissues. If the external compressive force exceeds pressure in the capillary bed, perfusion is halted and ischemia will ensue, leading to tissue hypoxia and bacterial colonization. Repeated episodes of compression will lead to ischemia—reperfusion injury that compounds the injury.

- **How long has the ulcer been present?** Ulcers of relatively recent onset may respond better to conservative measures, while more chronic ones tend to be more recalcitrant.

- **Is the patient ambulatory or wheelchair bound or bed bound?** For the patient with a trochanteric ulcer, chronic recumbence, specifically in the lateral decubitus position, can contribute to the etiology and persistence of the ulcer wound, along with placing the patient at risk for recurrence.

- **What type of mattress and turning regimen is the patient using?** Normal mattresses offer little protection against ulcer formation. Airflow mattresses that provide a pressure reducing support surface are better.

- **What options for closure, including surgical, have been tried?** Evidence of prior flap rotation in the regions of the lower extremity and buttock, that may have previously been used for the lateral thigh, should be sought since these options will likely not be able to be used again.

- **What comorbidities exist?** Any concomitant cardiovascular disease, acute neurologic disease, and orthopedic injury should be identified. In addition to medical problems, age is an associated factor. In terms of actual risk for pressure ulcer, the Braden scale is the most widely used method of assessing susceptibility.

2. A complete physical examination should characterize the wound, the surrounding soft tissues, and the appropriateness of the patient for either conservative or more aggressive therapy.

- **What is the extent of the lesion?** Characteristically the overlying skin only represents a small portion of the overall affected tissue. More significant than direct depth is the extent of circumferential undermining of the wound perimeter and the presence of subcutaneous tunneling radiating out from the central lesion. Both of these regions will harbor high concentrations of bacteria that impair healing.

- **How deep is the wound and what tissues are involved?** As mentioned, the presence of an eschar prevents adequate examination and staging of the wound. Debridement, either at the beside or in the operating room, and with or without the assistance of methylene blue dye as a marker for local spread, is vital.

- **Are the surrounding tissues edematous?** The role of edema in delineating the extent and severity of the infectious process seen in pressure sores must not be overlooked. Compressed, denervated skin is known to become edematous by several processes. Regional edema is often a sign of cellulitis extending beyond the wound, indicating the need for systemic antibiotics.

- **Are other sites ulcerated?** Ischial, trochanteric, and sacral regions are the most common sites for pelvic pressure sores. The loss of sympathetic tone in the blood vessels causes vasodilatation and leads to greater engorgement of the vessels and further, greater edema.

- **Does the patient lack sensation in the region of the wound?** Compounding the actual development of a trochanteric wound is the fact that the tissues are denervated. In the absence of protective sensation, patients will continue to traumatize their wound repetitively resulting in a failure to heal and a tendency to recur after treatment.

- The staging system most commonly accepted is that of the National Pressure Ulcer Advisory Panel Updated Staging System.

- **Is there associated infection?** Local wound infection around a trochanteric pressure ulcer is not uncommon and the presence of infection will certainly compromise healing. Bladder catheters, pulmonary sources, and bone involvement are all potential sources of infection.

- **How close to the anus is the ulcer?** While less of an issue than with a sacral or ischial ulcer, contamination of the wound with stool may be a problem in the postoperative period. While a dressing can temporarily protect the area, it may be advisable in grossly contaminated wounds to perform a temporary diverting colostomy.

- **Does the patient demonstrate involuntary spasm or contracture?** Spasm is common in patients with spinal cord injuries. It is believed that loss of supraspinal inhibitory pathways is the mechanism of spasm in these patients. The incidence varies with the level of injury. The more proximal the lesion, the higher the incidence of spasm (100% near the cervical region, approximately 75% in the thoracic region, 50% in the thoracolumbar region). If spasm is not eliminated prior to surgical wound closure, the pressure sore will be at high risk for recurrence as a result of the disruptive shear and traction forces. Contracture is seen with longstanding, unopposed tonic spasm. Because the hip flexors are so strong, contractures are common in the trochanteric region, contributing not only to the formation of ulcers, but also to ischial, knee, heel, and ankle ulcers.

3. Preoperative studies should document the patient's nutritional and overall health status as well as the wound's state of contamination.

- **What is the patient's nutritional status?** If the patient is suffering from protein-calorie nutrition, wound healing will not occur. If the patient is unable to take in adequate nutrition by mouth, supplemental means should be utilized. Tube feedings, either continuous or cycled, should be adjusted to minimize fecal incontinence and soiling of the wounds in many patients, are preferable to parenteral hyperalimentation. If malnutrition is suspected, calorie counts should be started, and visceral proteins measured. In addition, blood levels of critical micronutrients should be assessed and deficiencies corrected by supplements as part of the nutritional care.

  — Optimal healing exists when serum albumin is maintained above 3.0 gm/dL. Assuming there are no other stress factors, 25 to 35 cal/kg of nonprotein calories should be delivered daily. Daily protein requirements will be 1.5 to 3.0 gm/kg, depending on the size of the ulcer and the starting protein and albumin levels.

  — Vitamins A and C are important in wound healing.

  — Zinc is specifically involved with epithelization and fibroblast proliferation.

  — Calcium is a cofactor for many enzymatic pathways.

  — Ferrous iron and copper are necessary for normal collagen metabolism.

- **What are the resident bacterial flora in the wound?** Culture of the wound, even in the absence of cellulitis or abscess, should be obtained prior to surgical intervention to screen for drug-resistant species colonization.

4. Conservative treatment measures should be instituted early to minimize existing damage and avoid further progression of the sore by relieving the source of the pressure.

- A simple program of turning the patient at frequent intervals will allow for adequate circulation in the affected areas while avoiding repeated episodes of ischemia. In addition, various available mattress systems are designed to relieve pressure, including foam and static flotation mattresses (Group 1); alternating air, and low-air-loss mattresses (Group 2); and air fluidized beds (Group 3). The purpose of these surfaces is to more evenly distribute the patient's weight to minimize pressure in any one area. An air and sand bed is most effective at reducing the external pressure but is heavy and may cause pulmonary problems caused by the mandatory recumbence and/or electrolyte and water losses caused by the continuous warm dry air, especially in the elderly.

- Medications are available to reduce spasm.
  - Valium, 10 mg, may be given every 8 hours or in combination with baclofen.
  - Baclofen is usually started at 10 mg every 6 hours and may be increased to as much as 25 mg every 6 hours.
  - Dantrolene, 25 mg every 12 hours. Some caution should be used because hepatic toxicity has been reported, and serum transaminases should be monitored. If patients fail to respond to medical therapy, surgical intervention may be indicated.
  - The surgical management of spasm includes:
    a. Peripheral nerve blocks
    b. Epidural stimulators
    c. Implantable Baclofen pumps
    d. Surgical or medical rhizotomy uses subarachnoid blocks with phenol or Botox. Since clinical improvement can occur up to 18 months after injury, surgical rhizotomy is not performed during this period. In addition, some spinal cord lesions are not complete, and rhizotomy must be used with care to avoid exacerbating the injury.

- An aggressive program of physical therapy is important to avoid **contracture**, which occurs with unopposed contraction of flexor muscles and stiffening of joint capsules. Patients with significant hip and/or knee contractures should have an attempt made to treat the contractures prior to surgery. If not, the pressure sores are sure to recur. If the patient is placed in an alternate, but equally exaggerated posture, then the pressure will be unevenly redistributed again, and a different area will be at risk for breakdown. If physical therapy is unsuccessful at relieving the contractures, tenotomies may be performed. In mobile patients, however, releasing the hip contractures may lead to a flail extremity, which will interfere with transferring.

- It is always prudent to attempt ulcer closure without surgical means. There will usually be a period of time in which the ulcers can be observed. If during this time period the ulcer appears to be healing significantly, continuation of nonoperative treatment is indicated. Some patients may never be candidates for surgical correction because of significant medical problems. In these cases, avoidance of unrelieved pressure, control of infection (local and remote), control of incontinence, and improved nutrition may lead to successful ulcer closure or at least may allow for a stable wound that does not progress.

5. While the most successful treatment of pressure sores is prevention, recurrence is often inevitable. When planning a surgical strategy, the surgeon should consider not only the present surgery, but also the possible need for subsequent surgical procedures.

- In most cases, placing the patient in a flexed position to place the wound on tension during surgery is helpful for accurately determining the extent of the ulcer.

- The surgical management for pressure sores follows three main principles. First, **excisional debridement** of the soft tissue including the ulcer wall, its bursa, and any lateral extensions as well as abnormal bony tissue such as necrotic bone at the wound base and adjacent heterotopic calcification. Debridement should be performed in the operating room, where adequate light, assistance, and ability to control bleeding can be obtained.

- Prominent bony abnormality is treated by **ostectomy** to reduce the bony prominence and excise any osteitis or osteomyelitis. To minimize the creation of new problems, only a minimum amount of bone should be removed at the time of debridement. Radical ostectomy is avoided since it may lead to excessive bleeding, skeletal instability, and redistribution of pressure points to adjacent areas.

- When invasive infection is present, it is important that specimens be sent for culture to aid in postoperative antibiotic coverage and in the selection of the most effective topical antimicrobial agent. The infected wound should be left open and lightly packed with gauze soaked in saline; antibiotics such as silver sulfadiazine, or mafenide acetate; or antiseptics such as dilute iodine, or 0.025% Dakin's solution. Regardless of which agent is used, dressings are changed every 6 to 8 hours, and it is the mechanical debridement associated with dressing changes, as much as the solution employed, that may be responsible for decreasing the bacterial count.

- When infection is absent or has been resolved, **closure** of the wound is achieved with healthy, durable tissue. Flap design should allow coverage of the ulcer but should not prevent the use of other, secondary flaps for pressure sore recurrence. As a general rule, the largest flap of simplest design is the flap of choice as it allows rerotation if the lesion recurs.
  - Primary closure may be tempting, but it should be kept in mind that these ulcers represent an absence of tissue, and primary closure almost always leaves a subcutaneous "dead space." In addition, adjacent tissues are usually less compliant than would be necessary for a tensionless, primary closure.
  - Skin grafts are possible in the case of superficial ulceration but offer little durability and are prone to break-down even after complete healing.
  - Fasciocutaneous flaps offer an adequate blood supply with durable coverage and minimal potential for a functional deformity. The most commonly used flap for treatment of this location is the tensor fasciae

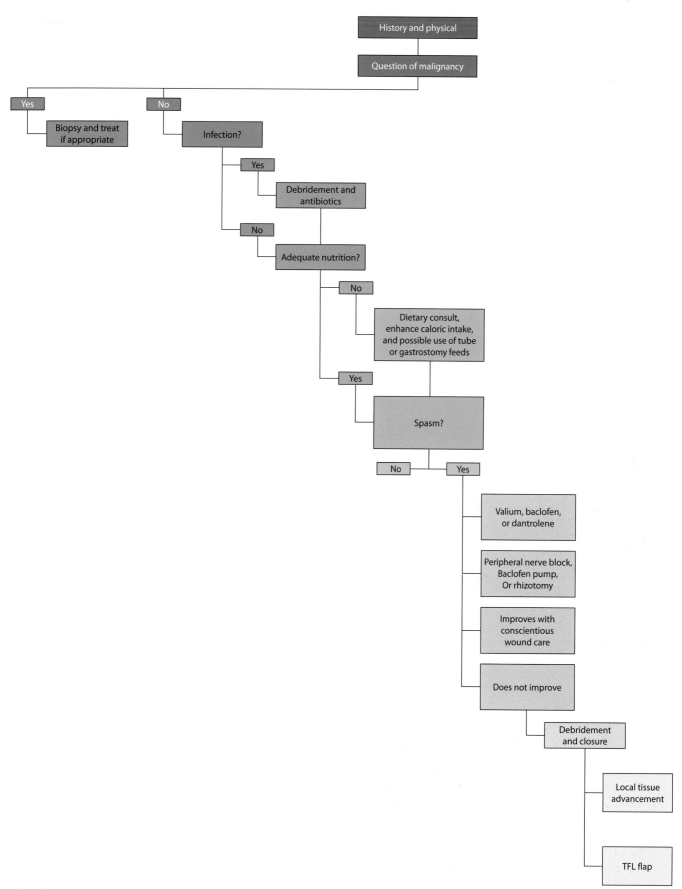

Algorithm 41-1 Algorithm for management of patients with trochanteric wounds.

latae (TFL) flap. It is a highly reliable flap, based on the perforating vessels from the TFL muscle. It pivots approximately 8 cm below the anterior superior iliac spine. Sensation from the nerve roots of L1, L2, and L3 by the lateral femoral cutaneous nerve makes this a potentially sensate flap in patients with spinal cord injury below L3. Its length also makes it useful for ischial and sacral ulcers. Caution should be advised, however, since the distal aspect of the flap is mostly a thin fascial sheet, and the bulk it can supply is limited. For this reason, it is probably best used for trochanteric ulcers only.

— An alternate source of tissue is the rectus femoris muscle which lies in the central portion of the thigh. It is not used as a first option since harvest may arguably interfere with terminal extension of the leg at the knee.

— In patients who have multiple pressure sores or have undergone multiple previous procedures, there may not be any local options remaining. In extreme cases, it may be necessary to consider total thigh flaps, amputation, hemipelvectomy, or hemicorporectomy in order to obtain enough soft tissue to close the ulcer.

- Postoperatively, an absorptive, nonocclusive dressing should be used on the wound to keep it clean and dry. Overuse of topical emollients can cause maceration, and delayed closure of the suture line. Control of urine and stool is important and should have been addressed preoperatively. Drains are usually placed intraoperatively to remove serous drainage and to aid in apposition of the flaps to the wound bed. Drains are commonly left in place until drainage is diminished to a negligible amount and collagen deposition in the wound is anticipated to be sufficient to maintain flap adherence to wound base, usually approximately 14 days after surgery. The surgery usually induces a bacteremia so antibiotics should be continued during the perioperative period. Since most pressure sore cultures are polymicrobial, broad-spectrum antibiotics are used (these may be tailored according to preoperative culture and sensitivity results, if available). Patients are kept in a protective position postoperatively for a minimum of 3 weeks. Positioning must not concentrate pressure in a different location. A fluidized air (group 3) bed is the best option for protecting the patient and the flap from excess pressure. After 3 to 4 weeks, most patients have progressed enough to allow monitored weight bearing on the affected site for 15- to 30-minute intervals, which progresses to 2 hours as tolerated after 6 weeks.

6. In addition to recurrent infection and fluid collection beneath the reconstruction, recurrence of the ulcer is the most common and undesirable Complication. Complications:

- Infection is minimized by the use of appropriate parenteral antibiotics and serial debridements.

Closure should be entertained only when the wound is deemed clean enough for coverage.

- Hematoma is often related to the patient's underlying comorbidities and current medical regimen. The formation of a postoperative hematoma may be minimized by taking the patient off anticoagulant medications around the time of surgery (if possible) and correcting any hematologic problems with replacement colloid (if necessary). Large drains—either open or self-suctioning—should be used liberally.

- Prevention and avoidance of **recurrence** require cooperation and motivation of the patient and those who provide the care of the patient. The reasons for the high rates of recurrence are multifactorial. The underlying medical problems that contribute to etiology often persist after surgery. Nursing care remains labor-intensive (turning, local wound care, avoidance of urine and fecal contamination). As stated above, it warrants repeating that unless the predisposing factors can be modified (e.g., alter behavior, eliminate spasm, release contractures), there is no reason to provide surgical treatment to a clean wound in an otherwise untreated patient with continuing cause for ulceration. Management of the recurrence often begins with local wound care and assessing which factors caused the ulcer. When all have been addressed satisfactorily, a second attempt at closure—using either the same flap or a different flap—may be entertained.

PRACTICAL PEARLS

1. It is far more important to treat the cause than the disease.

2. The search for causative factors is the first step in treatment.

3. Surgery should be postponed until the patient and the wound have been optimized and the wound has failed to progress to healing.

4. While the bone at the base of the wound contributes to the pressure, it is not advisable to perform radical bone resection.

5. Recurrence should be anticipated in planning the surgical approach and determining which patients are candidates for closure.

References

1. Mustoe TA, O'Shaughnessy K, Kloeters O. Chronic wound pathogenesis and current treatment strategies: A unifying hypothesis. *Plast Reconstr Surg.* 2006;117(Suppl 7):35S-41S.

2. Kring DL. Reliability and validity of the Braden scale for predicting pressure ulcer risk. *J Wound Ostomy Continence Nurs.* 2007;34(4):399-406.

3. National Pressure Ulcer Advisory Panel. Information available at: http://www.npuap.org/pr2.htm.

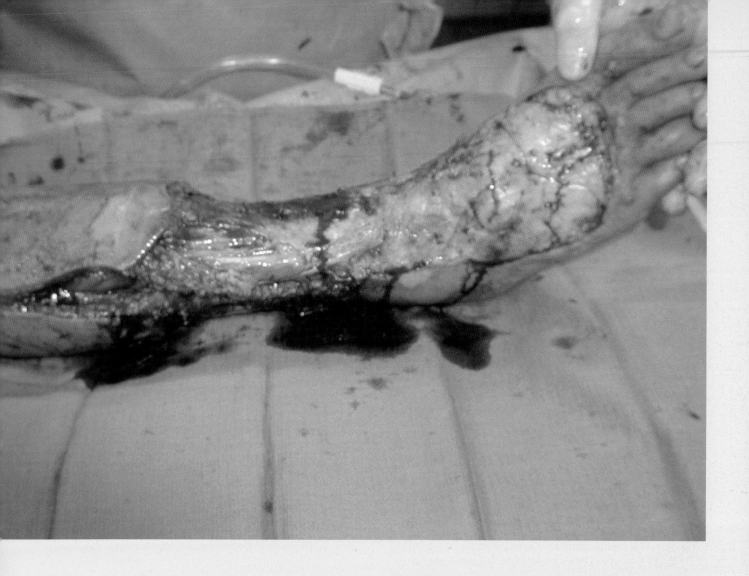

A trauma service asks you to evaluate a 20-year-old patient who sustained an avulsion injury to the lower leg from a motorcycle accident.

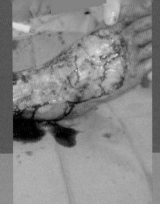

CHAPTER 42

Lower Extremity Injury

Babak J. Mehrara

1. The priority in the treatment of multisystem injury is to salvage the patient, not necessarily the limb. Patients should be initially seen and triaged by the trauma service. A thorough history and physical examination is important in these cases to identify risk factors that might compromise the reconstructive effort. ABCs always take precedence in cases of trauma.

- **How old is the patient?** While age is certainly not an absolute criterion for or against a more aggressive approach to limb salvage, extremes in age in either direction may contribute to the ultimate management decision. Children, for example, tend to recover from nerve injury better than adults and therefore efforts to salvage a mangled leg may be more exhaustive.

- **When did the trauma occur?** A lengthy time between injury and treatment may increase the amount of tissue damage and wound colonization.

- **Was there a mechanism of crush injury?** Crush injury to the leg, where there are closed fascial compartments, may lead to increased tissue pressure from edema and development of compartment syndrome.

- **Is there a history of preexisting peripheral vascular disease?** Patients with an existing problem with blood supply to the lower extremity can fare worse with subsequent trauma and further vascular injury, either primary or secondary.

- **Is there a history of diabetes?** In patients with diabetes, there is a higher morbidity, but equal mortality, to nondiabetic patients. Specifically, the results of flap anastomoses are equal to those of nondiabetics.

- **Is there a history of smoking?** Smoking will adversely affect both wound and bone healing.

2. A thorough physical examination should be performed to determine the extent of injury and the tissue types involved.

- **Where is the wound located?** Wounds of the thigh are often easier to manage than wounds of the proximal leg, which in turn may be easier to manage than those of the distal leg where there is a paucity of muscle and soft tissue.

- **How much soft tissue injury exists?** The size of the wound, including any surrounding necrotic tissue is important to identify since free tissue transfer is often required for larger defects (>25 cm^2). For the same reason, any underlying dead space should be noted.

- **Is there any exposure of hardware, bone, or tendon?** Reliable coverage of such structures is imperative to achieve healing and prevent infection. The Gustilo classification (1984) described the escalating severity of open lower extremity wounds.

- **Are distal pulses palpable?** An ischemic limb does *not* imply a vascular injury. The vessels may be in spasm or may be kinked secondary to the injury. Pulses may return after fracture reduction. Questionable manual examinations may require Doppler examination of the vessels. Angiograms are usually necessary to evaluate thoroughly the vascular status of a mangled extremity that remains ischemic or requires a microvascular free flap for later reconstruction.

- **Is there any evidence of compartment syndrome?** This should be suspected in any crush injury to a closed compartment to prevent tissue necrosis. The

Table 42-1 Gustilo classification of open tibial wounds

Type	Description
I	Open fracture with a wound <1 cm
II	Open fracture with a wound >1 cm
III	Open fracture with extensive soft tissue injury:
III A	Open fracture with adequate soft tissue coverage.
III B	Open fracture with tissue loss, periosteal stripping, or bone exposure.
III C	Open fracture with arterial injury requiring repair.

Others: (MESS, LSI, PSI, NISSSA, HFS-97) Low test scores were useful in predicting which limbs could be salvaged, high test scores could *not* predict which limbs could *not* be salvaged.

cardinal signs of compartment syndrome are pain out of proportion to the injury, pain on passive flexion or extension, a palpably swollen or tense compartment, and/or absence of pulses, which is usually a late sign. Measurement of the compartment pressure makes the definitive diagnosis. The presence of clinical suspicion with/without a compartment pressure >30 mm Hg is an indication for emergent fasciotomy.

- **Is there complete distal sensation?** Loss of posterior tibial nerve function, as noted by absent sensation on the plantar aspect of the foot, is a relative contraindication for lower extremity salvage. The results of nerve repair and grafting in the lower extremity have been poor because of the long distance from the spinal cord and the motor end plates, the complex distribution of nerve fascicles, and the long distance required for the nerve to grow to the motor end plate, resulting in end organ atrophy.

  — **Peroneal nerve** disruption results in foot drop and loss of sensation of the dorsum of the foot. Although not crippling, lifelong foot splinting or tendon transfers are required to offset the foot drop. The loss of sensation of the dorsum of the foot does not cause much morbidity.

  — **Posterior tibial nerve** disruption results in the loss in plantar flexion of the foot, which facilitates step-off during ambulation. The most devastating loss is the loss of sensation of the plantar aspect of the foot. It results in the loss of some position sense and chronic injury to the plantar aspect of the foot.

- **Is there evidence of associated injury?** While the trauma to the extremity in the photograph is certainly severe, potentially life-threatening injuries involving the head, chest, or abdomen pose a greater problem.

3. Studies as part of the workup and management are important and should be arranged in a timely fashion to minimize wound contamination.

- For bony injury, the pattern of the fracture is best evaluated with **plain X-rays**. Extensive periosteal stripping, comminution, and marrow obliteration require coverage with vascularized soft tissue. Posterior dislocations of the knee are prone to disruption of the popliteal vessels and represent a vascular emergency.

- **Angiography** are important in the evaluation of the vascular supply to the distal extremity in the presence of suspected disruption and/or in anticipation of free tissue transfer. Noninvasive angiography is becoming increasingly popular with MR angiograms and CT angiograms; however, these may not be available emergently. On-table angiograms can also be performed if an unacceptable delay in obtaining a formal angiogram of an ischemic leg is unavoidable.

4. Important consults should be arranged as their needs arise during the trauma workup.

- Patients should be admitted to the **trauma surgery** service to identify and/or manage concomitant injuries.

- Fracture of the long bones, such as the femur, tibia, and/or fibula will require stabilization and management by the **orthopedic surgery** service.

- Major arterial injury will require evaluation and reconstruction by the **vascular surgery** service.

- Other consultations can be obtained as necessary in the polytrauma patient who may have preexisting medical conditions.

5. The goal in treating open fractures of the lower extremity is to preserve a limb that will be more functional than an amputation. If the extremity cannot be salvaged, the maintenance of maximum functional length is important. This is particularly important with respect to the knee joint. If the knee is salvageable, amputation below this level should be performed. Although the ideal below-knee amputation stump has >6 cm of tibia below the tubercle, any length of tibia should be preserved as the benefits of a below-knee amputation are great compared to above-knee amputation. The work of ambulation is significantly reduced in patients with below-knee amputations as compared to patients with above-knee amputations (25% increased energy and oxygen consumption requirement with ambulation versus 65% for patients with above-knee amputations). The patient must understand that a severely mangled extremity may take multiple operative procedures and months to years before it can be used for weightbearing and the patient can return to employment.

- Indications for salvage include:
  — Pediatric patients.
  — Adults with preserved plantar sensation.
  — Reasonable hope that the patient will regain the ability to ambulate within 1 year.
- Absolute indications for primary amputation include:
  — Crush injury with warm ischemia time >6 hours.
- Relative indications for primary amputation include:
  — Serious associated polytrauma.
  — Unstable patient who cannot tolerate prolonged salvage operations.
  — Severe ipsilateral foot trauma.
  — Anticipated protracted course to obtain soft-tissue coverage and tibial reconstitution.
  — Segmental tibial fractures.
  — Multiple zones of injury.
  — Transection of the posterior tibial nerve.
- Initial management includes antibiotics and tetanus prophylaxis.
- Debridement with pulsed lavage and skeletal stabilization in the operating room is important soon after arrival and may be repeated until definitive soft tissue coverage is accomplished. If the patient has other life-threatening injuries, treatment should be limited to stabilization of the extremity and control of bleeding. Amputation of a mangled extremity in a clinically unstable patient may be more prudent than an extensive reconstructive course and should be considered in the initial evaluation of the patient.
  — Closed treatment of the bony injury is acceptable for low-energy, closed wounds (internal fixation has a faster time to union and a lower malunion rate).
  — **External fixation** is ideal in a severely traumatized lower extremity with massive soft tissue and bone injury. It allows rigid fixation without additional soft tissue trauma and minimal bone devascularization. It also allows easy access to the wound for additional debridement. External fixators can be utilized with the Ilizarov technique for bone lengthening in situations of bone gaps (>6 cm), or they may be left in place after cancellous or vascularized bone grafting until additional stability of the fracture is obtained.
  — **Internal fixation**, such as by intramedullary nailing, is useful only for minimally comminuted fractures without significant bone loss. Reamed nails obliterate the entire endosteal blood supply to the bone by stripping out the medullary canal and may not be indicated for the massively traumatized lower extremity. Nonreamed nails are advocated because they do not take up the entire intramedullary canal, they do not require complete stripping of the endosteal blood supply. Hardware exposure runs the risk of a progressive infection rapidly up the intramedullary canal, thus serial debridements and delayed soft-tissue coverage are contraindicated with this technique.

- The timing of soft tissue coverage is determined by the need to cover vital structures and the risk of infection. Early coverage is associated with a lower complication rate. In the 1980s, it was noted that complications worsen when an open tibial fracture is allowed to enter the subacute phase of healing (1 to 6 weeks). The reconstructive options are dictated by the site of the injury.
  — Recent reports have described the use of negative pressure therapy in open extremity wounds. Although these results are encouraging, additional data and prospective studies (if feasible) would be extremely helpful. The technique serves as an excellent dressing prior to definitive coverage as well as a means of salvaging a flap loss or treating patients in whom free tissue transfer is otherwise contraindicated.
  — In general, tissue expansion is often avoided in the lower extremity because of the high morbidity (infection rates of 5% to 30%). If used, should be placed above muscle fascia. The surgeon should plan for transverse advancement, not longitudinal, and the pocket for the implant should be dissected completely. Bed rest and elevation following placement are imperative.
  — In the thigh, local tissue advancement or skin grafts are usually available and sufficient for coverage. For extensive injuries, the large anterior thigh muscles may be mobilized to fill the defect. A **rectus femoris flap** may be based on its lateral femoral circumflex pedicle to provide muscle with an arc of rotation ranging from the midthigh to the greater trochanter and lower abdomen. The use of this flap may be associated with a decreased strength of knee flexion. The **tensor fascia lata flap** based on the lateral branch of the lateral femoral circumflex vessels can provide a larger skin paddle that can durably cover anterior wounds of the thigh.
  — In the proximal third of the leg, use of the **medial gastrocnemius flap** is frequently the best option. It has a proximal pedicle and a broad muscle belly that originates on the tibia and inserts into the calcaneus as part of the Achilles tendon. Its reach may be increased by release from its origin and insertion and by scoring the fascia. The **lateral gastrocnemius flap** is useful for coverage of lateral knee defects; however, care must be taken to avoid injury to the peroneal nerve during harvest. An alternative option is the **reverse anterolateral**

thigh flap based on a collateral circulation arising from the geniculate vessels with anastomoses to the descending branch of the lateral femoral circumflex artery and vein. A sizable skin paddle can be harvested and transferred to provide durable coverage. Harvest can be tricky, however.

— In the middle third of the leg, the **soleus flap** is frequently the best option. It is arises from the tibia and also inserts in the calcaneus as part of the Achilles tendon. Other options include the medial and lateral gastrocnemius muscle. The **flexor digitorum longus (FDL) flap** has a small muscle belly useful only for small defects. Sacrifice leads to minimal functional loss [toe flexion supported by flexor digitorum brevis (**FDB**)]. An **extensor digitorum longus (EDL) flap** or **extensor hallucis longus (EHL) flap** can also be used, but again only for small defects. The former is supplied by branches of the anterior tibial artery and harvest must avoid injury to superficial peroneal nerve. In dissecting the latter, the surgeon must leave the distal tendon attached to the **extensor digitorum communis (EDC)** to prevent great toe drop. The *flexor hallucis longus (FHL) muscle is necessary for push off and should not be sacrificed.* Fasciocutaneous flaps have been used. They are usually random pattern flaps with a length:width of roughly 3:1.

— In the distal third of the lower leg and ankle, free tissue transfer is frequently the best option. Recipient vessels include the anterior tibial artery and vein, which are approached laterally between tibialis anterior and EDL (EHL originates low in the leg) and the posterior tibial artery and vein, which are approached medially above the soleus. The "zone of injury" around the defect should be avoided to minimize vessel friability and perivascular scar formation. Vessels distal to the zone of injury may be used successfully. Here, reliable, flaps should be chosen. The **rectus abdominis flap** (either myocutaneous or muscle alone) based on the deep inferior epigastric pedicle, has an acceptable pedicle length and is of significant volume. Easily harvested in a supine position and covered by a skin graft. The **serratus muscle flap**, based on the serratus branch of the thoracodorsal pedicle, has a long pedicle. It may be harvested with the upper body in a lateral decubitus position and combined with the latissimus for large wounds. The **latissimus dorsi muscle flap**, based on the thoracodorsal pedicle, has a long pedicle and large bulk to fill dead space. It may be harvested with the upper body in a lateral decubitus position. Added size may be achieved with a combined latissimus-serratus flap. The use of this flap should be considered carefully because of its importance in crutch walking. Thus, if the odds of limb salvage are lower than normal (i.e., crush injury, etc.) with resultant amputation, then

alternative tissue coverage may be more suitable. The **gracilis muscle flap** is a smaller muscle but has little donor site morbidity and a hidden scar. Also, the pedicle is shorter. The **anterolateral thigh flap** can be harvested from the same thigh either as a fasciocutaneous flap or as a musculocutaneous flap. The fasciocutaneous flap is an excellent option for weight-bearing areas, as it will hold up to loading better than skin grafts. Also, the ALT skin flap facilitates future surgery since skin-to-skin closure can more easily be performed than skin grafted muscle flaps. The **vastus lateralis flap** can be transferred as a muscle flap based on the same pedicle (descending branch of the lateral femoral circumflex artery and vein). Local muscle flaps have limited usefulness since they are often in the zone of injury. Local fasciocutaneous flaps can also be in the zone of injury and are more useful in nontraumatic wounds. These include the saphenous flap and the reversed sural neurocutaneous flap.

— For the heel, free flaps are often required but local flaps are more useful in nontraumatic wounds. An **instep fasciocutaneous (medial plantar) flap** is harvested between plantar fascia and FDB (which lies between abductor hallucis and abductor digiti minimi). It is based on medial or lateral plantar artery. Donor site requires skin graft coverage. The **lateral plantar flap** is a medially based durable rotation flap elevated superficial to the plantar fascia. Sensation preserved by including the medial calcaneal nerve. It is *unable* to reach the distal heel. The **FDB flap**, mobilized on the lateral plantar vessels, is useful for heel, Achilles, and medial and lateral malleolar defects.

— In the forefoot, incisions on weight-bearing surfaces should be avoided. Skin grafts for non–weight-bearing areas. Local flaps include the instep fasciocutaneous flap and the toe fillet flap. A free flap option is the radial forearm flap which lacks undesirable bulk.

— On the dorsum of the foot, a skin graft is best if an adequate bed is available.

● Postoperative care following surgery in the lower extremity can be as important as the surgery itself in achieving commendable results.

— The gold standard for monitoring flaps postoperatively is clinical examination. Doppler examination can be performed frequently during the early postoperative period then weaned as necessary over the next several days. This practice reflects the fact that most vessel thromboses occur early (i.e., within the first 2 to 3 days). Temperature probe is occasionally helpful in the lower extremity; however, it can be difficult to assess. In general, a difference in temperature of the flap from a control area on the leg of more than 3°C warrants investigation. This

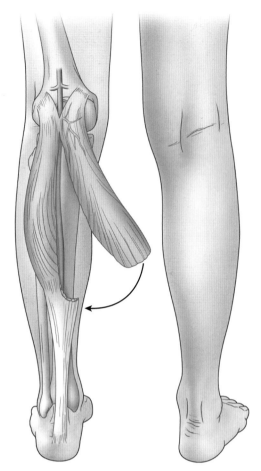

Figure 42-1 Schematic drawing highlighting gastrocnemius muscle flap reconstruction.

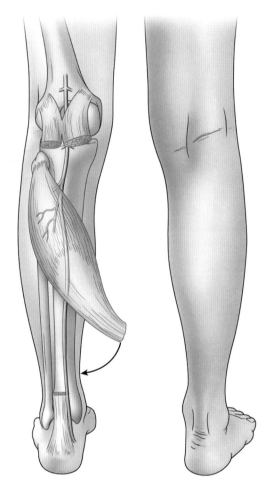

Figure 42-2 Schematic drawing highlighting soleus muscle flap reconstruction.

difference may be because of hypovolemia or other causes; however, if no other causes can be identified it is usually considered an early indicator of venous insufficiency.

— The use of anticlotting medication depends on the preference of the surgeon and the condition of the vessels. In general, **heparinization** prior to cross clamping an end artery is prudent. Many surgeons administer a dose of 3000 to 5000 units 2 to 3 minutes prior to clamping the vessels to avoid distal thrombosis. Postoperative heparinization is usually reserved for patients with intimal injury or crush injuries with wide zones of damage. Subcutaneous heparin or low molecular heparin is useful for prevention of deep venous thromboses (DVT) that may complicate the postoperative care of patients kept at bed rest. Many microsurgeons use an **antiplatelet agent**, such as baby aspirin administered either immediately preoperatively or postoperatively for prevention of thrombosis. Although this practice is somewhat routine, its efficacy has not been proven with prospective studies. **Dextran** has also been used to improve

flap circulation. However, its use has been associated with the development of pulmonary edema and with an anaphylactic response in a small percentage of patients. Because of these limitations, dextran may have limited indications in limb salvage.

— Patients treated with free flaps or local flaps are kept at bed rest for the first 1 to 2 days followed by a progressive regimen of sitting and standing. The extremity is kept elevated to avoid venous congestion. After 10 to 14 days, limited dangling of the extremity can be started (i.e., no more than 5 minutes at a time). If healing is otherwise uncomplicated, the lower extremity can be wrapped lightly with an ace bandage starting on postoperative day 21 to minimize swelling when the foot is dependent. Weight-bearing status is dictated by the bony injuries and is individualized.

6. Complications following coverage of lower extremity wounds resulting from trauma can be significant.

● Some degree of **bleeding** following soft tissue reconstruction is not uncommon and is often related to the

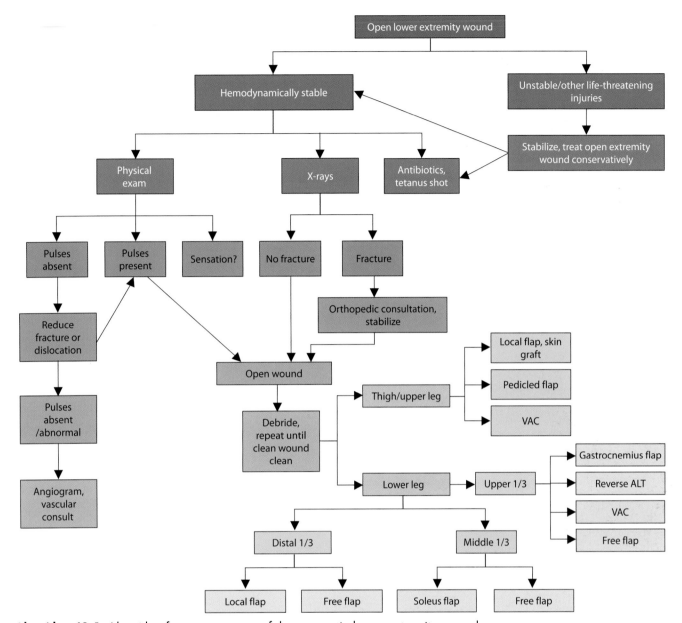

Algorithm 42-1 Algorithm for management of the traumatic lower extremity wound.

administration of postoperative anticoagulation. In the face of bleeding, the medication should be discontinued and any sources identified.

- Similarly, **infection** is not uncommon and is related to the initial insult, which never occurs in a sterile environment. Adequate debridement of all nonvital tissue and coverage with appropriate antibiotics should be routine.

- **DVT** are related to the interruption in normal venous flow through the lower extremity. Patients who are then kept at bed rest postoperatively are at further risk for clotting. Prophylaxis with ab intraoperative compression device for the contralateral extremity and postoperative anticoagulation are important.

- The most worrisome complication following pedicled or free tissue transfer to reconstruct a defect in the lower extremity is **flap loss**. A review of 304 patients after posttraumatic microvascular reconstruction of the lower extremity (75% below the midtibia) found an 8% failure rate (vs. 3% for nonlower extremities), which doubled with vascular trauma, tripled with large bony defects, and quintupled if vain grafts were required. Flap loss should be addressed by repeat free tissue transfer noting any problems with technique from the initial procedure or by leaving the necrotic flap in place as a biologic dressing that is not infected with the hope that later skin grafting will be possible on top of any granulation tissue that remains ("Crane principle"). A cross-leg flap (**lifeboat**) is reserved as a last resort. It is based on the posterior descending subfascial cutaneous branch of the popliteal artery. Length to width ratio should be 3 to 4:1. Its use carries up to 40% local flap necrosis and 20% infection rate.

PRACTICAL PEARLS

1. Dissect recipient vessels prior to harvesting flap as the location and length of these vessels may change your flap design.

2. Obtain as accurate a picture of the zone of injury and extent of injury prior to surgery. If this is not possible, then perform all debridement and tissue assessment prior to harvesting flap for coverage.

3. Soft tissue coverage of open bone fractures or exposed hardware should be performed as soon as feasible. Prolonged exposure significantly increases rates of infection and flap loss.

4. Not all wounds with exposed bone require flap coverage. If the bone is intact then conservative management (i.e., dressing changes or VAC) may be a viable alternative.

5. Try to plan for future operations if necessary or for potential flap failures. What are the potential backup vessels? Will the patient require additional surgery in the future that may necessitate reelevating the flap?

References

1. Mackenzie DJ, Seyfer AE. Reconstructive surgery: Lower extremity coverage. In: Mathes S, ed. *Plast Surg*. Philadelphia, PA: W. B. Saunders, 2006;1355-1381.

2. Bose MJ, Mackenzie EJ, Kellem JF, et al. An analysis of outcomes of reconstruction or amputation after leg-threatening injuries. *N Engl J Med*. 2002;347:1924-1931.

3. Khouri RK, Shaw WW. Reconstruction of the lower extremity with microvascular free flaps: A 10-year experience with 304 consecutive cases. *J Trauma*. 1989;29;1086-1094.

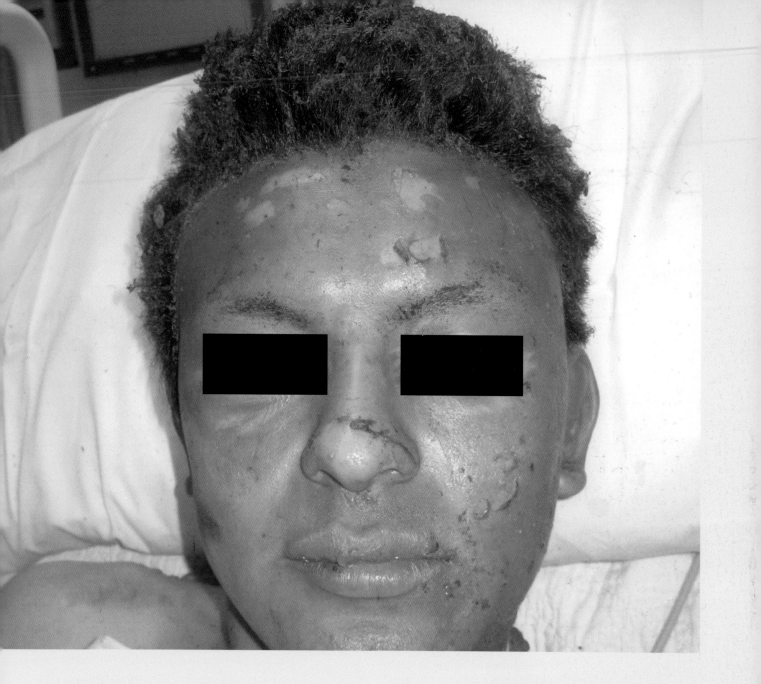

A 20-year-old man presents to the emergency department following an explosion in the backyard from lighting gasoline.

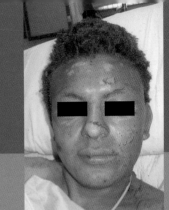

CHAPTER 43

Flame Burn

Lily F. Lee and Warren L. Garner

1. Thermally injured patients, like all other trauma victims, should be evaluated systematically. This starts with a systematic **primary survey** that focuses on the critical ABCs.

- **Does the patient have a patent airway?** Endotracheal intubation should be considered on patients who have suffered severe burns or where there is any question of an inhalation injury or an upper airway burn. An easy intubation on arrival in the emergency department may become difficult or impossible with the development of local airway swelling caused by burn edema and/or the administration of large amounts of resuscitation fluid. Singed nasal hairs, facial or oropharyngeal burns, and expectoration of carbonaceous sputum are signs that inhalation injury may be present. Signs of upper respiratory obstruction—such as a hoarse voice, stridor, or air hunger mandate immediate intubation. During intubation, the operator should make note of any soot, edema, or sign of injury to the laryngopharynx and vocal cords.

- **Is the patient breathing adequately?** Smoke injury to the lungs caused by "toxic products of combustion" can make effective ventilation and oxygenation problematic. This pulmonary injury should be treated with mechanical ventilation. Once an airway is established, the patient should be supported with mechanical ventilation. High flow percussive ventilation has been noted to be a successful adjunct. This device has many advantages. It allows for sufficient oxygenation without increasing FIO_2, increases the ease of clearing secretions, and the ability to stack breaths for improved ventilation. The diagnosis of inhalation injury often is not clinically obvious. The physician must maintain a high degree of suspicion of its presence. Bronchoscopy is the gold standard for establishing the diagnosis of inhalational injury.

  — Circumferential eschar over the torso can cause a decrease in chest wall excursion sufficient to result in respiratory embarrassment. If present, escharotomies should be performed in the anterior axillary lines, using an electrocautery current or scalpel to incise the entire length and depth of the eschar. If chest excursion is still not adequate, additional incisions can be joined with a chevron-shaped connection over the costal margin.

  — Most patients should have spontaneous respiratory drive, even on the ventilator. If the patient is unable to breath for himself, a neurological assessment is needed to determine the cause for a depressed respiratory drive.

- **Does the patient have adequate circulation?** This may be determined by confirming that distal pulses are present and capillary refill is adequate. Burn patients can become hypothermic and inadequately perfused easily. Increasing a patient's core body temperature can be accomplished using warm intravenous fluids, external airflow mattresses, warm blankets and increasing the room temperature. Establishment of large bore intravenous lines is necessary for fluid resuscitation.

  — Circumferential burns third-degree burns with inexpansive eschar can be a life- or limb-threatening problem in the extremities. Do not wait for a loss of pulses. In an awake patient, excessive pain with passive range of motion is an early sign that the extremity will benefit from escharotomy. Other signs of impending vascular compromise are paresthesias, firm compartments to touch, and cool digits that do not transmit at pulse oximeter.

  — Extremity escharotomies are performed in the midlateral lines of the affected extremity, taking care in the arm to avoid the ulnar nerve posterior to the medial epicondyle, and in the lower extremity to avoid the common peroneal nerve posterior to the fibular head. If the fingers are severely burned, digital escharotomies should be performed along their midlateral lines, preferably on the ulnar aspects of the second, third, and fourth digits and the radial aspect of the fifth. This procedure minimizes scars on the primary working surfaces of the fingers. Escharotomy of the thumb is best performed along the midlateral radial aspect. The thenar and hypothenar muscle compartments are often involved in severe hand burn injuries. Eschar and, if necessary, fascia over these compartments should be incised. In deep hand burns, dorsal escharotomies with interosseous compartment fasciotomies should also be performed. It is important to extend escharotomies from normal skin through the eschar to normal skin.

2. Once a patient has been stabilized, a thorough **secondary survey** is vital. It is important to diagnose and treat concomitant life-threatening injuries. Many of these patients will have also suffered blunt or penetrating trauma. All consequences of such trauma can be present in "burn" patients, including closed head injury, pneumothorax and other thoracic trauma, spinal injuries, intra-abdominal injuries, pelvic and long bone fractures, and significant blood loss. To perform a thorough physical examination, the patient should be completely undressed and all body surfaces examined.

- **Where did the burn occur? Was it indoors or outdoors?** The circumstances of the injury can be quite valuable in directing the search for associated trauma, and can indicate the possible presence of inhalation injury.

- **Were chemicals present?** Toxic smoke can produce injury to the lungs caused by "the products of combustion" and make effective ventilation and oxygenation problematic. This should be treated with early intubation and mechanical ventilation.

- **How large is the burned area?** The classic "Rule of Nines" and the Lund-Browder chart are easy to use. The patient's palm (wrist to fingertips) represents approximately 1% total body surface area (TBSA). Only second-and third-degree (not first-degree burn) should be included in the calculation.

- **How deep is the burn?**
  - **First-degree burns** are easy to diagnose. The most familiar example is a sunburn with erythema and mild edema. The skin is tender and warm and refills rapidly after pressure is applied. All layers of the epidermis and dermis are intact so no topical antimicrobial is necessary. Uncomplicated healing is expected within 5 to 7 days. It is important to stress the importance of moisturizers during the healing process.
  - **Second-degree burns** encompass a wide spectrum of dermal or partial thickness injury. The hallmark of the partial-thickness burn is blister formation. Blistering denotes at least some element of viable dermis beneath the blister fluid. Confusion may result, however, when partial-thickness burns are examined after blisters have been ruptured and uncovered. These burns are described as wet and exquisitely tender, although deep-partial thickness injuries may be insensate. Blanching with pressure and capillary refill are other signs of dermal integrity, but may be absent with deep partial-thickness injury. Hair is generally present in these burns. Healing of partial-thickness burns is variable. If the wound appears to be healing spontaneously within 2 to 3 weeks, conservative treatment may be applied. Should the wound be slow to heal, either as a result of the depth of the burn or poor nutritional status, the wound may require excision and grafting.
  - **Third-degree (full-thickness) burns** have a characteristic appearance. With complete destruction of all epidermal and dermal elements, they are insensate and create little discomfort for the patient. The appearance of the skin is often dull and leatherlike. Thrombosed vessels beneath translucent skin are pathognomonic for full-thickness injury.

- **Is the patient up to date with their tetanus immunization?** The tetanus status of the burned patient with open wounds should be determined and brought up to date.

- **Does the patient have any preexisting medical conditions, medications, or have any allergies?** All these are necessary information to obtain at the time of the initial evaluation.

3. Numerous diagnostic tests may be required in the acutely burned patient.

- Expeditious radiologic examination of the cervical spine, chest, and pelvis are often required to exclude the possibility of associated blunt trauma.

- Basic laboratory tests frequently reveal disorders of **blood and electrolytes**. Red blood cell destruction in large burns may be up to 40% of the circulating volume. It is believed that 8% to 15% of the volume is destroyed initially by the thermal insult, with eventual loss of another 25% secondary to decreased survival time. Glucose intolerance may be seen in the early

281

postburn period secondary to massive catecholamine release.

— Persistent metabolic acidosis may indicate inadequate perfusion; however, these parameters are sometimes slow to catch up with fluid balances. End organ perfusion, such as urine output in a patient with normal renal function, should be used to titrate fluids for resuscitation.

● With a suspected inhalation injury, arterial blood gases and **carboxyhemoglobin** (CHgb) levels should be obtained. If the CHgb is elevated (>10%), 100% oxygen must be administered.

● The mainstay of diagnosing inhalation injury to the oropharynx, hypopharynx, larynx, and upper airway is fiberoptic bronchoscopy. It is easy to perform during resuscitation of an unstable burn patient. Significant findings in the hypopharynx and larynx include vocal cord edema and charring, sloughing, or edema of the hypopharyngeal and upper tracheal mucosa.

4. Nonoperative management should begin with establishing intravenous access to handle the often voluminous fluid resuscitation requirements determined by the Parkland Formula, which is calculated in burns >20% TBSA.

● It is preferable to establish vascular access through unburned skin as catheters through burn wounds will be more vulnerable to infection. Intravenous access can be performed through burned tissue if necessary for adequate volume delivery.

● If adequate perfusion is maintained during resuscitation, plasma volume loss decreases substantially by 12 to 18 hours post injury. Blood volume remains low for days in severe burns unless aggressively corrected. The Parkland Formula is widely used in the United States. In the second 24 hours, there is ongoing debate over the use of colloid such as albumin in patients who require greater than 150% to 200% of the initially calculated crystalloid volume to maintain a urine output of 0.5 cc/kg per hour during the first 24 hours post burn.

● The modified Parkland Formula provides resuscitation with Ringer's lactate at a volume of 4 cc/kg of body weight per percent surface area burned. One-half the calculated volume is replaced in the first eight hours after the burn and the second half is replaced in the next 16 hr. The rate is then adjusted as necessary to keep the urine output around 30 to 50 cc/hr for adults and 1 cc/kg per hour for children.

● Nutritional support should be started for all burn patients upon admission. If the patient is not able to feed himself, enteral diet of naso- or oro-gastric tube feedings should be initiated for a goal of 30 to 40 kcal/kg per day.

● A Foley catheter should be inserted and urine output measured hourly. With crystalloid resuscitation regimens such as the Parkland Formula, urine output remains an excellent guideline for the adequacy of resuscitation. To accurately reflect perfusion, the urine must be nonglycosuric and not produced by an osmotic load (e.g., dextran, hypertonic saline).

● Analgesics and sedatives must be given to relieve pain and anxiety. This should be dispensed via the intravenous route only: intramuscular absorption is erratic. Continuous pain relief is more effective in the acute setting than catching up with breakthrough pain.

● The patient must be kept warm using warm intravenous fluids, warm gases if the patient is intubated, and adequate coverings. Hypothermia is a frequent and often serious problem in these patients. The patient's core temperature should be monitored continually.

● The ABA has identified the following injuries as those usually requiring a referral to a burn center.

— 2-degree and 3-degree burns >10% body surface area (BSA) in patients <10 or >50 years of age.

— 2-degree and 3-degree burns >20% BSA in other groups.

— 2-degree and 3-degree burns with serious threat of functional or cosmetic impairment (face, hands, feet, genitalia, perineum, and major joints).

— 3-degree burns >5% TBSA in any age group.

— Electrical burns, including lightning injury.

— Chemical burns with serious threat of functional or cosmetic impairment.

— Inhalation injury with burn injury.

— Circumferential burns with burn injury.

— Burn injury in patients with preexisting medical disorders that could complicate management, prolong recovery, or affect mortality.

— Any burn patient with concomitant trauma (for example, fractures) in which the burn injury poses the greatest risk of morbidity or morality.

● Topical antibiotics are the single most important factor in minimizing infection. In the untreated burn wound, cultures will be negative for the first few hours. Deep wounds become colonized in 24 hours by gram-positive cocci, and in 3 to 7 days by gram-negative aerobes. It is therefore important to institute topical antibiotic therapy as soon as possible.

— Silver-based products have become increasingly popular in the treatment of burn wounds. Because of the unsightly staining caused by silver nitrate solutions used in the past, many companies have produced silver dressings in the form of sponges, foams, hydrofibers, and fabrics. Application of silver is neither painful nor toxic. It is a broad-spectrum agent with minimal absorption from the burn wound, making toxicity virtually unknown. It is an excellent prophylactic agent, but it is not indicated for established wound sepsis. Development of resistance to the silver ion is distinctly uncommon. **Silver sulfadiazine (Silvadene)** is the most frequently used topical agent because it causes minimal pain and does not stain the skin. It is supplied in a water-soluble base at a concentration of 1%, which is sufficient to inhibit growth of most sensitive microorganisms in vitro. It is applied every 12 to 24 hours and is active against gram-positive and gram-negative bacteria, as well as Candida albicans. It forms a thin pseudoeschar over the wound 2 to 3 days after application, which may confuse an examiner attempting to determine wound depth. Wound penetration is intermediate and should not be used on full-thickness burns that are already exhibiting signs of infection. Systemic absorption does occur, but documented episodes of toxicity have been quite rare. Leukopenia is not infrequently seen after 2 to 3 days of treatment with this silver sulfadiazine, which usually resolves without discontinuing the drug. Leukopenia rarely depresses the white count to <2,000 white blood cells/mm^3. There have been reports of induction of resistant organisms, mainly Enterobacteriaceae and Pseudomonas aeruginosa.

— **Mupirocin (Bactroban)** is an antibiotic with improved coverage of gram-positive cocci. It is dispensed as an ointment which allows it to stay without a dressing over the face.

— **Mafenide sodium (Sulfamylon)** is a broad-spectrum antibiotic with the best eschar penetration of any agent, allowing it to efficiently penetrate cartilage. It is an excellent choice for use on burned ears and noses. Useful for control of established burn wound infection because of its excellent penetration. It can be used as a 10% cream, similar to Silvadene, or in a 5% solution usually mixed with Nystatin powder and irrigated into bandages to keep moist. It is a strong carbonic anhydrase inhibitor and results in an alkaline diuresis. Use can lead to acid-base abnormalities when used on >20% of the BSA. Polyuria can lead to a hyperchloremic metabolic acidosis, which, if then compensated for by hyperventilation, may eventually lead to pulmonary failure in the compromised patient. This is a clear indication to discontinue the drug. With drug stoppage, this effect should reverse in 24 to 36 hours. Its use may cause significant pain, probably because of its high osmolarity.

● Some type of nutritional supplementation will be required in the majority of patients with burns >20% TBSA. The hypermetabolic state induced by a major burn is similar to the stress response to trauma or sepsis, but it is stronger and longer lasting. There is evidence that the hypermetabolic state in a major burn lasts for up to 1 year after the burn. A 40% burn causes a metabolic effort equal to twice the basal energy expenditure. Alimental nutrition should be used if possible. Oral intake is often limited by compliance, palatability, and general energy level.

— The Curreri Formula quantitates adult daily caloric requirements as 25 cal/kg + 40 cal/TBSA. For children, 60 cal/kg + 35 cal/TBSA. It is accurate for moderate-sized burns in young healthy patients, but overestimates the need in large burns or in the older adults.

— Harris-Benedict equation is useful in predicting the basal energy expenditure (BEE) for a given patient. An alternate method of computing calorie requirements in the burn patient is simply to double this BEE for a burn of greater than 30% TBSA.

— Serum albumin has a long half-life and is therefore insensitive to acute changes in nutritional status. The mainstay of our clinical monitoring is a twice-weekly prealbumin value because of its shorter half-life. A nitrogen balance study, which is calculated from a 24-hour urine collection for urinary urea nitrogen can also be obtained. The goal is a positive nitrogen balance.

● Gastrointestinal bleeding from a Curling's ulcer was formerly a common complication in burned patients, but it is virtually nonexistent today. Gastric and duodenal mucosal lesions have been shown to occur within 48 hours post injury. Antiulcer prophylaxis should be used if the patient is unable to tolerate full enteral feedings.

● If the carboxyhemoglobin level is elevated, the patient should immediately be administered 100% oxygen. This will decrease the washout time of the carbon monoxide from 250 minutes (T 1/2 on room air) to 40 to 50 minutes (T 1/2 with FIO$_2$ of 1.0). Hyperbaric oxygen has not been shown to be of additional significant benefit compared to 100% oxygen in these patients.

5. Prompt burn wound **excision and autograft** closure is the treatment for patients with burns that are unlikely to heal spontaneously. Larger areas may require staged treatment.

● Initial debridement by tangential excision is done in the burn center in a warmed room with general anesthesia. Areas of function and cosmetically sensitive areas (such as the extremities and neck) are given priority for excision and autograft. Once the inflammatory load of the burn eschar has been removed, closed wounds will be able to heal faster with a better functional and cosmetic outcome. This is because of a calming of the inflammatory cytokines that lead to edema and overhealing. Excision to fascia has limited indications. It offers the advantages of a more reliable bed for grafting and may be performed on the extremities with decreased blood loss. Disadvantages include the fact that excised fat does not regenerate and a permanent cosmetic deformity is guaranteed, especially in obese patients. With circumferential excision, there is a risk of distal edema and a 100% risk of damage to superficial nerves and tendons. The fascia over joint surfaces such as the elbow, knee, and ankle is relatively avascular, and eventual flap coverage may be required in these areas.

- In all areas but the face, immediate autografting should be performed if sufficient donor sites are available. Most skin grafts are taken at a thickness of 0.010 to 0.012 inches and secured with either sutures or staples. While sheet grafts should be used whenever possible, skin meshed at 1:1.5 and minimally expanded can yield excellent cosmetic results. Meshed grafts allow egress of fluid, even with minimal expansion. They can be used with excellent results in all areas except the face where the use of sheet grafts is preferred.

- The use of **artifical dermis** to stage the closure of a wound can be performed in large burns where donor sites are limited. Integra is one dermal regeneration template composed of a bilayer of collagen-glycosaminoglycan matrix and a silicone semipermeable membrane which in effect acts like artificial skin. The "dermal" matrix allows cells to grow into the matrix forming a "neodermis" over the excised wound bed. Once the "neodermis" has formed, usually 2 to 3 weeks, the silicone membrane can be removed and a thin split thickness skin graft can be grafted over the "neodermis."

  — Integra is used when there is not enough unburned donor site or if the patient may not be able to handle a large donor site burden.

  — Because Integra does not depend on the imbibition that an autograft needs, it has been successfully used to graft over poorly vascularized structures such as calvaria/bone and tendons.

  — The contour deformities or scale-like appearance of aggressively debrided regions which have been autografted can be mitigated by the neodermis which forms better contour over a wound bed.

6. There are numerous surgical and nonsurgical complications that can result from burn injury and the necessary interventions.

- **Hypovolemia** has been replaced by burn **edema** as a significant postresuscitation problem in many survivors of initial fluid therapy. While not as immediately lethal as burn shock, burn edema can decrease tissue oxygenation and blood flow.

- There are several types of **inhalation injury** and any one may be present or absent in a given victim of inhalation injury. All should be searched for, diagnosed, and treated independently and appropriately. In general, a firm diagnosis of inhalational injury adds approximately 20% the TBSA when calculating for fluid resuscitation.

  — **Carbon monoxide inhalation** is odorless and tasteless but impairs tissue oxygenation by preferentially binding to hemoglobin by a factor above 200 and displacing oxygen from the hemoglobin molecule.

  — **Direct thermal injury** to the lower airway is uncommon because of the great heat-dissipating capacity of the oropharynx. An exception is inhalation of steam, which has 4000 times the heat-carrying capacity of air. The increase in airway edema parallels the generalized burn edema in any given patient, peaking at 18 to 24 hours postburn and resolving more than 4 to 5 days. In addition to the direct effect of mucosal edema, mucosal swelling also impairs clearance of secretions in the airway compounding the problem. Inhalation of products of combustion.

  — By far the most common and significant component of inhalation injury is the **inhalation of products of combustion**. Aldehydes, ketones, cyanide, and organic acids are all produced from combustion of these materials. All cause significant chemical injury to the respiratory tract. While an initial dramatic clinical response may be absent in these injuries, the result may be very similar to that seen in aspiration of acidic gastric contents. Mucosal ciliary function may be markedly and almost instantaneously depressed, causing marked impairment of secretion clearance. With severe damage to the airways and sloughing of the bronchial mucosa, plugging and secondary infection begin to supervene at 72 hours postburn.

- The risk of **death** for a burn patient without a significant inhalation injury is highest from systemic **sepsis**. Clinically, any change in the patient's general status should lead to a high suspicion. By far the most common sites of primary infection in burn patients are the blood stream, the burn wound, the lower respiratory tract, and the urinary tract. Careful serial clinical and laboratory monitoring of the patient is the most sensitive method of diagnosing sepsis before disastrous hemodynamic effects occur. Biopsies for quantitative culture of the burn wound can be performed. Wound colonization with >100,000 organisms/gram of tissue is an indication that a wound bed will not be able to accept or heal a graft. Expedient excision or reexcision is indicated. The development of hypothermia and leukopenia are particularly ominous signs in the patient who is clinically becoming septic and demand aggressive intervention. Pseudomonas aeruginosa and Staphylococcus aureus are the dominant pathogens in burn centers. Candida species are the most commonly isolated fungal organisms recovered from burn patients; other fungal infections are uncommon. Viral infections, particularly with cytomegalovirus, are reported with increasing frequency, although their clinical impact is undetermined. There is little place for prophylactic antibiotic usage in burn patients.

- **Myocardial depression** is well described and is most evident in deep burns of 40% TBSA. A myocardial depressive factor has been postulated in the serum of burn patients but has never been identified. Cardiac

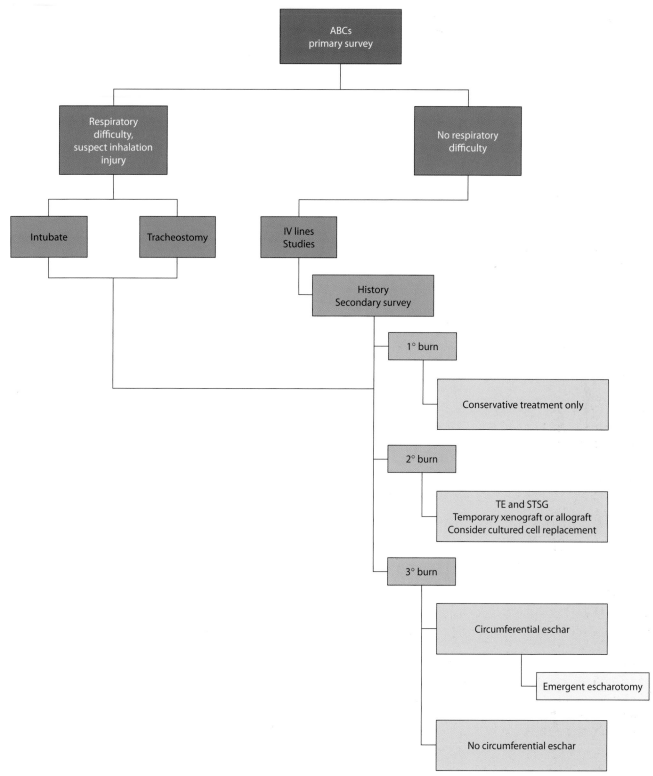

Algorithm 43-1 Basic algorithm for management of the burned patient.

output returns to near normal levels before restoration of a normal plasma volume. Clinically, low central venous pressures and pulmonary artery pressures in the face of adequate cardiac output and peripheral perfusion are often seen.

PRACTICAL PEARLS

1. Fluid resuscitation must not be solely formulaic but rather be titrated to end organ perfusion.

2. Burn wounds must be covered with a moist antimicrobial to minimize the risk of wound infection and resultant sepsis.

3. Expedient excision of burn wounds decreases inflammation and improve overall healing.

4. Artificial dermal dressings can be utilized to more judiciously use existing donor sites.

5. Quantitative culture of burn wound must be used to decide if a wound is infected.

References

1. Cone, JB. What's new in general surgery: Burns and metabolism. *J Am Coll Surg*. 2005;200(4):607-615.

2. Sheridan RL, Tompkins RG. What's new in burns and metabolism. *J Am Coll Surg*. 2004;198(2):243-263.

3. Dougherty W, Waxman K. The complexities of managing severe burns with associated trauma. *Surg Clin North Am*. 1996;76(4): 923-958.

4. Singh V, Devgan L, Bhat S, Milner SM. The pathogenesis of burn wound conversion. *Ann Plast Surg*. 2007;59(1):109-115.

5. Namias, NM. Advances in burn care. *Curr Opin Crit Care*. 2007;13(4):405-410.

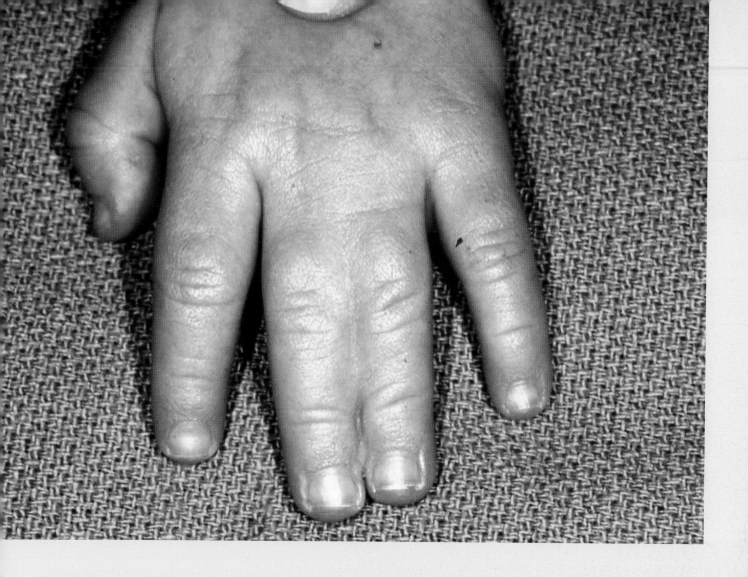

A local pediatrician asks you to evaluate the
patient depicted in the photograph above.

CHAPTER 44

Syndactyly

Neil Ford Jones

1. Fusion of the fingers—termed syndactyly—is easy to diagnose based on appearance of the hand alone. It represents a failure of differentiation or separation and is the commonest congenital hand deformity seen in 1 in 2000 live births. It is more commonly isolated and unilateral but may be hereditary in 10% to 40%, which are usually bilateral. There is a male predominance by 2:1. A thorough history is still important to answer several important questions.

- **How old is the patient?** Syndactyly is a congenital anomaly seen at birth but often may not be treated until the patient is older. It is never acquired although scar formation from burn injury, for example, can mimic congenital fusion of the digits.

- **How is the patient limited by the deformity?** Generally, in children, the anomaly does not cause dysfunction. Problems arise if growth of one digit is compromised by fusion to another shorter digit.

- **Are there any other congenital anomalies?** Numerous syndromes have syndactyly of either the hand, foot, or both as part of the clinical spectrum.

  - In addition to craniosynostosis, midface hypoplasia, and cleft palate, **Apert syndrome** presents with characteristic hand anomalies of which three types have been described. Type I involves a central mass of digits with the thumb and finger free. Type II involves union of the thumb or small finger to the central mass. Type III is the most severe. All three components share a single nail. Patients develop repeated nail infections. Similar associations are seen with **Pfeiffer** and **Saethre-Chotzen syndromes.**

  - The classic features of **Poland syndrome** include absence of sternal head of the pectoralis major, hypoplasia and/or aplasia of breast or nipple, deficiency of subcutaneous fat and axillary hair, abnormalities of the rib cage, and brachysymphalangism. Additional features include hypoplasia or aplasia of serratus, external oblique, pectoralis minor, latissimus dorsi, infraspinatus, and supraspinatus muscles, total absence of anterolateral ribs, herniation of the lung, and syndactyly.

- **Down's syndrome** is a chromosomal disorder caused by duplication of chromosome 21 as a result of nondisjunction during duplication. It is characterized by mental retardation, limited growth, downslanting palpebral fissures, protruding tongue, syndactyly of the hands.

- **Holt-Oram syndrome** is an inherited disorder caused by mutations in the transcription factor TBX5. It is characterized by abnormalities of the upper limbs and heart, specifically aplasia, hypoplasia, fusion, or anomalous development of the bones of the hands as well as atrial and ventricular septal defects. The hand anomalies can produce a spectrum of phenotypes, including triphalangeal thumbs, absent thumbs, or phocomelia, otherwise seen with thalidomide use.

- **Oral-facial-digital (and oro-palato-digital) syndrome** is inherited as an x-linked disorder affecting transcription of the *OFD1* gene. It is usually seen in females and is characterized by corpus callosum and/or cerebellar agenesis, hypertelorism or telecanthus, cleft palate, micrognathia, dental abnormalities, brachydactyly and syndactyly, and polycystic kidney disease.

- **Popliteal pterygium syndrome** is an autosomal dominant disorder affecting the IRF6 gene on chromosome 1 and most reported cases are sporadic. Of note, van der Woude syndrome is caused by a different mutation of the same gene. The clinical manifestations of popliteal pterygium syndrome include web formation behind the knee down to the heel, webbed toes, cleft palate with or without cleft lip, fibrous bands in the mouth known as syngnathia, and malformations of the genitalia.

- **Prader-Willi syndrome** is an autosomal dominant disorder caused by deletion or disruption of one or more genes on the proximal long arm of the paternal chromosome 15 or maternal uniparental disomy 15. It is characterized by low muscular tone, obesity, mental retardation, short stature, hypogonadotropic hypogonadism, and small hands and feet.

- **Smith-Lemli-Opitz syndrome** is an autosomal recessive genetic condition caused by deficiency of the final enzyme in the synthesis of cholesterol. It is characterized by microcephaly and micrognathia, strabismus and cataracts, cleft palate, cardiac and pulmonary defects, polydactyly and syndactyly of the toes, as well as genital anomalies.

- **Does the trait appear in any other family members?** Since several hereditary syndromes present with syndactyly as a component of the clinical spectrum, these should be sought in family members.

2. Examination of the hands should focus on which parts of the digits are involved and the extent to which fusion has occurred. Of the numerous possible syndromic associations with syndactyly, many can be uncovered by a careful physical examination. The treating physician must look at both hands as well as both upper and lower extremities for associated findings.

- **How are the digits involved?** The hand findings are classified into simple (soft tissue only) or complex (bone and cartilage), partial or complete. Digits with syndactyly are joined on either their ulnar or radial aspects (or both) and are generally not deviated in an abnormal direction. *Camptodactyly* refers to a flexion deformity of one or more digits, while *clinodactyly* refers to ulnar or radial deviation of the digits.

- **Is there a simple syndactyly of the soft tissues or is there a bony union?** Gentle palpation of the space between each of the fusion digits can determine whether or not there is a bony union between neighboring digits. Bony union is important to identify since it may make the reconstruction effort more difficult.

- **Which digits are involved?** Common locations in the hand include the 3rd web space followed by the 4th and 2nd web spaces in order of frequency. Digits with a greater natural length discrepancy warrant earlier release to avoid growth disturbance in the longer digit.

- **Which parts of the digits are involved?** Acrosyndactyly represents fusion of the distal portions (fingertips) of the digits, which occurs sporadically (*not* hereditary) but may be seen in Apert syndrome where it is usually symmetrical.

- **Is the union between the digits skin and soft tissue or is bone also involved?** Two or more partially or completely fused digits which may involve skin webbing (simple) or bony fusion (complex).

- **Are there other unrecognized anomalies in the hand and wrist?** Symphalangism represents failure of IP joint separation with absence of the PIP joint. There is no joint capsule or synovial cavity. The flexor and extensor tendons are missing. There is no proven treatment, but free vascularized joint transfers have been considered.

- **Are there other anomalies in the upper extremity?** Poland syndrome, most notably, involves syndactyly and hypoplasia of the pectoralis major muscle as well as underdevelopment of the chest wall structures, including the breast.

- **Are there other congenital anomalies elsewhere in the body?** In addition to abnormalities listed with the syndromes above, syndactyly of the foot should be sought since these similar distal anomalies occur simultaneously.

3. **Plain radiographs** of *both* hands are, usually, sufficient for the workup. More complicated studies are generally not warranted. Patients with concomitant syndromes require additional studies based upon the associated findings. The plain films of the hands do not need to be done at the time of birth but are often deferred until prior to any reconstructive efforts. Important considerations include:

4. Consultation with a **geneticist** may be offered (1) to determine whether other congenital anomalies are present and (2) to estimate the chance of having a subsequent child with similar findings. Postoperative consultation with a certified **hand therapist** who has experience treating children is of even greater importance so as to optimize the results of surgical intervention.

5. Surgical reconstruction of the hand is generally performed before prehension develops at 2 years and usually around 6 months. One finding that would expedite the repair would be a digit length discrepancy in which case earlier repair is advocated to avoid growth disturbance in the longer digit.

- Reconstruction of the simple syndactyly involves separating the digits while providing adequate skin coverage and creating a new web space. Opposing skin flaps from each of the involved digits, as well as full-thickness skin graft, provides coverage. One flap design uses a pentagonal island based at the distal extent of the metacarpals, where the skin is dimpled. The surgeon must identify the neurovascular

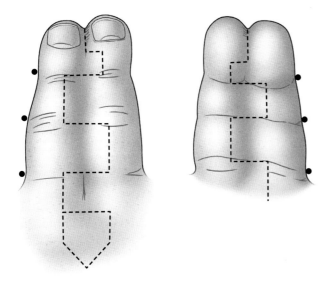

Figure 44-1 Schematic drawing highlighting the dorsal and volar soft tissue flaps for syndactyly reconstruction.

bundles on either side of the fusion. The junction of the nerve distal to the web space warrants intraneural separation of the nerve and possibly division of the artery. Before division of the artery, the tourniquet should be released and the digits inspected for ischemia. The digits are then lined with the skin flaps and full-thickness skin grafts from the groin, where the donor site can be closed primarily. Dressed with gauze and a cast with the elbow in 90-degree flexion and the fingertips exposed.

- Separations involving digits with fusion on either side are staged every 4 to 6 months to minimize devascularization of the central digit.

- Complex syndactyly requires separation of bone as well as soft tissue coverage and may require reconstruction around the nail.

6. Complications are related to vascularity of the involved digits and ultimate healing following surgery.

- **Contracture** is perhaps the most common and can be lessened by well-coordinated postoperative therapy. Some surgeons note a 10% reoperation rate.

- **Digital necrosis** is the most devastating. It should be considered prior to separation of the digits as well as in the postoperative period. Any question about the

viability of the digits warrants a removal of the cast and the sutures and a return to OR for inspection and vein graft if necessary.

- **Skin graft loss** is the most common complication following syndactyly release and may be related to infection.

- **A shallow web space** may develop. The normal web space slope is approximately 35 to 45 degrees. The most important is the first since it allows opposition of the thumb. It may be deepened by several described methods, including:
  — "4-flap Z-plasty"
  — "Butterfly flap"
  — Dorsal, proximal flap

- **Nail deformity** may occur in cases where the nail plate is united and must be divided. In such cases, a horizontal flap of skin from the most distal portion of the finger tip may be rotated inferiorly to create a lateral nail fold.

PRACTICAL PEARLS

1. Design the proximal palmar extent of the web space between the involved digits by projecting its position from the position of the adjacent normal web spaces.

2. Use dorsal or dorsal and palmar skin flaps to reconstruct the new web space.

3. Separate the fingers after identifying the digital nerves, and if necessary separate the bifurcation of the common digital nerve more proximally to allow insetting of the web space flap.

4. Careful defatting of the fingers and skin flaps.

5. Attempt to cover the "dominant" finger (the one that opposes to the thumb) with zigzag flaps or rectangular flaps. Cover remaining raw areas with full thickness skin grafts harvested from the groin, hypothenar eminence, or instep of the foot.

6. Do not separate both sides of the same finger at the same operation to avoid devascularizing the finger.

7. Use an above-elbow sugar-tong splint with the elbow flexed greater than 90 degrees to immobilize the hand for 10 to 14 days to prevent movement of the skin grafts and possible loss.

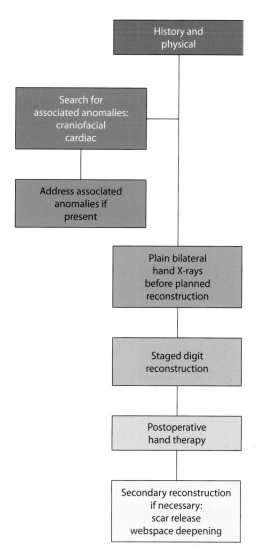

Algorithm 44-1 Algorithm for management of syndactyly.

References

1. Flatt AE. Webbed fingers. *The Care of Congenital Hand Anomalies*. St. Louis, MO: Quality Medical Publishing; 1994:228-275.

2. Bauer TB, Tondra JM, Trusler HM. Technical modification in repair of syndactylism. *Plast Reconstr Surg*. 1956;17:385-392.

3. Colville J. Syndactyly correction. *Br J Plast Surg*. 1989;42:12-16.

4. Deunk J, Nicolai JP, Hamburg SM. Long-term results of syndactyly correction: Full-thickness versus split-thickness skin grafts. *J Hand Surg [Br]*. 2003;28:125-130.

5. Moazzam A, Butt FS. A training model for designing flaps for release of syndactyly. *Plast Reconstr Surg* 2003;112:1743.

6. Upton J. Apert syndrome. Classification and pathologic anatomy of limb anomalies. *Clin Plast Surg*. 1991;18:321-355.

7. Chang J, Danton TK, Ladd AL, Hentz VR. Reconstruction of the hand in Apert syndrome: A simplified approach. *Plast Reconstr Surg*. 2002;109:465-470.

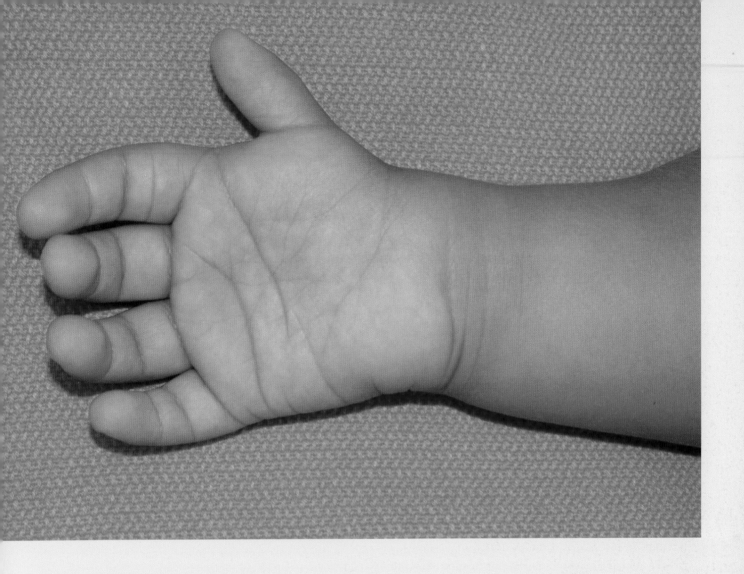

A 2-year-old boy presents to the office with
the deformity shown above.

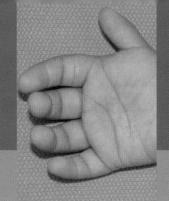

CHAPTER 45

Thumb Hypoplasia

Shelley Noland and James Chang

1. Careful examination of the digits of the hand reveals the thumb to be less developed than expected. For the patient with digit hypoplasia, especially of the thumb, a thorough history should be obtained as part of the work-up. Key questions to ask as related to this congenital anomaly include:

   • **When the deformity first noted?** As mentioned, this represents a congenital deformity present since birth. Although smaller than normal, the thumb should grow roughly commensurate with the child and not demonstrate any "catch-up" growth.

   • **How old is the patient?** The ideal age for treatment of thumb hypoplasia ranges from 1 to 5 years depending on the necessary procedure. For example, pollicization is best performed at 1 to 2 years of age. It may also be important in older patients to note why no interventions had been performed as yet.

   • **What is the patient's family history, prenatal history, and birth history?** This information may provide clues to the etiology of the malformation which may have genetic, environmental, and/or teratogenic causes (i.e., diphenylhydantoin and thalidomide).

   • **Does the patient have other congenital anomalies?** Thumb hypoplasia may be associated with several congenital syndromes including:

     — Fanconi's anemia: Patients can develop all degrees of pancytopenia and is associated with thumb deficiencies at birth in more than half of patients.

     — Holt-Oram syndrome: defined by the presence of congenital heart disease and radial longitudinal defects.

     — Thrombocytopenia-absent-radius (TAR): Patients may be born with normal hematologic parameters, but develop a thrombocytopenia, which may worsen rapidly during the first year of life.

     — VACTERL: Patients present with a constellation of findings affecting several organ systems, including **V**ertebral malformations, **A**nal atresia or hypoplasias, **C**ardiac anomalies, **T**racheoesophageal fistula, **R**enal malformations, and **L**imb abnormalities (including radial dysplasia).

2. A thorough physical examination should be performed of both upper extremities from the shoulders proximally to the fingertips distally.

   • **Are the limbs of symmetrical length?** The spectrum of radial longitudinal deficiency includes deficiency of the radius, carpal abnormalities, and hypoplasia of the thumbs. If such a deficiency is present, correction should be addressed in advance of reconstruction of the more distal hypoplastic thumb.

   • **What is the comparative size of the digit?** The length and width of the thumb should be measured and recorded in reference to the contralateral thumb and remaining digits of the hand.

   • **Are the thenar muscles affected?** The presence or absence of thenar muscle development in the affected hand may help differentiate between type I and type II thumb hypoplasia (see below).

   • **Is the first web space open?** A narrow, tight first web space will require four-flap, or other, Z-plasty to open the web space and improve range of motion.

   • **Is the thumb CMC joint stable?** Using gentle motion, the stability of the CMC joint should be determined. A thumb with a stable CMC joint can be reconstructed, while one with an unstable CMC joint requires pollicization. This finding differentiates type IIIA from type IIIB thumb hypoplasia (see below).

   • **How does the patient grasp objects?** Using age-appropriate toys, the child should be observed during play. Preoperative inspection of the use of the hand may indicate the level of postoperative function. This can help differentiate type IIIA from type IIIB thumb hypoplasia (see below). In the former, the thumb is incorporated into object acquisition and manipulation activities, whereas in the latter, the thumb is often bypassed and prehension develops between the index and long digits. The hand then responds by widening the index-long finger web space with index finger pronation out of the palm.

   • **Are other digits involved?** The range of motion of the index finger should be noted with use of the hand. Adequate motion of the index finger MCP joint and PIP joint allows pulp-to-pulp pinch after pollicization.

3. Plain radiographs of the hand in three views (AP, lateral, and oblique) may help differentiate the type of thumb hypoplasia and plan for reconstruction.

- A tapered metacarpal without a base is characteristic of type IIIB hypoplasia.
- Unfortunately, there is no ossification of the carpal bones before 5 to 6 years of age so the involvement of the trapezium and trapezoid cannot be assessed.

4. A genetics consultation should be obtained to evaluate the patient and family for associated anomalies, since thumb hypoplasia may be associated with several congenital syndromes as listed above.

5. The overall goal of the treatment of thumb hypoplasia is to provide the hand with the best functioning thumb unit. Treatment is guided by the Blauth classification of thumb hypoplasia:

- A **type I** deficiency is characterized by minor generalized thumb hypoplasia with complete function. No treatment is generally required.
- A **type II** deficiency is characterized by thumb hypoplasia, the underdevelopment or absence of intrinsic thenar muscles, first web space narrowing, and metacarpophalangeal (MCP) joint ulnar collateral ligament (UCL) instability. Treatment of type II anomalies involves the following procedures:
  - Release of the first web space by four-flap Z-plasty provides the desired rounded contour in the first web space.
  - Opposition transfer will address the deficient or absent thenar muscles. The abductor digiti minimi (ADM) tendon is commonly utilized as a donor muscle.
  - Repair or reconstruction of the UCL is the standard intervention. This may not be sufficient, however, and additional chondrodesis of the MCP joint may be necessary.
- A **type III** deficiency has the characteristics of a type II deficiency as well as extrinsic muscle and tendon abnormalities and skeletal deficiency including a hypoplastic metacarpal and hypoplastic or aplastic carpal bones. Type III is further classified into **type IIIA** which has a stable CMC joint and **type IIIB** which has an unstable CMC joint.

— Type IIIA hypoplasia requires transfers to overcome the extrinsic musculotendinous abnormalities of EPL and/or FPL tendons. The transfer of adjacent extensor indicis proprius can consistently replace EPL function. However, reconstruction of FPL is more difficult as the flexor tendon sheath may be deficient which requires pulley reconstruction combined with tendon centralization or tendon transfer.

— Type IIIB hypoplasia requires **pollicization** because of the unstable CMC joint. Pollicization is generally performed around 1 to 2 years of age, before the development of oppositional pinch. This avoids the development of compensatory side-to-side pinch pattern between adjacent fingers. Incisions should avoid scarring in the web space. The standard technique is as follows (Figure 1):

a. The dorsal veins are carefully isolated and preserved.

b. The proper digital artery on the ulnar side of the index finger is identified and the branch to the long finger is divided.

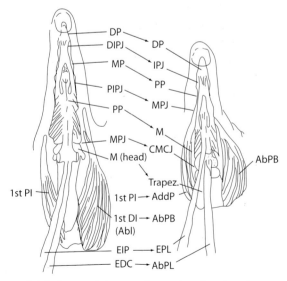

Figure 45-1 Second digit pollicization for thumb reconstruction.

c. The digital nerves to the index finger are identified and dissected free.

d. The extensor tendons are dissected from adjacent structures.

e. The first dorsal and palmar interossei muscles are elevated from the index metacarpal and MCP joint.

f. The index metacarpal is shortened, leaving only the metacarpal head as the new trapezium. The index MCP joint is placed in hyperextension.

g. The index finger is positioned into 45 degrees of abduction and 100 to 140 degrees of pronation.

h. Power after pollicization is as follows: for flexion, the native flexors are left intact and shorten as tone normalizes; for extension, the EIP acts as the new EPL (it is usually shortened the length of the metacarpal shortening); for abduction, the first dorsal interosseous muscle acts as the abductor pollicis brevis and the EDC acts as the abductor pollicis longus; for adduction the first palmar interosseous muscle acts as the adductor pollicis.

- A **type IV** deficiency is also known as a "floating thumb" (pouce flotant). The hypoplastic thumb is connected by only a skin bridge. It usually contains two rudimentary phalanges, a complete neurovascular bundle, and a nail bed. Proximal to the constriction, the thumb unit is severely hypoplastic with involvement of the metacarpal, trapezium, and scaphoid. No real thumb function is present. As a result, patients develop progressive pronation of the index finger with widening of the second web space and broadening of the index pulp. This deficiency also requires pollicization (see above).

- A **type V** is complete aplasia of the thumb. This also requires pollicization (see above).

6. Aside from the usual complications of bleeding and infection, which are usually rare, congenital thumb reconstruction may be complicated by any of the following:

- MCP or CMC joint instability, which is usually related to the adequacy of joint reconstruction. There may be a need for further opposition transfer.

- **Ischemia** of transferred digit in pollicization.

- First web space **contracture**.

- **Weakness** of the thumb.

- **Stiffness** following pollicization.

- **Excessive length** may require secondary shortening of the reconstructed digit.

- **Malrotation** may occur at the time of the initial reconstruction or result from early movement around the osteotomy site and healing in a less than desirable position. Secondary correction requires repeat osteotomy and improved fixation.

PRACTICAL PEARLS

1. When performing the physical examination, assess for evidence of radial longitudinal deficiency.

2. Thumb hypoplasia is classified into five types according to the Blauth classification. This classification is important because it dictates the necessary treatment.

3. Four-flap Z-plasty is the preferred method for release of the first web space.

4. Remember to examine the index finger for stiffness because this will translate when pollicization is performed.

5. Early good results in childhood persist into adulthood.

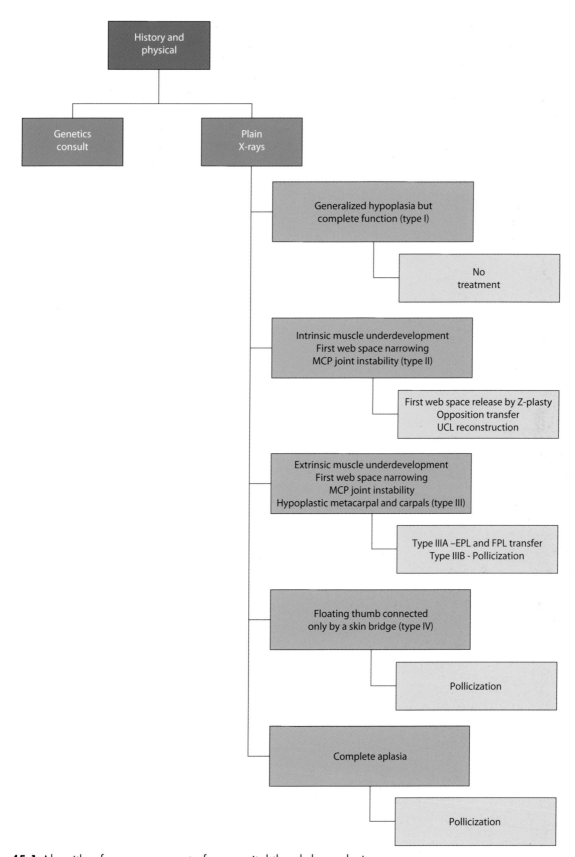

Algorithm 45-1 Algorithm for management of congenital thumb hypoplasia.

References

1. James MA, McCarroll HR Jr, Manske PR. The spectrum of radial longitudinal deficiency: A modified classification. *J Hand Surg [Am]*. 1999;24(6):1145-1155.

2. Buck-Gramcko D. Pollicization of the index finger: Method and results in aplasia and hypoplasia of the thumb. J *Bone Joint Surg Am*. 1971;53(8):1605-1617.

3. Littler JW. The Neurovascular pedicle method of digital transposition for reconstruction of the thumb. *Plast Reconstr Surg*. 1953;12(5):303-319.

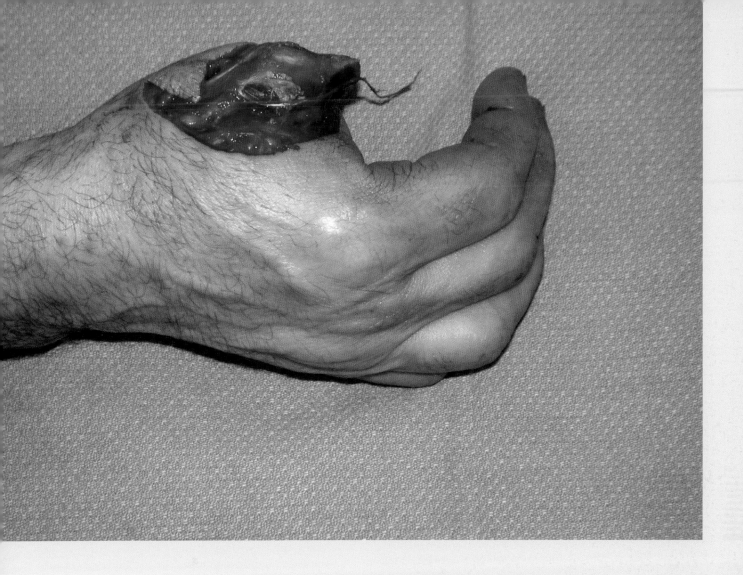

A 43-year-old man presents to the emergency department following traumatic injury from a log splitter to the thumb.

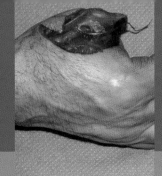

CHAPTER 46

Thumb Amputation

Kodi K. Azari and W.P. Andrew Lee

1. For the patient who presents acutely to the emergency department with a complete or partial amputation of the thumb (or any other digit), a thorough history should be expeditiously obtained to work up the patient who may be a candidate for emergent surgical reconstruction.

   - **What was the mechanism of the injury?** Injuries secondary to sharp instruments such as knives create more favorable wounds for replantation. Crush injuries tend to produce greater areas of tissue damage which adversely affects vessel and nerve function. Finally, avulsion type injuries tend to detach the tendons from their musculotendinous junction and devascularize long segments of nerve important in the functional reconstruction.

   - **At what time did the injury occur?** Although there are no definite limits to ischemia, the length of cold and warm ischemia following amputation is important. Twelve hours of warm and 24 hours of cold ischemia are generally considered limits for replantation attempts of digits. Cooling can extend the window of opportunity for replantation or revascularization. One hour of warm ischemia is roughly equal to 6 hours of cold ischemia.

   - **Where did the injury occur?** Farm and garden injuries carry a higher infection risk and require broader antibiotic coverage.

   - **Which is the patient's dominant hand?** There is always greater concern for regain of function when the dominant hand is involved.

   - **What is the patient's occupation and avocation?** A virtuoso concert violinist has different requirements than a self-employed laborer. The latter requires faster return to gross function than the former who may tolerate a longer rehabilitation schedule in the hopes of regaining more precise motor function.

   - **Does the patient have coexisting medical conditions?** Major medical comorbidities such as heart disease, peripheral vascular disease, diabetes, kidney failure, etc. should be noted.

   - **Is the patient's tetanus status to date?** Any open wound can be infected with tetanus if oxygen is unable to reach the injured tissues. The disease may follow trivial puncture wounds, as well as highly contaminated tissue injury. Some individuals may be protected for life against tetanus after a primary series of vaccinations but in most people, antitoxin levels fall with time. Current recommendations for tetanus prophylaxis in adults include a booster dose every 10 years. Because antibody levels may fall too low to provide protection before 10 years have passed, patients who sustain a deep or contaminated wound should receive a booster dose if it has been more than 5 years since the last dose.

2. A thorough physical examination of both upper extremities from the shoulder to the digits should be performed.

   - **Does the patient have an adequate airway, breathing, and circulation?** In the trauma patient, it is paramount to diagnose and treat concomitant life-threatening injuries. Many of these patients will have also sustained nonhand trauma. The consequences of such trauma, such as intracranial injury, pneumothorax and other thoracic trauma, spinal injuries, intra-abdominal injuries, pelvic and long bone fractures, and significant blood loss should be considered.

   - **Which digits are involved?** Injury to the thumb may coexist with injury to other digits that may go undiagnosed in the obtunded patient. Radial digits are more important in fine motor control, including pinch. Ulnar digits are more important for gross motor strength.

   - **At which level is the amputation?** Surgical options for thumb reconstruction depend on the level of the amputation. Plain X-rays will assist in determining whether the amputation is through a bone (proximal or distal phalanx or metacarpal) or through a joint (interphalangeal or metacarpophalangeal).

   - **Is there evidence of crush or avulsion injury?** Crush injury will demonstrate a wide zone of injury proximal and or distal to the amputation site. Avulsion injury might present with detachment of the flexor and/or extensor tendons at the more proximal tendon-muscle junction. In crush or avulsion injuries, the success of either replantation or revascularization is poorer and vein grafting may be necessary.

3. All hand trauma patients should have radiographic studies of the hand and amputated parts.

4. There are no specific consults to arrange. Postoperatively, these patients will require carefully controlled **occupational therapy** to maximize return of function.

- Plain X-rays of the intact hand and amputated part in three views (AP, lateral, and oblique) are imperative to identify bony injury. Important findings include the level of bony injury, comminution, and joint involvement.

- Specific laboratory studies that should be obtained include baseline hemoglobin and/or hematocrit level, prothrombin time, and platelet count to assess for a preexisting coagulopathy, type and cross-match for 2 to 4 units of packed red blood cells if there was a history of significant blood loss.

- An ECG should be obtained in older patients and in those with a history of cardiac ischemia or arrhythmia.

- Similarly, a preoperative chest X-ray may be indicated in certain patients.

5. There are many treatment options that have been devised for the reconstruction of traumatic thumb injuries. By definition, replantation refers to the reattachment of a *completely* severed body part. Revascularization refers to reattachment of an *incompletely* amputated body part that requires vessel reconstruction to maintain viability. Management begins with checking the tetanus status of the patient and giving a booster dose if not up-to-date.

- The simplest, albeit not always the best option, is shortening of the remaining bone and primary closure of the skin.

- Other surgical options for thumb reconstruction depend on the level of the amputation and the time since injury. For injury at or distal to the interphalangeal joint (IP) joint level, reasonable options for treatment include:

  — **Replantation or revascularization** is done with the patient in the supine or prone position and under tourniquet control. In most instances, bone shortening is performed followed by osteosynthesis with K-wires, 90-90 interosseous wiring, or a combination of an interosseous wire and a crossing K-wire (Lister technique). Repair of the tendons, arteries, veins, and nerves is performed in sequential fashion. Vascular anastomosis is performed outside the zone of injury following serial sectioning under the high power magnification of the operative microscope. There should be a low threshold for interposition vein grafting. Skin closure should be very loose and unmeshed partial-thickness skin grafts or allografts should be used when necessary to avoid excessive tension. Following replantation or reconstruction with free tissue transfer, pulse oximetry can be used to document arterial flow to the replanted part to monitor perfusion.

  — **Metacarpal lengthening.** Distraction osteogenesis technique is used to provide 2 to 3 cm of metacarpal length. This requires K-wiring of the joint to prevent flexion deformity, postoperative intensive therapy, and may require secondary bone grafting.

  — **Deepening of the first web space.** The four-flap Z-plasty is an excellent technique for maximizing the length of the first web space.

  — No reconstruction at all.

- For injury within the proximal phalanx:

  — **Great toe transfer** has the best motion and strength. It is indicated for amputation from the proximal phalanx proximally. The flap is based on the first dorsal metatarsal artery off the dorsalis pedis system. It may also be based on the larger first plantar metatarsal artery, which is absent in one-third of patients. The procedure requires intact thenar muscles. Advantages include a single-stage procedure, retention of growth potential, motion at the IP and MP levels, and the potential for sensibility. Disadvantages include a large digit, long operative time, and donor site morbidity.

  — The **wrap around procedure** provides the best appearance. It is a free soft tissue (and distal portion of the distal phalanx) flap from the first or second digit that is placed around a free bone graft (usually iliac crest). Advantages include a single operation, good strength, and less donor site morbidity. Disadvantages include the absence of growth potential and the potential for graft loss.

— **Second toe transfer** provides the least satisfactory appearance and IP joint function is weak. This flap is based on the first dorsal metatarsal artery. Advantages include a single-stage procedure, retention of growth potential, and adequate mobility. Disadvantages include small appearance, long operative time, and donor site morbidity.

- For injury at the metacarpophalangeal joint (MCP) level, distraction, web space deepening, or wrap-around procedures are reasonable options.

- For injury at the level of the metacarpal, toe-to-thumb, osteoplastic thumb reconstruction (such as an osteocutaneous reversed radial forearm flap) can be utilized.

- For injury at the carpometacarpal joint (CMC) level, **pollicization** is the only option in the absence of thenar musculature. It is used for total or subtotal defects of the thumb. It narrows the palm and is less effective in adults.

6. Complications following more complex reconstructions of the thumb may be challenging to manage.

- **Infection** is a potential complication with any open wound. As such antibiotics are generally administered prophylactically.

- **Malunion or nonunion** of bone is possible at the site of reattachment. In the face of documented malunion or nonunion, secondary bone grafting across the defect is likely required to obtain rigid support for the digit.

- The development of a symptomatic **neuroma** may warrant secondary excision and burying the proximal nerve stump in soft tissue or bone.

- **Chronic pain** in the reattached digit not attributable to a specific cause is perhaps the most difficult to manage postoperatively and may require consultation with a specialist in pain management.

- **Stiffness** may be related to scarring in one or more tissue types, including skin, tendon, and/or joint capsule. Secondary tenolysis may be required to maximum postoperative digital function.

- **Digit loss** is perhaps the most worrisome complication. Early evidence of ischemia often warrants return to the operating room and inspection of the arterial and venous anastomoses for patency. Thrombosis may be because of the technical problems at the suture line, kinking of the vessel, or compression from external structures. Many surgeons employ a postoperative regimen of anticoagulation to minimize the risk of thrombosis.

PRACTICAL PEARLS

1. The level of amputation and the patient's functional needs dictate reconstruction technique.

2. The most satisfactory reconstruction techniques provide some element of sensation.

3. Liberal use of vein grafts rather than anastomosis under tension improves replantation success.

4. Skin closure following replantation should be loose and unmeshed skin grafts can be considered.

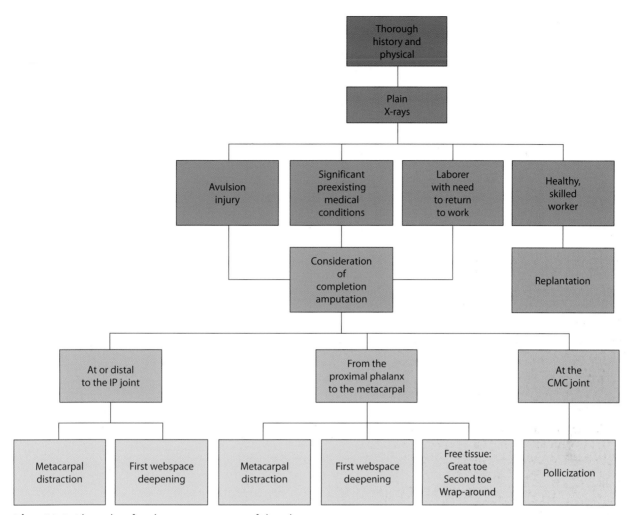

Algorithm 46-1 Algorithm for the management of thumb amputation.

References

1. Matev IB. Thumb reconstruction through metacarpal bone lengthening. *J Hand Surg [Am]*. 1980;5:482.

2. Stern PJ, Lister GD. Pollicization after traumatic amputation of the thumb. *Clin Orthop Relat Res*. 1981;155:85-94.

3. Wei FC, Chen HC, Chuang CC, et al. Microsurgical thumb reconstruction with toe transfer: Selection of various techniques. *Plast Reconstr Surg*. 1994;93:345.

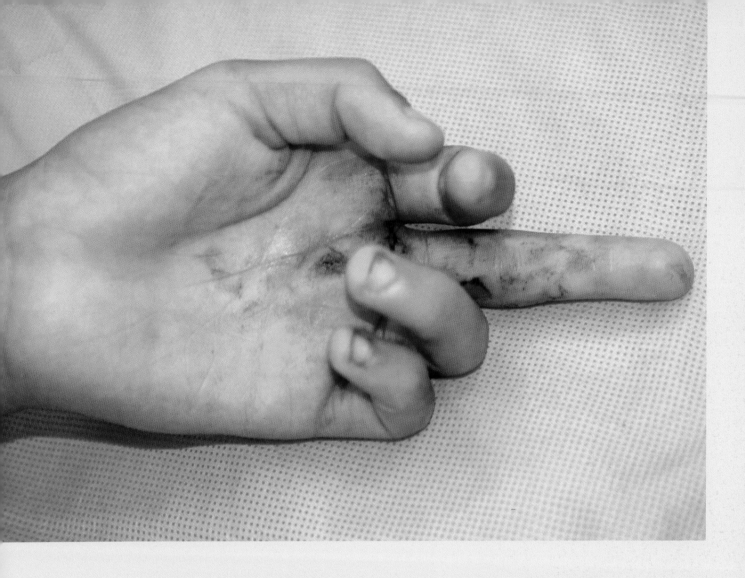

A 22-year-old right-hand-dominant chef presents to the emergency department after cutting his left hand with a cooking knife.

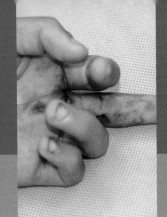

CHAPTER 47

Flexor Tendon Laceration

Michael W. Neumeister

1. Based upon a history of penetrating trauma and a posture of the hand characterized by an absence of a natural flexion cascade, the patient appears to have transection of the flexor tendons to the middle finger. A thorough history of the injury is important to direct the surgeon to the specific injuries and options for management. Important questions for the surgeon to ask the patient include:

   - **What was the mechanism of injury** (i.e., was this a crush or was this a sharp laceration)? Crush and mutilating injuries often involve multiple tissues including neurovascular bundles of soft tissue and bone as well as flexor tendon lacerations. Devitalize the contaminated tissue mandate the thorough debridement and irrigation. Clean lacerations require minimal debridement of the flexor tendon ends and often permit a more anatomical repair.

   - **When did the injury occur?** Most tendon repairs should occur within the first 24 to 48 hours, however, it is acceptable to repair the tendons within the first 10 days. Prolonging the repair of the tendons results in a greater inflammatory phase that may lead to a worse outcome because of secondary adhesion formation as result of the inflammation. Delayed repairs may also lead to collapse of the fibro-osseous canal mandating a staged reconstruction instead of a primary repair. Finally, delayed repairs result in retraction of the tendon which may not be advanced as easily.

   - **How was the finger positioned at the time of injury?** Lacerations to the flexor tendons while the finger is in active flexion results in a greater retraction of the tendon ends relative to those injuries that occur with the finger in extended position. This adds information to the surgeon so that appropriate exposure and incisions can be planned.

   - **Which hand is dominant?** Injury to the flexor tendons of the dominant hand may lead to greater dysfunction but the rehabilitation is the same.

   - **What is the patient's occupation?** Lacerations to the flexor digitorum superficialis (FDS) and flexor digitorum profundus (FDP) tendons result in serious dysfunction of the proximal interphalangeal (PIP) joint and distal interphalangeal (DIP) joints, respectively. Laborers, typists, and musicians may have different needs of their fingers to perform their daily occupation. Although primary repair is performed in every patient, delayed repairs require specific attention to patients' occupation. In the laborer where intricate function of the distal phalanx may not be a requirement of his job, staged reconstruction may not be the best option. Instead, an arthrodesis of the DIP joint or tenodesis or simple observation may be a better option. On the other hand, for musicians who require an intricate movement of their fingers including the DIP joint, staged reconstruction may be warranted.

2. Physical examination of the injured hand and digit should be thorough to evaluate all functions of the hand.

   - **Does the resting cascade of the fingers appear normal?** In a resting position, the normal cascade of the fingers involves a greater degree of composite flexion in the little finger relative to the ring finger. As one moves from the ulnar to radial aspect of the hand, the amount of composite flexion of the fingers decreases such that the thumb has the least amount of composite flexion. Loss of the normal cascade in any one of the fingers is an indication that the flexor tendons have been transected (an exception to this rule is if there is a fracture to the finger that may result in the abnormal position of the digit).

   - **Is there any evidence of ischemia to the digits?** It is very common to injury the neurovascular bundles on volar lacerations of the finger. The hand surgeon should identify the normal color, turgor, capillary refill and temperature of the involved digit. The devascularized finger mandates immediate revascularization.

   - **Is the distal neurologic supply to the digits normal?** Lacerations of the volar aspect of the digit may often involve the neurovascular bundles resulting in diminished sensibility distal to the laceration. Patients should be assessed for gross sensation and two-point discrimination prior to the use of local anesthetic.

   - **Do the individual tendons that power the digit function properly?** The FDS muscle originates from two sources: the ulnar head arises from the medial epicondyle of the humerus and the medial collateral ligament of the elbow joint and the radial head arises distal to the radial tuberosity. Its tendon inserts at the volar base of the middle phalanx. The FDP muscle originates along the proximal, medial and anterior surfaces of the ulna and interosseous membrane and its tendon inserts at the distal phalanx. Unless the patient has significant pain or apprehension, an independent evaluation of the FDS and FDP tendons will help identify the severity of the injury. Injuries that have significant trauma to the fingers or the patient has had significant pain, a passive tenodesis test of the wrist or forearm compression test (squeezing the volar forearm muscles results in flexion of the fingers if the musculotendinous units are in continuity) can identify intact tendons.

- **Are each of the joints stable?** An assessment of the joint stability including the joint dislocation should be performed. In delayed reconstruction, a supple joint is mandatory prior to embarking upon reconstruction of the tendon pulley system.

- **Is the soft tissue of the digit intact?** Assure that the overlying and subcutaneous structures are adequate to allow repair of the tendons and subsequent rehabilitation.

3. Preoperative studies are important in cases of trauma to the hands.

4. There are no imperative preoperative consults that need to be arranged.

- **Plain X-rays** of both hands should be performed on most cases of trauma. The images may identify associated bony defects that would require reduction and fixation. Often, the insertion of a tendon remains attached to bone but the bone fractures.

5. The ideal tendon repair should involve easy placement of sutures, secure knots, anatomical tendon end approximation, minimal interference with blood supply, and strength to permit early motion protocols. Prior to surgical intervention, it is important for the surgeon to obtain adequate and informed consent for a tendon repair/reconstruction. The patient must be fully aware of the functional goals after the treatment, the importance of rehabilitation and therapy, the expected time off, and possible complications including, infection, bleeding, hematoma, stiffness, tendon rupture, skin loss, need for revision surgery, and need for staged reconstruction.

- Surgical exposure is obtained through zigzag Brunner type incisions or through incisions along the mid-axial line of the digit.

- The tendon should be handled only at the severed end to minimize trauma to the uninjured aspect of the tendons.

- Suture material should be nonreactive, small caliber, appropriate strength with excellent knot handling characteristics; 3-0 core sutures are significantly stronger than 4-0 core sutures. Similar strength is noted between Ticron, nylon, Prolene, Ethilon, and Mersilene sutures. Prolene and nylon sutures glide through the tendon easier with minimal trauma to the substance of the tendon.

- The number of strands across the severed ends of the tendon injury site influences the strength of the repair. 8-strands are greater than 6-strands, which are greater than 4-strands, which are greater than 2-stands. A 2-strand core suture technique is not strong enough to permit an active range of motion protocol during rehabilitation. A 4-strand or greater repair is strong enough to initiate an active range of motion protocol in the rehabilitation.

- Specific treatment options by zone of injury:

  — **Zone I injuries** are distal to the FDS insertion. Options for repair include:

    a. Primary repair by advancement of the severed ends if the gap is less than 1 cm.

    b. Tendon graft if the gap is greater than 1 cm.

    c. Tenodesis

    d. DIP arthrodesis

  — **Zone II injuries** are the most challenging. They occur between the FDS insertion distally and the distal palmar crease proximally ("no man's land"). The tight pulley system exists in this region and important variables for return of optional range of motion include an active range of motion protocol, patient age, edema formation, presence of composite tissue injury, presence of associated fractures, zone of injury, adequate repair of the A-2 and A-4 pulleys, the use of epitendinus suture, and the avoidance of gap formation. The FDS should be maintained to preserve vincular blood supply to

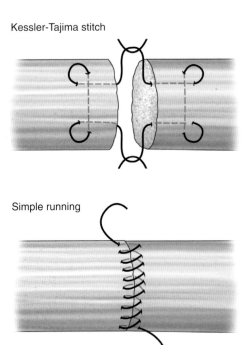

Kessler-Tajima stitch

Simple running

Figure 47-1 Schematic drawing highlighting the core suture and epitendinous suture for tendon repair.

FDP. The FDS repair also provides independent PIP joint flexion. Absolute contraindications include gross infection, human bite injuries, and cellulitis. Choices for reconstruction include the following:

a. Primary repair should be performed whenever possible. The injury site may be closed in the emergency department and reopened at the time of definitive repair 1 or more days later. Various suture techniques have been described in the literature, including Bunnell (single shoelace style with three crosses per tendon half), Kessler, Kessler-Tajima (two-suture Kessler), Tsuge, 1- and 2-suture Taras (twice-grasped Kessler), Becker (beveled edges), modified Becker for nonbeveled edges, McLarney (four core—two straight and two crossed—with running epitendinous), and Silva (eight core sutures), among others. Subtle differences are observed between the different repair techniques. 3-0 core sutures are significantly stronger than 4-0 core sutures.

b. Delayed primary repair may be indicated for grossly contaminated wounds. Second- or third-look surgeries are performed to offer further debridement. Once the wound has been adequately debrided, delayed primary repair is preferred.

c. Secondary repair is performed weeks after the initial injury. It is often unsuccessful for a variety of reasons necessitating different strategies.

d. Profundus advancement is used distal to the FDS insertion when more than 1 cm of tendon is lost. Excessive shortening will cause flexion in the repaired digit and with limited flexion in the remaining digits ("quadriga effect").

e. While tendon grafts have been shown to grow with the host, some have advocated *not* grafting children if they cannot comply with therapy. A specialized postoperative regimen involves 3 to 4 weeks of immobilization followed by unrestricted motion.

f. Tendon transfer often utilizes the FDS tendon to the ring finger.

g. Arthrodesis of the DIP joint accounts for a loss of only 15% of the total arc of rotation of the digit.

h. The proximal end of the cut profundus tendon may be looped around the FDS insertion (dynamic tenodesis).

i. A pulley reconstruction techniques may be performed in which a slip of FDS tendon or a portion of the wrist extensor retinaculum is used.

— **Zone III injuries** occur distal to the palmar crease to the level of the carpal canal. Within this area, the lumbricales originate from the FDP tendon. Primary repair is advocated. The functional results usually depend more on the nerve repair (median and/or ulnar nerve) than on the tendon repair.

— **Zone IV injuries** (carpal tunnel). Primary repair is advocated. The functional results usually depend on repair of the median nerve repair rather than the tendon.

— **Zone V injuries** occur proximal to carpal tunnel. Primary repair is advocated. The results are similar to zone IV and are usually excellent. The presence of median or ulnar nerve injury (and thus denervation of the intrinsic muscles) warrants maintenance of the PIP joint in extension during the postoperative period. Tenolysis is required in approximately 15%.

• Early controlled mobilization as an integral component of the postoperative rehabilitation protocol improves the repair process and decreases adhesion formation. Immobilization is reserved for noncompliant cases, such as small children and patients mentally incapable of following therapy.

— Early controlled passive motion as advocated by the Duran protocol or the Kleinert or Brooke Army Hospital protocols is as follows:

a. 0 to 4 weeks—passive flexion with the elastics and active extension by the patient/therapist. A dorsal blocking splint keeps the wrist held flexed 20 to 30 degrees, the MP joints 40 to 60 degrees, and the IP joints straight.

b. 4 to 6 weeks—active range of motion 4 to 6 times per day and scar massage within the splint.

c. 6 to 8 weeks—active and passive range of motion is allowed with removal of the blocking splint.

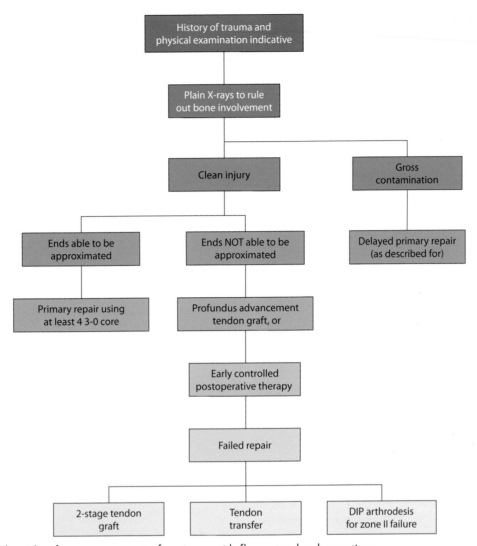

Algorithm 47-1 Algorithm for management of patients with flexor tendon lacerations.

d. 8 to 12 weeks—resisted flexion exercises.

e. 12 weeks—full use.

— Mayo Clinic synergistic dynamic tenodesis split permits wrist extension.

- An active mobilization protocol has also been proposed in which the patient is placed in a dorsal blocking splint with a wrist tenodesis splint. The digit is exercised by passive flexion within the splint. It requires at least a 4-strand or greater repair to prevent early rupture. Edema control—splinting for joint contractures and scar remodeling therapy proceeds after 8-weeks of therapy if needed.

  a. 4-weeks—active exercise without tenodesis splint.

  b. 6-weeks—removal dorsal blocking splint.

  c. 8-weeks—add light resistance.

6. In addition to the usual complications of bleeding and infection, limited postoperative function and tendon rupture are the most concerning complications. The American Society for Surgery of the Hand (ASSH) has adopted a range of motion scale that measures total active composite range of motion (TAM) to evaluate outcomes.

- A suspicion of **tendon rupture** may be confirmed by clinical examination, ultrasound, or MRI. The rate of rupture averages 5% regardless of suture technique or therapy protocol. It is higher with FPL repairs. Treatment involves prompt repair.

- **Adhesions** are promoted by numerous factors, including tendon and composite tissue damage, loss of tendon sheath, gap formation, ischemia, immobilization, persistent inflammation, and secondary trauma. Treatment options for adhesions include:

  — Tenolysis, which is indicated following the repair if the amount of passive range of motion exceeds the amount of active range of motion despite aggressive hand therapy. It is considered 3 or more months after repair if therapy has reached a plateau with no further gains.

  — One-stage, pulp-to-palm graft is appropriate in the digit with minimal scarring, supple joints, and an adequate pulley system. The palmaris longus may supply 13 cm of tendon length and is present in 75% to 85% of all patients. The plantaris tendon graft may be as long as 31 cm and is present in 80% to 90% of patients. The long extensors of the central three toes may supply 30 cm of length. The EIP and EDM may supply 10 cm and 11 cm of tendon graft length, respectively.

  — Staged reconstruction is used as a salvage procedure, following an attempt at one or more other reconstruction options. A silicone rod can be sutured or screwed to the distal phalanx with the A2 and A4 pulleys reconstructed on top. This is followed by a period of therapy to maintain maximal passive range of motion and scar massage. The second stage is performed 2 to 3 months later. The distal attachment is secured into a hollow made in the bone (distal phalanx) with a pullout suture. The proximal end is secured with a Pulvertaft weave. Complications include too-tight graft (quadriga effect), too-loose graft (lumbrical-plus deformity), stiffness, adhesions, and rupture. Prompt re-exploration is again mandated for ruptures.

— Salvage techniques include arthrodesis or amputation.

PRACTICAL PEARLS

1. Irrigation and debridement of all nonviable ends will improve healing rates and minimize rupture.

2. Meticulous, atraumatic involves handling the tendons only at the severed ends to minimize trauma to the remainder of the tendon.

3. Repair with at least four core strands to permit an early active range of motion protocol that does not risk early rupture.

4. Things to avoid in tendon repair include: tendon bunching, exposure of suture knots, trauma to uninjured portions of the tendon, gap formation, and trapping of the suture line behind a pulley.

5. Strict adherence to rehabilitation protocols.

References

1. Lutsky K, Boyer M. Flexor Tendon Injury. In: Trumble TE, Budoff JE, eds. *Hand Surgery Update* IV. American Society for Surgery of the Hand. 2007.

2. Boyer MI, Taras JS, Kaufman RA. Flexor tendon injury. In: Green's Operative Hand Surgery. Vol. 1. Philadelphia, PA: Elsevier Churchill Livingstone. 2005:219-276.

3. Gelberman RH, Siegel DB, Woo SL, Amiel D, Takai S, Lee D. Healing of digital flexor tendons: Importance of the interval from injury to repair. A biomechanical, biochemical, and morphological study in dogs. *J Bone Joint Surg Am.* 1991;73-1: 66-75.

4. Kleinert HE, Kutz JE, Ashbell TS, Martinez E. Primary repair of lacerated flexor tendon in no man's land. In: Proceedings of the American Society for Surgery of the Hand; *J Bone Joint Surg.* 1967;49A:577.

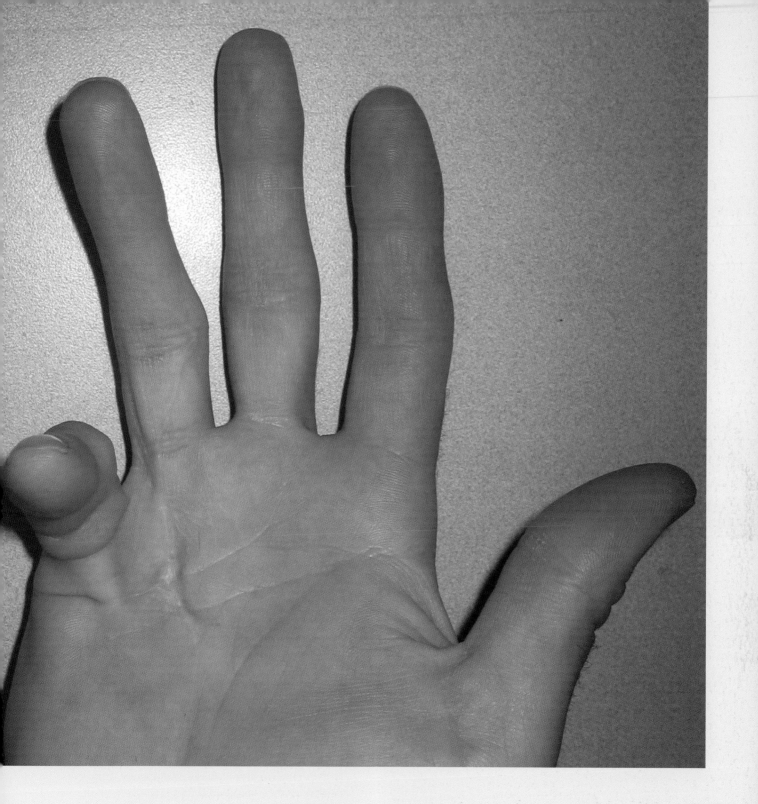

A 55-year-old man is referred to the office for difficulty in fully opening his fingers.

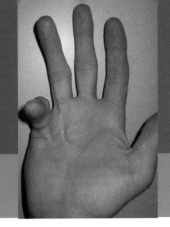

CHAPTER 48

Flexion Deformity of the Finger

John Ko

1. Chronic flexion of the digits may be related to any of the structures present within the finger. Joint injury, tendon scarring, and/or skin contracture can all lead to difficulty with extension and flexion. In addition, Dupuytren's disease, one of the fibromatoses, affects the fascia of the skin leading to progressive flexion of involved digits. The etiology can often be diagnosed from a careful, directed history. It is vital to address several factors when determining prognosis of this disease and the treatment options available for each individual patient.

  - How did the problem begin? Patients who suffer from Dupuytren disease usually begin noticing asymptomatic thickening in the palm of their hands initially. It can then develop into nodules and cords which arise from the fascia of the hands. Although the disease itself does not affect the bony and tendinous structures, severe contractures of the fingers and restriction of hand function are symptoms.

  - **Was there a history of trauma to the finger?** Certainly, injury to any of the components of the finger mentioned above can result in limited range of motion.

  - **How old is the patient?** The incidence of Dupuytren's disease peaks between 40 and 60 years of age. It is less commonly seen in younger patients.

  - **What is the patient's gender?** The ratio of affected men to women is 2:1. In general, women have a less severe form of the disease. Men are seven to fifteen times more likely to require surgery.

  - **What is the patient's ethnicity?** Dupuytren's is largely confined to Caucasians. It is believed to be from Celtic origins and is more common in Scandinavia and the British Isles.

  - **Is the finger painful?** Contracture related to prior trauma is more likely to present with chronic pain, whereas Dupuytren's is a relatively painless condition.

  - **Are other family members affected?** It is inherited as an autosomal dominant with variable penetrance. An increased risk exists in other family members. There is an association with the HLA-DR3 gene.

  - **What is the patient's occupation or avocation?** No conclusive study has been able to correlate a patient's profession or hobby to the development of Dupuytren's disease.

  - **Does the deformity affect the patient's daily or weekly activities?** Often, the amount of deformity is a relative indication to proceed with intervention. More importantly, the patient's occupation as a causal factor in Dupuytren's disease is a controversial topic. There are, however, guidelines for Worker's Compensation, which include: younger age of onset (men younger than 40 years of age and women younger than 50 years of age), a documented single incident injury, and the time from injury to onset of disease is less than 2 years.

  - **Does the patient have concomitant medical issues?** A higher incidence of Dupuytren's disease exists in patients with other medical conditions including myocardial infarction, HIV infection, diabetes, and seizure disorder and in patients consuming significant quantities of alcohol and cigarettes or requiring prolonged use of barbiturates. Approximately 5% of patients with Dupuytren's are diabetic, with the frequency increasing with age and duration of diabetes. The incidence of seizure disorder in patients with Dupuytren's is roughly twice what it is in the general population. Occasionally, it develops following a Colles fracture or severe hand injury. Of note, there is a lower incidence in people with rheumatoid disease.

2. Dupuytren's disease affects the longitudinal layer of the palmar fascia and spares the deeper layers. Pretendinous bands (longitudinal extensions of the palmar fascia) become pretendinous cords at the metacarpophalangeal (MP) joint. Confluence of spiral bands, lateral digital sheath, and Grayson's ligaments become spiral cords at the proximal interphalangeal (PIP) joint. The spiral cord is suspected to cause PIP joint contracture. It may also be caused by the central cord (no precursor) or the lateral cord (from the lateral digital sheet). It causes the neurovascular bundle to be displaced medially. The natatory ligaments become natatory bands at the web space. These pass superficial to the neurovascular bundles. The thumb is *not* commonly involved. Distal interphalangeal (DIP) contracture is rare and caused by the retrovascular and lateral cords. At the cellular level of Dupuytren's disease, there is increased expression of fibroblast growth factors and increased expression of type III collagen within the cords as opposed to the normal type I collagen. There are also prominent microtubules in fibroblasts from Dupuytren's

affected fascia. The skin plays no role in contraction. The physical examination should note key findings.

- **Which digits are affected?** The ring finger is affected most commonly, followed by the little and middle fingers. Approximately one-third of cases involve only one digit, one-third involve two digits, and one-third involve multiple digits. The thumb is *not* commonly involved.

- **Which joints are affected?** The disease begins as palmar nodules, progressing to cords, and affects the MP joints before the PIP joints. DIP contracture is rare and caused by retrovascular and lateral cords. Dupuytren's disease has been classified into phases: proliferative, involutional, and residual. The proliferative phase is heralded by nodule formation. Nodules form just distal or proximal to the distal skin crease of the palm. They are firm and adherent to the skin, not moving with flexion or extension of the digit. The involutional phase corresponds to the longitudinal band formation. The residual phase involves contraction of the cords and is the most quiescent phase.

- **Are both sides affected?** Bilateral disease is more common than either right- or left-sided disease.

- **Is the patient able to flatten his/her hand on a table?** As the MP joint contracture becomes greater than 30 degrees, the patient will not be able to flatten his/ her hand. This is a relative indication for surgery.

- **Are nodules seen in other areas of the body?** Several risk factors including an early age at onset, the presence of knuckle pads (Garrod's pads) or plantar fibromatosis (Ledderhose's disease) or penile fibrosis (Peyronie's disease), bilateral disease, or radial hand involvement all lead to a much more aggressive form called Dupuytren's diathesis and indicate a poorer prognosis.

3. Studies are of limited benefit in determining the etiology of the problem. **Plain X-rays** are obtained to rule out any bone or joint abnormalities. The presence of significant joint pathology may make resection of the diseased fascia of little benefit to regaining function of the digit.

4. There are no specific consultations that one needs to obtain.

5. There are nonsurgical as well as surgical strategies for the management of Dupuytren's disease.

- Nonsurgical treatment options include medications, enzymatic fasciectomy, and skeletal traction. The medic-

ations commonly used for Dupuytren's include allopurinol, colchicine, calcium channel blockers, interferon, vitamin E, and/or steroids. The latter should only be given a couple of times to relieve pain in mild cases, since they may lead to eventual tendon damage. No medications have shown proven benefit for established contractures. Skeletal traction therapy has been described in which the cords are lengthened approximately 2 mm per day for up to 2 weeks. A future direction that may be promising is the use of clostridial collagenase, which enzymatically degrades the contractures.

- Surgical treatment targets excision of the diseased tissue. There are no absolute indications for surgery. Relative indications include: functional disability, MP flexion greater than 30 degrees, PIP flexion of any degree, significant web space contracture, disturbed neurovascular function, articular cartilage loss, and concomitant trigger finger.

— There are several contraindications for surgery. Although none are absolute, caution must be used in dealing with patients who exhibit them.

a. One should not operate for pain alone.

b. Surgery should be delayed when skin maceration and infection are present.

c. Patients who are unlikely to comply with postoperative care instructions or continued physical therapy are often poor candidates for surgery.

d. Significant hand arthritis may be worsened with any type of surgery.

— Surgical release may be performed through linear or zigzag incisions in the digits and lazy S incision in the palm.

a Local fasciectomy excises a short segment of fascia through a transverse incision.

b Regional fasciectomy removes only diseased fascia and is often the first operation. This is the most common procedure performed for Dupuytren's disease and is more successful in the palm.

c. Extensive fasciectomy removes both diseased and normal fascia when the cords extend into the digit.

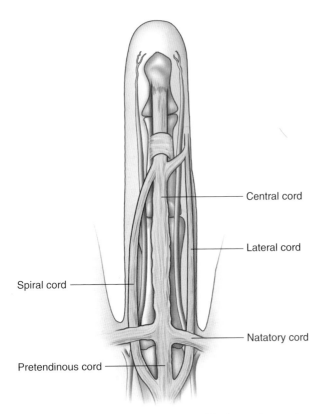

Figure 48-1 Schematic drawing highlighting the pathologic bands in Dupuytren's disease.

Labels on figure: Central cord, Lateral cord, Spiral cord, Natatory cord, Pretendinous cord

d. Dermatofasciectomy involves excision of the diseased fascia and the overlying skin. This procedure is reserved for treatment of patients with aggressive recurrent disease. Use of a full-thickness skin graft for coverage is often necessary.

— Wounds may be closed with suture, left open, or covered with a skin graft. Secondary healing of these wounds takes 4 to 6 weeks. Full-thickness skin grafts have been shown to decrease the formation of recurrent disease and may be a better option for severe or recurrent cases.

— For rehabilitation, the digits are splinted in extension. If the skin was left open, the splint is kept in place until the wounds have closed. At a minimum, the finger is splinted continuously for 3 to 4 weeks. Occupational therapy should be started after 1 week to minimize recurrence. A nocturnal extension splint may be used for three additional months.

— Complete correction of MP contraction can be achieved. The PIP is more resistant (especially the small finger), and thus results are more limited. This should be discussed preoperatively.

6. The overall rate of complications following surgical resection of the digital fascia approaches 20%. Patients should be carefully evaluated prior to discharge from the hospital or surgical facility.

- **Recurrence** caused by the incomplete excision of the affected tissues is by far the greatest complication. It can be seen in as many as 40% of all complications. This differs from extension, in which new areas of disease appear after resection of one area.

- **Hematoma, skin slough, and infection** account for up to 10% of all complications. Careful hemostasis following fasciectomy is important in minimizing morbidity.

- **Injury to the neurovascular bundle** is possible with excision of the diseased fascia and the abnormal position of the neurovascular bundle that occurs with fascial contraction. Suspicion of injury at the time of surgery or in the immediate postoperative period requires removal of the dressing and sutures, papaverine, rewarming, and possibly revascularization. Repair of the neurovascular bundle is required in some cases.

- **Cold intolerance** can result, especially in patients suffering from Dupuytren's diathesis. Careful protection in colder climates and possibly a move to a warmer environment may be recommended.

- **Reflex sympathetic dystrophy** occurs in roughly 5% of all patients who have surgical treatment and is twice as common in female patients. The cause is usually unknown.

PRACTICAL PEARLS

1. Pain should not be the sole indication for operative intervention since this is the least responsive to surgical management.

2. The skin over the volar surface of the digit can be colored with a surgical marker prior to starting the excision. Then, subdermal dissection can proceed with the purple color visualized from below. This minimizes the risk of leaving diseased fascia behind.

3. During the proliferative phase, the nodules are the primary abnormal structures since the cords have not formed yet. It is a mistake to excise only the nodules at this time because the disease progression will accelerate. Surgical correction should be delayed until cords are present.

4. The outcome of surgical release of the MP contractures is generally much better than at the PIP joint. For PIP contractures, only 20% of patients report immediate success after surgery. An additional 55% show some improvement, but 25% of patients report worsening of their symptoms. Think twice before operating on isolated PIP contractures.

5. The neurovascular bundle of the digits spirals from deep to superficial and back again. As the spiral cord forms, it displaces the bundle toward the midline and superficially. The location can be predicted preoperatively by finding a soft, pulpy mass of skin between the proximal finger crease and the distal palmer confluence. The bundle lies deep to this, so use caution when dissecting here.

6. The check rein ligaments, which span the PIP joint, often need to be released during the fasciectomy in order to allow the joint to fully straighten.

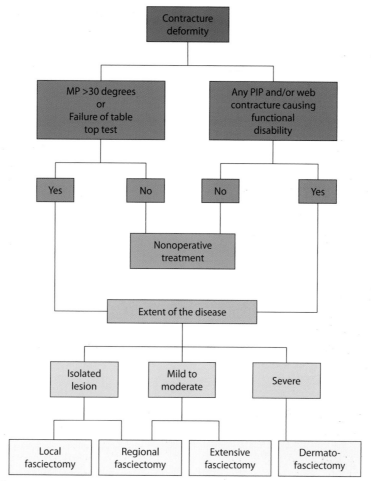

Algorithm 48-1 Algorithm for management of patients with Dupuytren's disease.

References

1. Hueston J, Dupuytren's contracture., *J Hand Surg [Br].* 1993;18(6):806.

2. Messina A, Messina J. The continuous elongation treatment by the TEC device for severe Dupuytren's contracture of the fingers. *Plast Reconstr Surg.*1993;92(1):84.

3. McFarlane R, Severe contractures of the proximal interphalangeal joint in Dupuytren's disease: Combined fasciectomy with capsuloligamentous release versus fasciectomy alone.*Plast Reconstr Surg.* 1996;97(3):567.

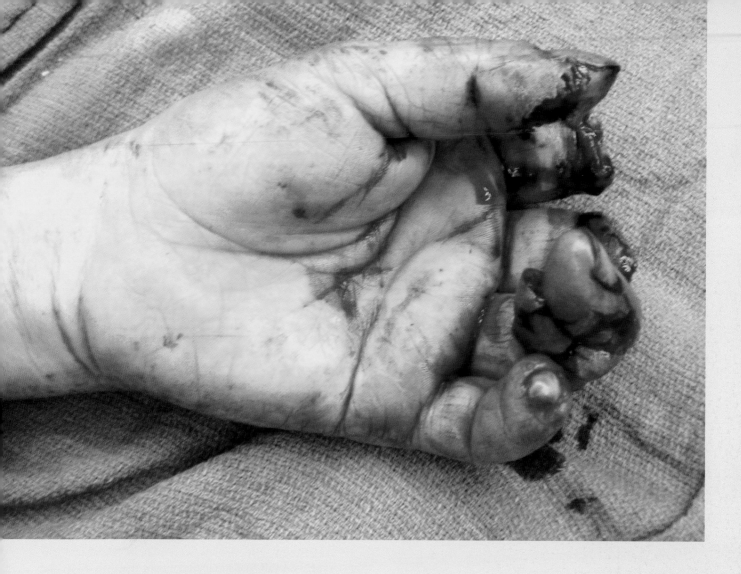

The emergency department calls you for a STAT consult to evaluate a 24-year-old man who sustained injury to the hand while at work.

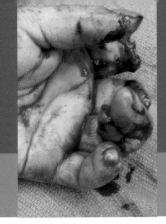

CHAPTER 49

Mangled Hand

Ernest Kirchman

1. The patient in question sustained significant injury to the right hand as a result of trauma. The priority in the treatment of traumatic injury is to rule out life-threatening conditions. Stabilization of the patient's airway, breathing, and circulation always takes precedence. Following this, a thorough history and secondary survey should be performed. The history may be elicited from the patient, but details may need to be obtained from observers, family members, or primary response providers (paramedics) if the patient is not able to respond.

- **What was the mechanism of injury?** The mechanism of trauma may provide clues to the types of injury sustained. Crush injury will commonly produce trauma to bones, soft tissues, and vessels. Injury to tendons is less likely. Avulsion-type injuries, on the other hand, can injure tendons, most frequently at the musculotendinous junction. Similarly, lacerating-type trauma will produce injury to vascular structures and tendons, but less commonly bone.

- **When did the injury occur?** While some intervention is necessary, it is important to determine when the injury occurred. Wounds that have been open for long periods of time are more prone to colonization and infection and thus less likely to be closed primarily.

- **Is the patient left-handed or right-handed?** Injuries to the dominant hand are considered more critical than injuries to the nondominant one and may warrant more aggressive attempts at reconstruction.

- **What is the patient's occupation and avocation?** Different professions may direct different goals of treatment. A laborer, who may need to return to construction-type work faster, may be better suited to amputation and wound closure than a pianist who relies on fine motor skills and thus be more tolerant of extensive rehabilitation.

- **Is there a history of smoking?** Smoking has an adverse effect on wound and bone healing. While little can be done at the time of injury, this is important to document and should be discontinued with ongoing therapy.

- **Is there a history of diabetes?** The presence of diabetes has a similar adverse effect on healing. Of note, the rate of flap anastomotic problems are equal those of nondiabetics.

2. A careful preoperative examination is critical to identify the extent of injury. In cases of hand trauma, several systems need to be assessed including the vascular status, the nervous innervation, as well as the skeletomuscular stability.

- **Are distal pulses palpable?** An ischemic limb does *not* always imply a vascular injury. The vessels may be in spasm or may be kinked secondary to the injury. Pulses may return after fracture reduction. Questionable manual examinations may require Doppler examination of the palmar arch and digital vessels.

- **What is the pattern of distal sensation?** Confirmation of gross median, ulnar, and radial sensation is important. The median nerve may be tested over the volar thumb, the ulnar nerve over the fifth digit, and the radial nerve over the dorsal first web space.

- **What is the level of function at the joints proximal and distal to the level of injury?** A thorough examination of the upper extremity should be begin at the neck and shoulder since injury in the distal extremity may have associated injury or causative factors more proximally. The examination should then evaluate the various axes and ranges of motion specific to each joint. In the forearm, supination and pronation should be evaluated as well as flexion and extension. In the hand, flexion and extension in the metacarpophalangeal joints should be evaluated separately from the proximal interphalangeal joints and distal interphalangeal joints, as well as abduction and adduction.

- **Is there any evidence of compartment syndrome?** This should be suspected in any crush injury to a closed compartment to prevent tissue necrosis. The cardinal signs of compartment syndrome are pain out of proportion to the injury, pain on passive flexion or extension, a palpably swollen or tense compartment, and/or absence of pulses, which is usually a late sign.

  — Measurement of the compartment pressure makes the definitive diagnosis. The presence of clinical suspicion with/without a compartment pressure >30 mm Hg is an indication for emergent fasciotomy.

- **How much soft tissue injury exists?** The size of the wound, including any dead space is important to identify since free tissue transfer is often required for larger defects (>25 cm^2).

- **Is there exposure of hardware, bone, or tendon?** Reliable coverage of such structures is imperative and likely requires free tissue transfer.

3. Preoperative studies are imperative in these patients to identify bony and/or vascular injury. Injury to tendons and nerves are best diagnosed by physical examination and examination of the wound at the time of operative exploration.

4. Important consults should be arranged as their needs arise during the workup. Significant injury to other organ systems usually mandates admission to a dedicated **trauma service** for management or observation prior to specialized surgical care. **Occupational therapy** will be critical in the postoperative management of these patients.

- For bony injury, the pattern of the fracture is best evaluated with **plain X-rays**, which may be obtained in conjunction with the trauma series. Extensive periosteal stripping, comminution, and marrow obliteration require coverage with better-vascularized tissue.

- **Angiography** is reserved for evaluation of the vascular supply to the distal extremity in the presence of suspected disruption and in anticipation of free tissue transfer.

5. The goal in treating severe open injuries of the hand, which include trauma to multiple anatomic structures is to preserve as much function as possible. If the extremity cannot be salvaged, the maintenance of maximum functional length is important.

- Initial, nonoperative management should include administration of antibiotics and tetanus prophylaxis (for those who are not up to date).

- If the patient has other life-threatening injuries, **initial treatment** of the extremity injury should be limited to control of bleeding, release of compartments, and stabilization of the extremity. Operative debridement of nonvital tissue and irrigation with pulsed lavage solution is similarly important and may be repeated until definitive soft tissue coverage is accomplished.

— Several compartments in the hand and forearm may need to be released:

  a. The forearm contains three anatomic compartments. An **anterior compartment** houses the flexors of the finger (flexor digitorum superficialis [FDS] and flexor digitorum profundus [FDP]), the thumb (flexor pollicis longus [FPL]), and the wrist (FCR, FCU, and palmaris longus), as well as the pronators (teres and quadratus). A **posterior compartment** houses the extensors to the fingers (extensor digitorum communis [EDC], extensor indicis proprius [EIP], extensor digiti quinti [EDQ]), the thumb (extensor pollicis longus [EPL] and extensor pollicis brevis [EPB]), and the ulnar wrist (extensor carpi ulnaris [ECU]), as well as the thumb abductor (APL) and wrist supinator. A third compartment houses brachioradialis, extensor carpi radialis longus [ECRL] and extensor carpi radialis brevis [ECRB].

  b. The hand contains ten compartments: 4 for the dorsal interossei, 3 for the palmar interossei, 1 for the thenar muscles, 1 for adductor pollicis, and 1 for the hypothenar muscles.

— Revascularization may be indicated for injury to either the arteries or veins.

— Reinnervation is required for injury to any of the major nerves in the hand or fingers. This should be identified preoperatively by physical examination noting sensory and motor deficits and the site of any lacerations cognizant of the course of the nerves.

— Skeletal stabilization at the initial procedure may range from nonoperative splinting to external stabilization to internal fixation. Closed treatment of the bony injury is acceptable for low-energy, closed wounds (internal fixation has a faster time to union and a lower malunion rate).

— Repair of tendon and ligaments should be performed when identified. Numerous suture methods have been described for tendon repair as defined by the number of core sutures that pass across the disruption of the tendon and the presence or absence of an epitendinous suture that encircles the repair.

— Early soft tissue coverage is associated with a lower complication rate. Definitive coverage may be performed later. Timing is determined by the need to cover vital structures and the risk of infection. The reconstructive options are dictated by the site of the injury. Tissue expansion is usually avoided in the extremities because of the high morbidity (infection rates of 5% to 30%).

   a. Skin graft

   b. Local flaps, if available (cross finger, kite, radial forearm).

   c. Regional flaps (groin flap).

   d. Free flaps (contralateral radial forearm, parascapular, anterolateral thigh).

— Amputation of a mangled extremity in a clinically unstable patient may be more prudent than an extensive course of reconstruction and should be considered in the initial evaluation of the patient.

● Secondary reconstruction may be needed for tendons, bone, or soft tissue. Tendon transfers specifically for low (or distal) nerve injuries are outlined below.

— For low median nerve injury (distal to the innervation of the extrinsic finger flexors and wrist flexors), motor deficits include loss of palmar abduction and thumb pronation (lumbricales to index and middle, opponens pollicis, abductor pollicis brevis, and flexor pollicis brevis). Common transfers to restore thumb opposition include EIP to APB (Burkhalter) or FDS of the ring finger to APB (Bunnell) or palmaris longus to APB (Camitz) or ADM to APB (Huber).

— For low ulnar nerve injury (distal to the innervation of the extrinsic finger flexors and ulnar wrist flexor), motor deficits include hyperextension at the MCP and hyperflexion at the DIP of the ring and small fingers ("claw deformity" caused by lumbrical loss and unopposed extension at the MCP by EDC) and unopposed flexion at the DIP by FDS. Common transfers to correct clawing include FDS of the middle finger to radial lateral bands of the middle, ring, and small fingers (Stiles-Bunnell) or ECRB extended by grafts to the radial lateral bands (Brand I) or ECRL extended by grafts to the radial lateral bands (Brand II).

— For low radial nerve injury, motor deficits include absent finger extension (EDC, EIP, and EDQ), wrist extension (ECRB, ECRL, and ECU), and thumb abduction (APL), and thumb extension (EPL and EPB). Common transfer groups to restore finger and thumb extension include:

   a. FCU to EDC and palmaris to EPL (Jones).

   b. FCR to EDC and palmaris to EPL (Starr).

   c. FDS of the middle finger to EIP and EPL and FDS of the ring finger to EDC of the middle, ring, and small fingers (Boyes).

6. Complications are understandably not infrequent following major hand trauma.

● Postoperative **ischemia** may have several etiologies. Initially, the hand should be inspected after the splint is released and the dressings removed. Examination with a hand-held Doppler may be necessary to confirm flow through the vessels. Reexploration, rewarming, papaverine, and possibly revascularization may all be indicated.

● **Malunion** or **nonunion** of bone may be particularly troublesome in the hand. Debridement and grafting may be required to stabilize the bone.

● In case of **flap loss**, a "lifeboat" should be considered. Loss of a free flap does not imply that another cannot be used. However, often a safer back-up plan is prudent, such as a groin flap.

● **Complex regional pain syndrome** (formerly called RSD) presents with sympathetic manifestations following even minor trauma. Three criteria are necessary for the diagnosis: (1) diffuse pain not related to the distribution of a peripheral nerve, (2) diminished function and stiff joints, and (3) skin and soft tissue changes. It is believed that tissue trauma likely leads to inappropriate release of norepinephrine at the end organ level. The diagnosis is made by clinical appearance, hypersensitivity to cold, temporary improvement with sympatholysis (parenteral phentolamine blocks alpha-1 receptors), and diffuse uptake on triple phase bone scan. Treatment involves early therapy to prevent stiffness, treatment of underlying nerve compression, and sympathetic interruption with phenoxybenzamine or bretylium.

PRACTICAL PEARLS

1. The injured hand should be splinted in the position of safety and elevated.

2. An external fixator should be considered for exposed fractures, which lack adequate soft tissue coverage to avoid infected internal hardware.

3. Use of a tourniquet in the operative room should be limited in the presence of extensive devitalized tissue or ischemia.

4. In degloving-type injuries, the skin flaps should be tacked down loosely, rather than attempting complete reapproximation, in anticipation of edema and demarcating necrotic areas.

5. When considering reconstruction, the patient's function should take precedence over the aesthetic appearance of hand.

6. Remember rehabilitation and hand therapy from day 1, to minimize joint stiffness.

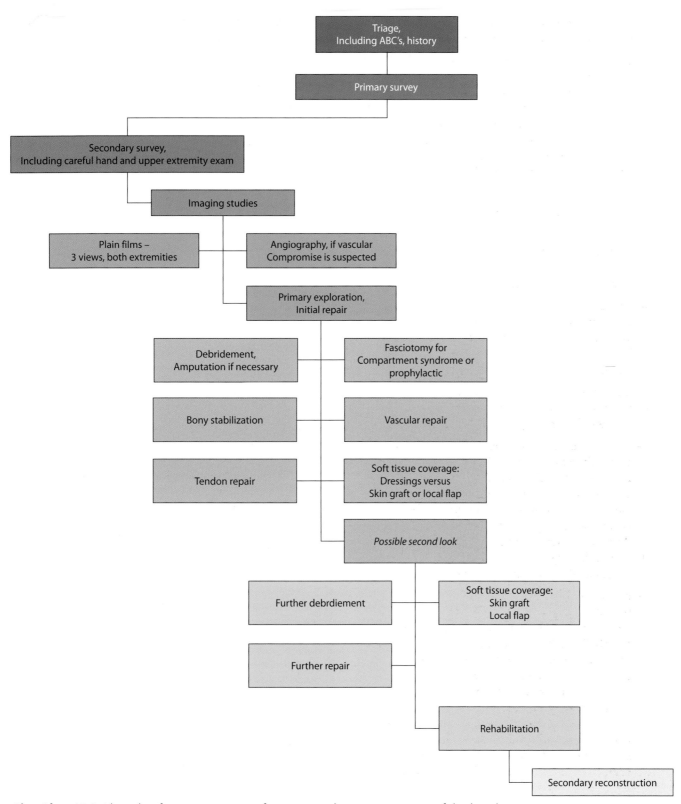

Algorithm 49-1 Algorithm for management of patients with traumatic injury of the hand.

References

1. Brown PW. Open injuries of the hand. In: Green DH, ed. *Operative Hand Surgery*. Vol. II. Oxford, UK: Churchill Livingstone, 1993.

2. Graham TJ. The exploded hand syndrome: Logical evaluation and comprehensive treatment of the severely crushed hand. *J Hand Surg*. 2006;31:1012-1023.

3. Weinzweig JW, Weinzweig N. The "tic-tac-toe" classification system for mutilating injuries of the hand. *Plast Reconstr Surg*. 1997;100:1200-1211.

4. Del Pinal F, Herrero F, Jado E, García-Bernal FJ, Cerezal L. Acute hand compartment syndromes after closed crush: A reappraisal. *Plast Reconstr Surg*. 2002;110(5):1232-1239.

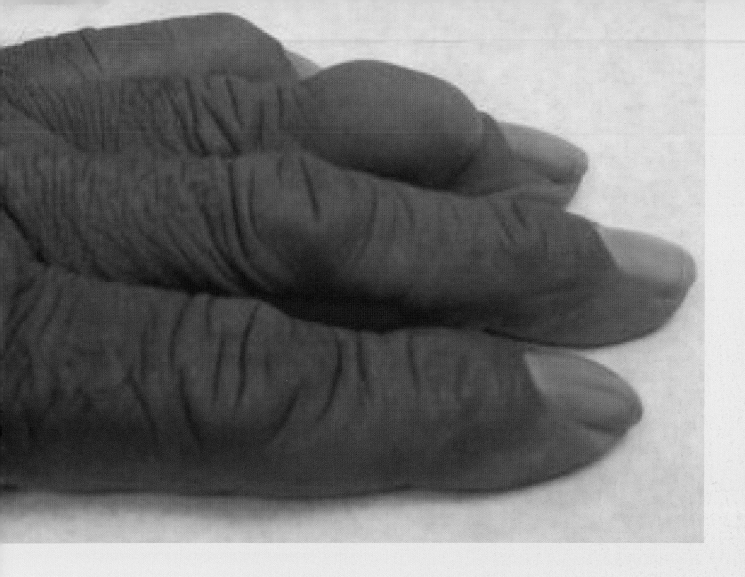

A primary care physician in the neighborhood asks you to see a patient with a new lesion on the dorsum of the finger.

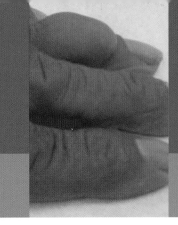

CHAPTER 50

Finger Mass

David T.W. Chiu

1. Numerous lesions can affect the hands and digits and range from benign infections and vascular lesions to malignant tumors. As with all lesions, it is important to establish a diagnosis. This is first performed with a directed patient history.

- **How old is the patient?** Certain entities tend to present in specific populations depending on age. Giant cell tumors, for example, have a predilection for patients 20 to 40 years of age while those of the tendon sheath appear in slightly older patients.

- **How long has the lesion been present?** Because of its exposed location, skin cancer is the most common malignancy of the hand. Risk factors for **basal and squamous cell carcinoma** include sun exposure, X-ray exposure, chronic wounds, and immune suppression. Squamous cell carcinoma often arises from preexisting actinic keratoses, commonly recognized by their scaly appearance and tendency to flake and bleed. Chronic wounds and scars can give rise to a subtype of squamous cell carcinoma called Marjolin's ulcer. This subtype is more aggressive and exhibits a higher rate of metastasis. Squamous cell carcinomas are generally locally invasive. **Melanomas** are less commonly encountered. Risk factors for the development of melanoma include sun exposure, fair skin, and a family history of similar lesions.

- **Was there a history of trauma?** Acute and chronic infections of the hand and digits result from breaks in the skin secondary to minor trauma and can cause masses as well. They are usually differentiated from other lesions by their acute onset, erythema, pain, and drainage. **Felons** are soft tissue infections of the pulp space of the digits. **Paronychiae** are infections of the soft tissue surrounding the nail. These are usually caused by *Staphylococcus aureus*. A chronic paronychia is usually caused by *Candida albicans* infection. Trials of topical steroids and antifungals can be attempted but are usually unsuccessful. Recalcitrant cases may require eponychial marsupialization.

- **How has the lesion changed?** Malignant lesions of the hand are less common than benign ones. However, when evaluating a lesion of the digits, the possibility that it is malignant should always be kept in mind.

Malignant tumors can be categorized as either primary or metastatic. Metastatic lesions to the digits are much less common than primary ones. When analyzing the different components of the hand, the skin is the most likely site of malignant lesions. Faster growth or changes in appearance might be a hallmark for change to malignancy.

- **Is the lesion painful?** Benign viral warts as well as giant cell tumors of bone and certain malignant lesions may be painful if there is involvement of nervous structures. **Glomus tumors** are tumors of the thermoregulatory system most often found in the fingertip. They are classically associated with nighttime paroxysmal pain and cold hypersensitivity. The most common solitary tumor of the peripheral nerves is the **schwannoma** or neurilemmoma. Overall, peripheral nerve tumors are uncommon accounting for less than 5% of hand tumors. The lesions, however, do not typically cause symptoms along the affected nerve distribution.

- **Does the lesion affect function?** The location of the lesion, such as over a joint space or tendon sheath, may give a clue to the structure from which the mass arises.

- **What is the handedness of the patient?** At times, the extent of the excision and reconstruction may be tailored based on the use of the hand. A right-handed person may not tolerate the same reconstruction option on his right hand as he does on his left.

- **What is the patient's occupation and avocation(s)?** Laborers require a quicker return to function than do persons who use their hands for more skilled tasks (musician). This may have implications on the type of reconstruction performed.

2. Benign tumors of the hand can also be thought of as arising from any of the varied anatomic structures in the digits. All components can give rise to abnormal or neoplastic growth. One of the most important distinctions to make regarding a mass is to determine whether it is benign or malignant. Benign lesions of the hand are far more common than malignant ones. The ganglion cyst is the most common mass found in the hand and is benign. Epidermal cysts, warts, giant cell tumors, and hemangiomas are also benign and follow in frequency.

- **Where on the digit is the lesion located?** Certain tumors, such as glomus tumors, tend to appear under the nailbed. Ganglion cysts, on the other hand, appear over joint spaces. Enchondromas typically affect the proximal phalanges.

- **What color is the lesion?** Red or purple lesions may be congenital hemangiomas, which can be found on the hands. Thirty percent are evident within the first week of life and that number reaches 70% to 90% within 4 weeks. Most hemangiomas run a course of proliferation for the first 10 to 12 months. Approximately 70% involute by 7 years of age but often leave residual sequelae, including loose, discolored skin, and soft tissue. Other vascular lesions including venous, lymphatic, and arteriovenous malformations may also be identified in the hand.

- **Is the lesion tender to palpation?** Most lesions on the digits are not painful. As mentioned, warts, glomus tumors, and malignant lesions may be painful and tender with palpation.

- **Is the lesion mobile?** Soft tissue lesions are usually mobile, while those arising from bone are not. There are a myriad of soft tissue sarcomas that can appear in the hand. However, these are seen quite infrequently. Again, most soft tissue types can give rise to a malignancy. Some of the soft tissue sarcomas include: synovial cell sarcomas, liposarcoma, fibrosarcoma, angiosarcoma, malignant nerve sheath tumors, lymphangiosarcoma, rhabdomyosarcoma, and malignant fibrous histiocytoma. Tumors involving the tendon sheath will characteristically move with flexion and extension of the digit. Malignant tumors arising from the bone are not very commonly found in the hand. The most frequent type is the chondrosarcoma. Chondrosarcoma arises from the cartilage. It is usually found in individuals older than 50 with men being affected twice as often as women. The lesion is usually locally invasive but can metastasize in approximately 10% of cases with the lung being the most likely affected site. Other bony tumors which can affect the hand are osteosarcoma and Ewing's sarcoma.

- **Are there any scars on the hands?** Scars may indicate damage to available flaps useful for reconstruction.

- **Is there laxity of the surrounding tissues?** If soft tissue reconstruction needs to be performed, the adequacy for donor sites needs to be assessed.

- **Are there any nerve deficits?** Involvement of nerves may be due to pressure from a mass effect or may indicate malignancy of the nerve sheath impairing its function.

- **Is there any palpable adenopathy in the axilla?** The axilla is the major lymph node draining basin for the upper extremity. As such, malignant tumors from the hand that spread via the lymphatics will pass through the lymph nodes in the axilla.

3. Only a few radiographic imaging studies are potentially valuable preoperatively. **Plain X-rays** of both hands in three views (AP, lateral, and oblique) are an important first modality to identify primarily osseous lesions and those with an osteophytic component, such as a mucous cyst.

    - **MRI** is the most sensitive study to image the soft tissues of the hands and digits.

    - **Biopsy** is reserved for lesions of the skin that suggest large basal or squamous cell carcinomas that may not be amenable to simple excision and melanomas where depth of invasion determines surgical margin and prognosis.

4. When dealing with hand lesions, one should take into consideration the need for other consulting specialists. For benign lesions, no specific preoperative consults are required. For malignant lesions, consultation with an **oncologist** is helpful to determine the need for adjuvant therapy and provide long-term follow-up. Multiple enchondromas of the phalanges are associated with Ollier's disease, which carries a 25% risk of conversion to chondrosarcoma. Ollier's disease along with the presence of soft tissue hemangiomas is likely Maffucci syndrome, which has an even higher conversion rate to malignancy.

    - Postoperatively, an **occupational/hand therapist** may be required for cases that require more extensive reconstruction and splinting.

5. Following an adequate workup, treatment of the finger lesion depends on its etiology.

    - Early infections can be treated with warm soaks and antibiotics. For more advanced lesions, drainage is required and may require removal of a portion of the nail to allow for egress of drainage.

- Most tumors of the hand are benign and may be treated with simple excision.

  — **Warts** are benign proliferations of the skin caused by infection with human papilloma virus (HPV). They have an endophytic growth pattern and can be painful. Treatment options include benign neglect, application of topical medications (podophyllin), laser, or excision.

  — **Mucous cysts** are the most common soft tissue tumors of the digits. They are better classified as pseudocysts because they lack a true epithelial lining. Mucous cysts are usually found at the level of the interphalangeal joint with the distal interphalangeal joint being the most common and a dorsal location being more common than a volar one. In the wrist, they are referred to as ganglion cysts. Treatment is directed at the source of the fluid rather than cyst lining. Decompression via aspiration or evacuation of the fluid is usually temporary and often leads to recurrence. Thorough treatment must include excision of the stalk extending to the joint and removal of any contributory exostosis.

  — **Epidermoid cysts** (also known as inclusion or epidermal cysts) result from the abnormal proliferation of epidermal elements within the confines of the dermis. The cause varies and may result from trauma, congenital defects in the pilosebaceous unit, or HPV infection. Their natural history is one of slow, asymptomatic growth until inflammation occurs or there is interference with function. Treatment is excision of the cyst and the entire cyst wall.

  — **Giant cell tumors of the tendon sheath** are commonly found in the hand in patients 30 to 50 years of age. They are usually painless and slow growing. They are associated with degenerative joint disease. There are two types: the more common localized type and the rarer diffuse type. The localized type is usually found on the volar aspect of the index and middle fingers near the distal interphangeal joint (DIP) joint, while the diffuse type usually affects the lower extremities. Excision is preferred treatment but can be difficult as the synovial capsule or tendon sheath can be involved. If the overlying skin is involved it should be removed, sometimes requiring grafting. Bony debridement may occasionally be required as well. Removal of all satellite lesions is important because recurrence rates range from 10% to 40%.

  — Treatment of **schwannoma** includes enucleation of the lesion with preservation of the nerve.

  — Since most **hemangiomas** involute with time, treatment is reserved for lesions which bleed or ulcerate. Depending on the lesion, treatment may be medical, laser, or surgical.

  — Treatment of **glomus tumors** is excision of the lesion. They usually present with pinpoint tenderness, paroxysmal pain, and cold hypersensitivity. On clinical examination, they may present as tender nodules near the fingertip. MRI is a useful adjunct in diagnosis. The lesions will appear dark on T1 weighted images and light on T2.

  — The most common bony tumor of the hand is the **enchondroma**. They account for 90% of bone tumors in the hand and most commonly arise from the proximal phalanx.

  — Large **giant cell tumors of the bone** may require joint fusions, arthroplasty, or bone replacement with a free flap. Smaller lesions may be amenable to curettage and packed with bone cement or bone graft. The lesions are more likely to recur without bone grafting. The recurrence rate with bone grafting can be as high as 10%.

- Treatment of malignant lesions is usually more radical and may involve adjuvant therapy in the form of radiotherapy or chemotherapy.

  — The standard nodular **basal cell carcinoma** can be removed by surgical excision with 2 mm margins with a 5-year cure rate of 90% to 95%. Radiation therapy, cryosurgery, or curettage yield similar results. Recurrent basal cell carcinoma should be treated more aggressively and monitored by careful pathologic evaluation to ensure adequate excision.

  — **Squamous cell carcinoma** should also be resected with a more aggressive margin. In general, excision with a 1-cm margin is recommended. Radiation, cryotherapy, or electrodessication are alternative treatment.

  — The treatment of **melanoma** depends on the depth of invasion. The staging is based on the pathologic depth of the lesion. In situ melanomas require a 0.5-cm margin. Lesions up to 1 mm in thickness require a 1-cm margin, lesions between 1 and 2 mm require a 1- to 2-cm margin, lesions between 2 and 4 mm require a 2-cm margin, while for those more than 4 mm in depth require at least a 2-cm margin. No benefit has been shown for taking margins above 2 cm.

- Prior to attempting reconstruction, negative tumor margins, including underlying cartilage and mucosa, must be obtained. Following removal of a hand lesion, multiple modalities are available for hand reconstruction.

  — **Skin grafts** can either be full-thickness or partial-thickness. Full-thickness grafts have the advantage of greater pliability and less contracture which should be kept in mind when reconstructing areas which require mobility. Skin grafts will take on the

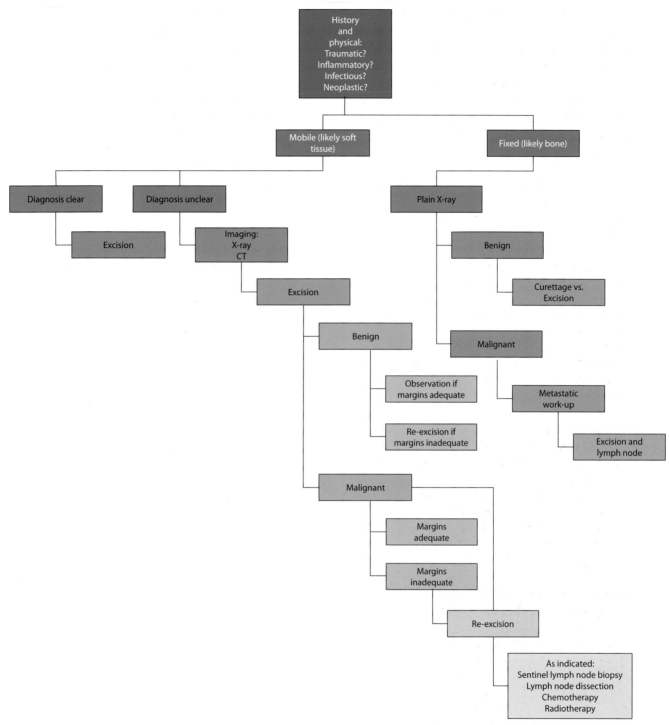

Algorithm 50-1 Algorithm for management of patients with masses of the hand and fingers.

surface of tendon or bone as long as the paratenon or periosteum is intact.

— **Local flaps** use adjacent tissue to reconstruct a defect. Examples include V-Y advancement of the volar pad for fingertip defects, rhomboid flaps, Z-plasty, and digital artery island flaps which are based on the digital vessels and are usually used to cover defects of the fingertip. Rotation flaps and advancement flaps may be designed to cover defects of the hand. They are random flaps, meaning they are not based on a specific vessel.

— **Regional flaps** are derived from nearby but not immediately adjacent tissue. Regional flaps with a random pattern blood supply have no named feeding vessel but are fed from the subdermal and subcutaneous plexus of arterioles and venules. A random flap usually requires two stages, one to inset the flap and a second to divide the pedicle. Since there is no axial vessel, attention should be paid to keeping the base of the flap as broad as possible. Cross-finger flaps and thenar flaps are examples of random pattern regional flaps. Axial flaps are fed by larger vessels and thus can be transferred in a single stage. Examples of axial regional flaps include the digital neurovascular island flap (also known as the Littler flap), the radial artery forearm flap, and the ulnar artery forearm flap. The most popular distant, axial pattern flap is the **groin flap**. It is based on the superficial circumflex iliac artery, which is relatively constant, and arises from the femoral artery in the femoral triangle. Flaps as wide as 12 cm can be closed safely. The flap can also be thinned prior to inset allowing for coverage with skin that is similar to hand and arm skin.

— Free tissue transfer from one area of the body to another. A free flap for reconstruction of hand defects should take into consideration the function of the given area and the need to have thin pliable skin in the area. Some free flaps can provide for reconstruction of other hand structures. For example, the dorsalis pedis flap can provide vascularized tendon for tendon reconstruction, or a free innervated gracilis muscle can be used to reconstruct function of lost muscles.

6. Complications should be addressed with the patient prior to intervention.

- **Decreased function** is particularly disturbing following reconstruction. Depending on the age of the patient and the site of the reconstruction, hand therapy by a certified hand therapist is important at some point in the postoperative period to restore function.

- **Infection** following reconstruction of hand defects is relatively uncommon as long as the defect is not in an infected field.

- **Flap loss** can occur when there is too much tension on the flap, kinking of a vascular pedicle, or if the flap is not designed correctly. Flap loss in microsurgery is due most commonly to thrombosis of the anastomosed artery or vein.

- In the setting of malignant lesions, **recurrence** is possible following resection for cure and surveillance should be continued to identify the new lesions.

PRACTICAL PEARLS

1. Benign lesions are found more commonly than malignant ones.

2. Ganglions are the most common hand masses.

3. If the extent of a lesion is unclear, the defect may be left open for later reconstruction pending negative pathologic margins.

4. An occupational therapist should be involved early in cases where return to functions seems slow or if the patient seems reticent to exercise the hand themselves.

5. For giant cell tumors, the key to lowering the recurrence is to take care in not entering the lesion which may seed the wound while still ensuring complete resection.

References

1. Strickland JW, Steichen JB. Nerve tumors of the hand and forearm. *J Hand Surg [Am]*. 1977;2(4):285-291.

2. Stern PJ, Dell PC. Benign and malignant tumors of the upper extremity. In: Peimer, CA, ed. *Surgery of the Hand and Upper Extremity*. New York: McGraw-Hill, Inc. New York) 1996:2231-2263.

3. Lister G, Pederson W. Skin flaps. In: Green DP, Hothkiss RN, Pederson WC, Wolfe SW, eds. *Green's Operative Hand Surgery*. New York Elsevier: New York 1999:1783-1850.

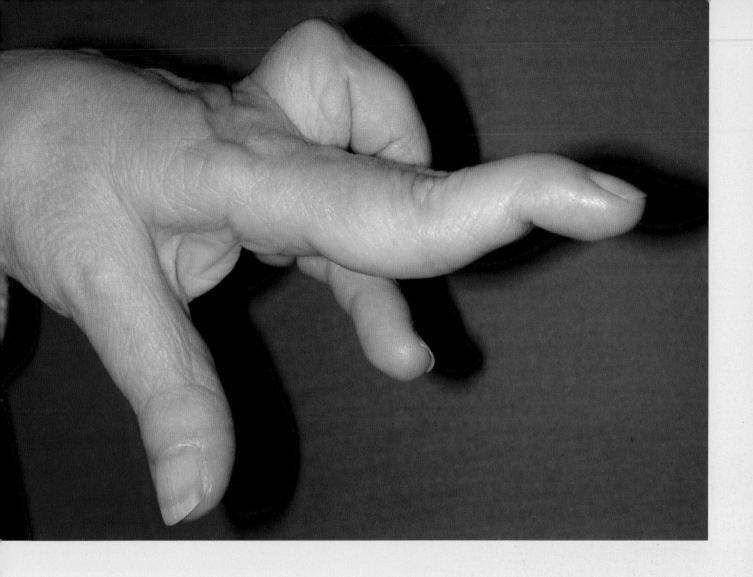

A 72-year-old woman presents with difficulty using the finger pictured above.

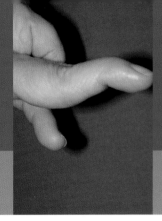

CHAPTER 51

Swan Neck Deformity

Aaron Daluiski

1. The patient in the photograph demonstrates joint deformity characterized by hyperextension at the PIP joint and flexion at the DIP joint. This is commonly referred to as a swan neck deformity solely because of its appearance. A swan neck deformity is caused by pathology at either the DIP or PIP joint (rarely the MP joint). At the DIP joint, the inciting event is disruption of the terminal extensor mechanism (e.g., mallet finger). This disruption in the extensor mechanism leads to secondary gradual hyperextension of the PIP joint. At the PIP joint, the primary pathologic structure is an incompetent volar plate, as seen in patients with rheumatoid arthritis. Volar plate laxity leads to hyperextension and dorsal displacement of the lateral bands. Once the lateral bands migrate dorsal to the axis of rotation of the PIP joint they accentuate the joint's hyperextension and cause the secondary DIP joint flexion. Rarer causes include rupture of the FDS tendon leading to hyperextension. Key points in the history when assessing this patient include:

   - **Was there a history of finger fracture?** Certainly fracture of the distal phalanx that contains the terminal extensor tendon may cause a mallet deformity and result in a swan neck posture. However, fracture of the middle phalanx that heals in hyperextension may also result in a swan neck deformity.

   - **How long has the deformity been present?** Acute onset on a swan neck deformity, although rare, indicates rupture of either the volar plate of the PIP joint or a traumatic mallet deformity, both of which can often be treated by splinting the primary affected joint.

   - **Does the patient have any preexisting or concomitant medical conditions?** Swan neck deformities are commonly seen in patients with rheumatoid arthritis. Synovitis as part of the condition may weaken the volar plate of the PIP joint and/or cause rupture of the terminal extensor tendon, both of which can lead to the deformity. In patients with rheumatoid arthritis, any flexion deformity of the MCP joint must be addressed first. Systemic ligamentous laxity will unbalance the tendon forces and lead to dorsal displacement of the lateral bands. This condition can also be secondary to conditions that lead to spasticity such as cerebral palsy.

   - **What is the patient's occupation/avocation and handedness?** The need to be aggressive with regards to surgical correction is determined partly by the patient's occupation and/or avocation and his/her handedness. Nonoperative splinting may be adequate in the older patient with a nondominant deformity, whereas ligament reconstruction may be more appropriate for a younger athlete with a dominant deformity.

   - **Does the deformity affect the patient's daily routine?** In many patients the deformity does not significantly interfere with daily function and may be left alone and observed.

2. As part of the thorough physical examination, both upper extremities, as well as the affected digit(s) should be inspected. Key findings to look for include the following:

   - **Which digits are affected?** Although the patient complains of one digit, similar pathology may be identified in other digits. This will also provide clues as to the etiology, since multiple, traumatic, mallet-type fractures are less likely.

   - **Is the PIP joint flexible?** The range of motion of the PIP joint is used for classification of deformity and should be noted prior to intervention.

     — In type I lesions, the PIP joint is flexible.

     — In type II lesions, PIP flexion is dependent upon position of MP joint (relaxation of the intrinsic).

     — In type III lesions, PIP joint is stiff with joint preservation on X-rays.

     — In type IV lesions, stiff PIP joint with destruction on X-rays.

   - **Is the DIP joint flexible?** It is important to ascertain whether there is function at the DIP joint prior to reconstruction of the more proximal PIP dysfunction.

   - **Is the MP joint flexible? Does MP flexion (relaxation of the intrinsic muscles) result in greater PIP laxity?** Intrinsic tightness should be identified prior to intervention since it should be addressed as part of the management strategy. Tight intrinsic muscles will prevent the digit from regaining a normal long-term posture and function.

- **What is the neurovascular status of the distal extremities? Is the capillary refill time prolonged?** Patients with poor blood supply to the fingers may not be candidates for surgical intervention so as to avoid creating secondary wounds that may not heal. Fortunately, these patients also have fewer indications for aggressive intervention.

- **Are there any scars on the hands?** Scars may indicate prior injuries and/or attempts at reconstruction. This information should be incorporated into secondary incisions to expose the vital structures or flaps to eventually cover them.

3. **Plain X-rays** of the hands in three views (AP, lateral, and oblique) should be obtained to rule out the presence of a phalangeal fracture and to evaluate the joint spaces. With a chronic deformity or in the presence of rheumatoid disease, the joint space will deteriorate over time. Good visualization of the MP, PIP, and DIP joints is necessary preoperatively.

4. In patients with established or suspected rheumatologic disorder, the overall care should be coordinated with a **rheumatologist**. Some patients may be in active treatment with immunosuppressant medications. These may or may not be able to be weaned prior to surgery or may make surgery contraindicated.

5. There are a number of conservative and invasive options described for the management of swan neck deformities.

- Conservative measures such as splinting are unlikely to permanently improve the patient's condition, but can be used to treat patients with supple deformities and minimal functional deficits.

  — DIP splinting should be used for primary mallet finger deformities.

  — If the primary pathology is PIP hyperextension, figure-of-eight PIP splinting can effectively prevent PIP hyperextension while allowing flexion.

- Surgical intervention for type I lesions can be managed with a combination of the following depending on the primary source of the deformity:

  — At the DIP joint, **repair of the Mallet deformity** may be performed with subsequent maintenance of the PIP joint in 20 degrees of flexion. The latter may be achieved either with a dorsal thermoplast splint or a Kirschner wire removed after 4 weeks followed by extension of the splint to 0 degrees at 6 weeks. The DIP joint may also be fused and PIP splinted at 20 degrees flexion.

  — At the PIP joint, a figure-of-eight or "silver ring" splint will prevent hyperextension while still allowing for flexion. **Volar plate repair**, **sublimus tenodesis**, or **PIP dermodesis** (which build in flexion contractures to the PIP joint by tightening the capsule/volar plate, using a slip of the FDS tendon or ellipsing volar skin from the finger, respectively) are surgical options. **Oblique retinacular ligament reconstruction**, in which the lateral band is detached proximally, rerouted volar to Cleland's ligament and reattached volar and proximal to the PIP joint is another option.

- Type II lesions require release of the intrinsic muscles and treatment of MP joint abnormalities (i.e., arthroplasties) if needed.

- Surgical intervention for type III lesions involves restoration of passive PIP motion. This is typically achieved by mobilization of the lateral bands and physical manipulation of the PIP joint.

- Type IV lesions usually require either **arthroplasty** or **arthrodesis**.

6. There are several potential complications following the various surgical interventions for swan neck deformity that should be addressed with the patient preoperatively. They include the following.

- Postoperative finger **stiffness** is perhaps the most common complication following ligamentous reconstruction. Fear for early disruption must be balanced with the need for early mobilization to prevent adhesion formation. The experience of the hand therapist may play an important role in this setting. In addition to careful range of motion, adjunctive techniques such as heat and massage may be valuable.

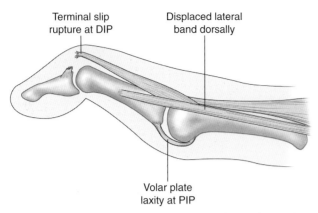

Terminal slip
rupture at DIP

Displaced lateral
band dorsally

Volar plate
laxity at PIP

Figure 51-1 Schematic drawing highlighting the pathology that results in a swan neck deformity.

- Postoperative **wound infection** is possible in all cases but should be infrequent with usual sterile technique and a dose of perioperative antibiotics.

- Any ligamentous reconstruction has the potential for **disruption**. This is why careful application of the postoperative dressing and explicit communication with the hand therapist is crucial to ensure a successful outcome. Early disruption may warrant a second attempt at rerepair. More delayed disruption may also warrant rerepair but may be considered for alternative options such as arthrodesis.

- For patients who are candidates for and wish to undergo arthrodesis of the joint, **nonunion** at the site is a potential complication.

PRACTICAL PEARLS

1. Treatment of the swan neck deformity is based on the functional deficit exhibited by the patient's deformity, not the deformity itself.

2. The key to treatment is the degree of passive flexibility of the PIP joint.

3. Figure-of-eight splinting can be used for patients with supple joint deformities.

4. The surgical treatment options should be decided by the location of the primary deformity and type of deformity.

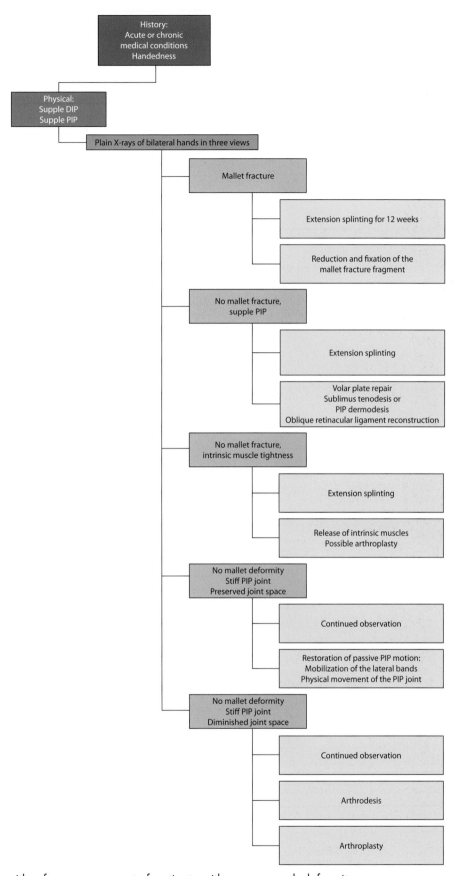

Algorithm 51-1 Algorithm for management of patients with a swan neck deformity.

References

1. Smith RJ. Balance and kinetics of the fingers under normal and pathological conditions. *Clin Orthop Relat Res.* 1974;104:92-111.

2. Littler JW. The finger extensor system. Some approaches to the correction of its disabilities. *Orthop Clin North Am.* 1986;17(3):483-492.

3. Nalebuff EA, Millender LH. Surgical treatment of the swan-neck deformity in rheumatoid arthritis. *Orthop Clin North Am.* 1975;6(3):733-752.

4. Lubhan JD and Cermak MB. Extensor mechanism reconstruction. In: Clayton AP, ed., *Surgery of the Hand and Upper Extremity*, New York, NY:McGraw-Hill; 1996: 1204-1215.

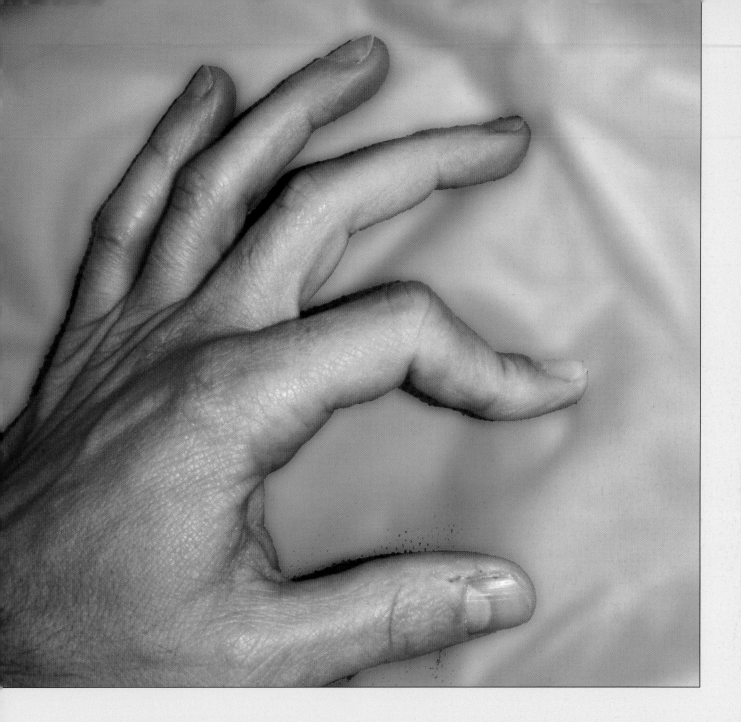

A 35-year-old man comes into your office

with difficulty getting dressed because

of his finger deformity.

CHAPTER 52

Boutonniere Deformity

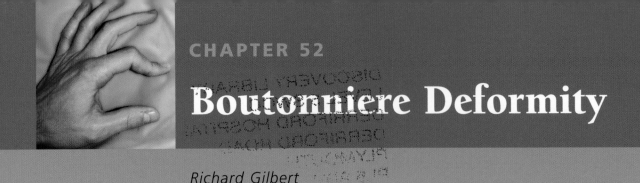

Richard Gilbert

1. The finger in the photograph demonstrates flexion at the proximal interphalangeal (PIP) joint and hyperextension at the distal interphalangeal (DIP) joint. (Figure 1). This abnormality is commonly referred to as a **boutonniere deformity** and is caused by disruption of the central slip of the extensor tendon. A thorough history should highlight several key points.

   - **Was there a history of trauma?** A boutonniere deformity is usually secondary to a closed injury, such as sudden forceful flexion of an extended PIP joint, or direct blunt trauma. They are classified as zone 3 extensor tendon injuries because of their location. Boutonniere deformities can also occur as a result of an open laceration or burn or be secondary to rheumatoid arthritis, other inflammatory arthropathies, ligamentous laxity, and rarely, advanced Dupuytren's disease.

   - **How long has the deformity been present?** Following disruption of the central slip of the extensor tendon, the triangular ligament and transverse retinacular ligaments stretch over time. The lateral bands are allowed to sublux volar to the axis of rotation of the PIP joint resulting in **PIP flexion** and dorsal to the axis of rotation of the DIP joint resulting in **DIP hyperextension**. A closed, acute injury to the central slip may initially be difficult to diagnose. This may be confused with a PIP joint sprain or a "jammed" finger. The boutonniere deformity may not develop until 10 to 14 days after the injury, when the lateral bands finally move volar to the axis of the PIP joint. Initially, active PIP joint extension is retained via the lateral bands. Many patients do not initially present until the actual boutonniere deformity develops. With time, the oblique retinacular ligaments (Landsmeer's ligaments) and volar plate contract, leading to a fixed PIP joint flexion contracture. In chronic cases, degenerative arthritis of the PIP joint can develop as well. Stages are noted below:

     - **Acute:** 0 to 2 weeks.
     - **Subacute:** 2 to 8 weeks.
     - **Chronic:** 8 weeks and longer, or when a fixed PIP joint flexion contracture has developed.

   - **Does the patient have any concomitant medical conditions?** Preexisting rheumatoid arthritis, lupus, or another inflammatory arthropathy can lead to systemic ligamentous laxity. The unbalanced tendon forces in the digits leads to subluxation of the lateral bands and a resultant boutonniere deformity.

   - **What is the patient's age, handedness, occupation and avocations? Does the deformity affect the patient's daily routine?** A boutonniere deformity may produce significant impairment in certain individuals and minimal functional impairment in others. A 20 degree PIP joint flexion contracture is usually well tolerated in most individuals.

2. A careful physical examination of the involved digit(s) should be undertaken to assess active and passive motion, the presence of fixed contractures and extensor tendon function.

   - **Are there any signs of trauma to the digit, especially over the dorsal surface?** Lacerations, open wounds, or healed scars may be clues to injury that has resulted in extensor tendon disruption.

   - **Is there swelling, ecchymosis, or tenderness over the dorsal base of the middle phalanx at the central slip insertion? Is there a palpable defect?** These may be signs of inflammation secondary to rheumatoid arthritis.

   - **How mobile are the individual joints?** It is important to preoperatively identify those patients in whom the joints are well preserved and those with more chronic findings who may have stiff ligaments and require more extensive reconstruction.

   - **Examination maneuvers:**

     — Passively flex the PIP joint to 90 degrees and hold pressure against the dorsal aspect of the middle phalanx. Then ask the patient to extend the PIP joint. If the patient can generate extension force at the PIP joint, the central slip of the extensor tendon is likely intact. Sometimes, a digital block can be helpful to eliminate pain as a cause of weakness. Normally, when the central slip is intact, the DIP joint cannot be extended, as the extensor force is primarily at the central slip directed to the PIP joint, not through the terminal extensor tendon to the DIP joint. In boutonniere deformities, the patient will be able to actively extend the DIP joint, because the central slip is disrupted, so the extensor force is primarily via the lateral bands to the DIP joint.

— Next, hold the PIP joint in full extension while the DIP joint is passively flexed. With a boutonniere deformity, there will be decreased passive DIP joint extension secondary to volar subluxation of the lateral bands and contracture of the oblique retinacular ligaments.

- **Does a psuedoboutonniere deformity exist?** A pseudoboutonniere deformity is secondary to a hyperextension injury to the PIP joint. The soft tissues volar to the PIP joint axis contract (primarily the volar plate), resulting in a PIP joint flexed position which can simulate a boutonniere deformity. In a pseudoboutonniere deformity, the DIP joint is not affected. The PIP joint flexion contracture usually develops more rapidly in a pseudoboutonniere injury.

- **How stable are the collateral ligaments of the PIP joint?** Central slip injuries can be secondary to a volar PIP joint dislocation, which often results in a concomitant collateral ligament injury.

- **What is the stage of the injury (as described by Zancolli)?**
  — *Stage I*: Weak PIP joint extension and resting flexion of the PIP joint. The weak PIP joint extension is retained via the lateral bands. The PIP joint can be passively corrected to full extension.
  — *Stage II*: Loss of active PIP joint extension, secondary stretching of the triangular ligament, and subluxation of the lateral bands volar to the axis of the PIP joint.
  — *Stage III*: Progressive hyperextension of the DIP joint occurs via the subluxed lateral bands. Hyperextension of the metacarpophalangeal (MCP) joint may also occur.
  — *Stage IV*: Fixed PIP joint flexion contracture secondary to contracture of the oblique retinacular ligaments and PIP joint volar plate.
  — *Stage V*: Fixed boutonniere deformity with secondary PIP joint arthritis (diagnosed on X-rays).

3. **Plain X-rays** of the involved digit in two or three views (AP, lateral, and oblique) should be obtained. The MCP, PIP, and DIP joints of the involved digit must be visualized.

- In **acute boutonniere deformities**, one must rule out an associated avulsion fracture off of the dorsal aspect of the middle phalanx. Congruity of the PIP joint should also be assessed, as boutonniere deformities can develop as a result of a volar PIP joint dislocation. In a pseudoboutonniere deformity, an avulsion fracture of the PIP joint volar plate may be visualized.

- In **chronic boutonniere deformities and in rheumatoid arthritis**, radiographs may demonstrate degenerative changes and subluxation of the PIP joint.

4. Specific consultations may be helpful and even necessary in the treatment of patients with Boutonniere deformity.

- Preoperative evaluation by an **occupational therapist** may be useful to document baseline function and/or assist with fabrication of a splint.

- Consultation with a **rheumatologist** should be arranged if the patient has suspected rheumatoid arthritis.
  — In **rheumatoid digits** (other than the thumb), PIP joint synovitis results in either attenuation or rupture of the central slip and triangular ligament, producing subluxation of the lateral bands and a boutonniere deformity. In rheumatoid arthritis, the MCP joint is usually hyperextended as well. With time, the PIP joint degenerates secondary to the rheumatoid synovitis and the deforming unbalanced extensor tendon forces.
  — In the **rheumatoid thumb**, the disease initially affects the MCP joint. MCP joint synovitis results in secondary rupture of the extensor pollicis brevis (EPB) tendon. The extensor pollicis longus (EPL) tendon subluxes volar and ulnar to the axis of the MCP joint, resulting in flexion of the MCP joint, and dorsal to the axis of the IP joint, resulting in hyperextension. This produces the "Z collapsed" boutonniere thumb deformity. With time, these joints subluxate and further degenerate.

5. The majority of closed boutonniere injuries can be successfully treated nonoperatively with splinting.

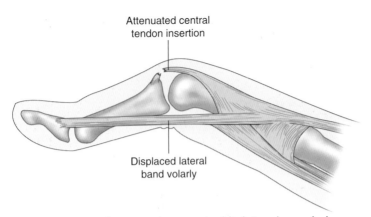

Attenuated central
tendon insertion

Displaced lateral
band volarly

Figure 52-1 Schematic drawing highlighting the pathology that results in a boutonniere deformity.

- The most common type of splint used is a static extension splint which holds the PIP joint in extension and leaves the MCP and DIP joints free. The patient must wear this full time for at least 6 weeks. The patient is instructed to actively flex the DIP joint, as this helps to advance the central slip distally to its insertion, via tension on the lateral bands.

- In more chronic cases, when there is an established PIP joint flexion contracture, the PIP joint is first treated with either serial extension casts or dynamic extension splints, to regain PIP extension. Once PIP extension is obtained, the PIP joint is statically splinted for an additional 6 weeks in extension.

- Surgery may be indicated in both acute and chronic boutonniere deformities. Specific indications for an acute boutonniere deformity include:

  — Displaced, nonreducible avulsion fracture of the dorsal base of the middle phalanx.

  — Boutonniere deformity secondary to a laceration or open wound.

  — Boutonniere deformity associated with lateral and axial instability of the PIP joint.

  — Failure of splinting.

- Surgical options for the **acute boutonniere deformity** include:

  — Open reduction-internal fixation (ORIF) of displaced avulsion fracture of the middle phalanx.

  — If the boutonniere deformity is secondary to an open laceration or wound, the tendon is repaired with a nonabsorbable suture, taking care not to shorten the tendon. The central slip can also be fixed to the dorsal base of the middle phalanx using an anchored suture. The lateral bands must be relocated and sutured dorsal to the axis of the PIP joint. The PIP joint is immobilized for 4 to 6 weeks in full extension with either an oblique transarticular Kirschner wire or a static splint. The DIP joint is left free and active DIP joint flexion is encouraged to prevent tendon adhesions.

  — If the central slip cannot be primarily repaired, the lateral bands can be released and mobilized dorsally to reconstruct the central slip and rebalance the extensor tendon at the PIP joint.

  — Before undertaking surgery in a chro**nic boutonniere deformity**, an established PIP joint flexion contracture must be corrected with either serial casting or dynamic extension splinting. If this does not restore full PIP extension, the joint can be surgically released and then the central slip can be reconstructed at a second stage procedure.

  — One surgical option is to excise the scar tissue at the distal aspect of the central slip and then reattach the central slip to its insertion through bone holes or with an anchored suture. Care must be taken not to shorten the central slip, as this will lead to reduced PIP flexion. The PIP joint is then immobilized for approximately 6 weeks in full extension with an oblique transarticular Kirschner wire.

  — If the central slip cannot be repaired by direct reattachment to the dorsal base of the middle phalanx, other reconstructive procedures have been described.

  — The lateral bands can be released and mobilized dorsal to the PIP joint axis to reconstruct the central slip and rebalance the extensor mechanism (Salvi procedure).

  — A turndown procedure or V-Y advancement of the central slip to regain length has also been described.

  — Many other reconstructive procedures using local tissue (Matev and Littler procedures) or tendon grafts (Nichols procedure) have been described to reconstruct a nonrepairable central slip rupture.

  — The Fowler extensor tenotomy procedure releases the extensor mechanism at the junction of the proximal and middle thirds of the middle phalanx. This allows the extensor force to be concentrated at the PIP joint and lessened at the DIP joint, improving the Boutonniere deformity. Care must be taken to avoid releasing the oblique retinacular ligaments, preventing a full mallet deformity from occurring.

  — Resultant PIP joint arthritis is a relative contraindication to soft tissue reconstructive procedures alone.

  — PIP joint arthrodesis is a viable option in laborers and low-demand individuals with a chronic boutonniere deformity associated with a degenerative PIP joint. It is also indicated in the setting of a degenerative PIP joint with an un-reconstructable extensor tendon.

  — In younger patients, a PIP joint arthroplasty and extensor tendon reconstruction can be considered.

- Even in the presence of significant boutonniere deformities, patients with rheumatoid arthritis may continue to function quite well, not requiring any type of intervention. The treating surgeon must evaluate the whole upper extremity and the medical status of the patient, prior to undertaking surgical treatment for a boutonniere deformity in a patient with rheumatoid arthritis. Treatment depends upon the function of the patient, the extent of the PIP joint flexion contracture, whether or not it is fixed, and the extent of degeneration of the PIP joint articular surfaces. Treatment options include: Static/dynamic PIP joint extension splinting, PIP joint synovectomy, extensor tendon reconstruction, Fowler extensor tenotomy, PIP joint fusion, and PIP joint arthroplasty. In rheumatoid arthritis, the MCP joint often requires surgical treatment as well. In the rheumatoid boutonniere thumb deformity, both the MCP and IP joints usually require concomitant treatment.

6. Complications as a result of treating a boutonniere deformity include the following:

- Probably the most common "complication" in this regard is **failure to properly diagnose and treat the injury** before a fixed PIP joint flexion contracture develops. As stated earlier, initially these can be subtle injuries which can be misdiagnosed as a sprained or "jammed" PIP joint.

- Failure to fully correct the PIP joint flexion contracture (either with splinting or surgical release), prior to performing the extensor tendon reconstructive procedure, resulting in a **persistent contracted boutonniere deformity**.

- **Skin necrosis** or breakdown may also occur secondary to pressure from a splint.

- Many of the surgical reconstructive procedures for chronic boutonniere deformity have a high failure rate of the ligamentous reconstruction and a high recurrence rate of the PIP joint flexion contracture.

- Repairing or reconstruction of the central slip too tight, resulting in **limited PIP joint flexion**.

- Kirschner-wire related complications, such as **pin-tract and joint infections**, or bending or breakage of the wire.

- **Nonunion** of the fracture in the setting of an ORIF of an avulsion fracture.

PRACTICAL PEARLS

1. A closed, acute injury to the central slip may initially be difficult to diagnose, and may be confused with a PIP joint sprain. The boutonniere deformity may not develop until 10 to 14 days after the initial injury, when the lateral bands sublux.

2. X-rays should always be taken to rule out an avulsion fracture off of the dorsal aspect of the middle phalanx.

3. The majority of closed, acute boutonniere deformities can be successfully treated with approximately 6 weeks of full-time PIP joint extension splinting, encouraging active DIP flexion.

4. Many of the surgical reconstructive procedures for chronic boutonniere deformity have a high failure rate of the ligamentous reconstruction and a high recurrence rate of the PIP joint flexion contracture.

5. Failure to fully correct the PIP joint flexion contracture with splinting, serial casts, or surgical release, prior to performing extensor tendon reconstruction, is a relatively common cause of poor outcomes in chronic boutonniere deformities.

References

1. Baratz ME, Schmidt CC, Hughes, TB. Extensor tendon injuries, In: Green DP, Hotchkiss RN, Pederson WC, Wolfe SW, eds. *Green's Operative Hand Surgery*, 5th ed. Philadelphia, PA: Elsevier Churchill Livingstone, 2005; 199-206.

2. Coons MS, Green SM. Boutonniere deformity. *Hand Clin.* 1995;11(3): 387-402.

3. Curtis RM, Reid RL. Provost JM. A staged technique for the repair of the traumatic boutonniere deformity. *J Hand Surg.* 1983;8(2):167-171.

4. Rockwell WB, Butler PN, Byrne BA. Extensor tendon: Anatomy, injury, and reconstruction. *Plast Reconstr Surg.* 2000;106(7):1592-603.

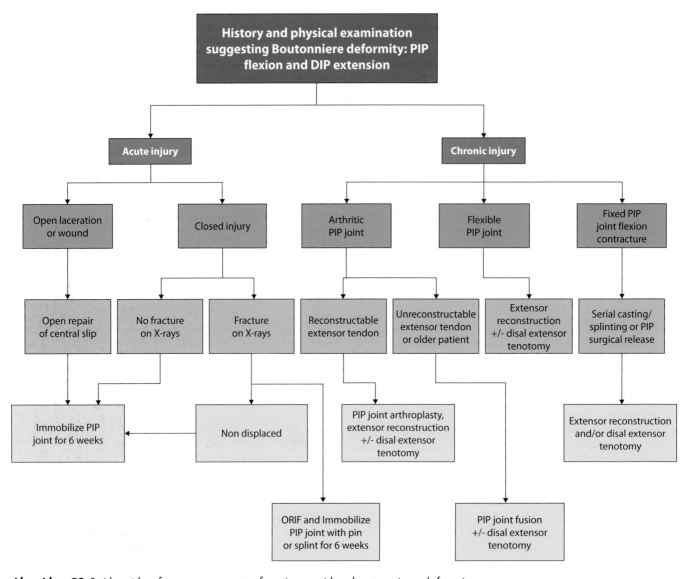

Algorithm 52-1 Algorithm for management of patients with a boutonniere deformity.

Index